ADVANCES IN NEUROLOGY
Volume 76

ADVANCES IN NEUROLOGY
Volume 76

Antiepileptic Drug Development

Editors

Jacqueline A. French, M.D.
Associate Professor
Department of Neurology
University of Pennsylvania
Philadelphia, Pennsylvania

Marc A. Dichter, M.D., Ph.D.
Professor
Department of Neurology and Pharmacology
University of Pennsylvania
Philadelphia, Pennsylvania

Ilo E. Leppik, M.D.
MINCEP Epilepsy Care
Minneapolis, Minnesota

Lippincott - Raven
PUBLISHERS
Philadelphia • New York

Acquisitions Editor: Mark Placito
Manufacturing Manager: Dennis Teston
Production Manager: Lawrence Bernstein
Production Editor: Lawrence Bernstein
Cover Designer: Patricia Gast
Indexer: Dorothy Jahoda
Compositor: Lippincott-Raven Electronic Production
Printer: Maple Press

Printed in the United States of America

9 8 7 6 5 4 3 2 1

ISBN: 0-397-51848-x
ISSN: 0091-3952

Advances in Neurology

Advances in Neurology Series

Vol. 76 Antiepileptic Drug Development: *J. French, M.A. Dichter, I. Leppik,, editors,* 304 pp., 1998.
Vol. 75 Reflex Epilepsies and Reflex Seizures: *B.C. Zifkin, F. Anderman, A. Beaumanoir, A.J. Rowan, editors,* 336 pp., 1998.
Vol. 74 Basal Ganglia and New Surgical Approaches for Parkinson's Disease: *J.A. Obesso, M.R. DeLong, C. Ohye, and C.D. Marsden, editors*, 286 pp., 1997.
Vol. 73 Brain Plasticity: *H.J. Freund, B.A. Sabel, and O.W. White, editors*, 448 pp., 1997.
Vol. 72 Neuronal Regeneration, Reorganization and Repair: *Frederick J. Seil, editor*, 416 pp., 1997.
Vol. 71 Cellular and Molecular Mechanisms of Ischemic Brain Damage: *B.K. Siesjo and T Wieloch, editors,* 560 pp., 1996.
Vol. 70 Supplementary Sensorimotor Area: *H.O. Luders, editor*, 544 pp., 1996.
Vol. 69 Parkinson's Disease: *L. Battistin, G. Scarlato, T. Caraceni, and S. Ruggieri, editors,* 752 pp., 1996.
Vol. 68 Pathogenisis and Therapy of Amyotrophic Lateral Sclerosis: *G. Serratrice and T.I. Munsat, editors*, 352 pp., 1995.
Vol. 67 Negative Motor Phenomena: *S. Fahn, M. Hallett, H.O. Luders, and C.D. Marsden, editors*, 416 pp., 1995.
Vol. 66 Epilepsy and Functional Anatomy of the Frontal Lobe: *H.H. Jasper, S. Riggio, and P.S. Goldman-Rakik, editors,* 400 pp., 1995.
Vol. 65 Behavioral Neurology of Movement Disorders: *W.J. and A.E. Lang, editors*, 368 pp., 1995.
Vol. 64 Neurological Complications of Pregnancy: *O. Devinsky, E. Feldman, and B. Hainline, editors*, 288 pp., 1994.
Vol. 63 Electrical and Magnetic Stimulation of the Brain and Spinal Cord: *O. Devinsky, A. Beric, and M. Dogali, editors*, 352 pp., 1993.
Vol. 62 Cerebral Small Artery Disease: *P.M. Pullicino, L.R. Caplan, and M. Hommel, editors,* 256 pp., 1993.
Vol. 61 Inherited Ataxias: *A.E. Harding and T. Deufel, editors*, 240 pp., 1993.
Vol. 60 Parkinson's Disease: From Basic Research to Treatment: *H. Narabayashi, T. Nagatsi, N. Yanagisawa, and Y. Mizuno, editors*, 800 pp., 1993.
Vol. 59 Neural Injury and Regeneration: *F.J. Seil, editor*, 384 pp., 1993.
Vol. 58 Tourette Syndrome: Genetics, Neurobiology, and Treatment: *T.N. Chase, A.J. Friedhoff, and D.J. Cohen, editors*, 400 pp., 1992.
Vol. 57 Frontal Lobe Seizures and Epilepsies: *P. Chauvel, A.V. Delgado-Escuerta, E. Halgren, and J. Bancaud, editors*, 752 pp., 1992.
Vol. 56 Amyotrophic Lateral Sclerosis and Other Motor Neuron Diseases: *L.P. Roland, editor,* 592 pp., 1991.
Vol. 55 Neurobehavioral Problems in Epilepsy: *D.B. Smith, D.Treiman, and M. Trimble, editors*, 512 pp., 1990.
Vol. 54 Magnetoencephalography: *S. Sato, editor*, 284 pp., 1990.
Vol. 52 Brain Edema: Pathogenesis, Imaging, and Therapy: *D. Lang, editor*, 640 pp., 1990.
Vol. 51 Alzheimer's Disease: *R.J. Wurtman, S. Corkin, J.H. Growdon, and E. Ritter-Walker, editors*, 308 pp., 1990.
Vol. 48 Molecular Genetics of Neurological and Neuromuscular Disease: *S. DiDonato, S. DiMauro, A. Mamoli, and L.P. Rowland, editors*, 288 pp., 1987.
Vol. 47 Functional Recovery in Neurological Disease, *Stephen G. Waxman, editor*, 640 pp., 1987.
Vol. 46 Intensive Neurodiagnostic Monitoring: *R.J. Gumnit, editor*, 336 pp., 1987.
Vol. 45 Parkinson's Disease: *M.D. Yahr and K.J. Bergmann, editors*, 640 pp., 1986.
Vol. 44 Basic Mechanisms of the Epilepsies: Molecular and Cellular Approaches: *A.V. Delgado-Escueta, A.A. Ward, Jr., D.M. Woodbury, and R.J. Porter, editors*, 1120 pp., 1986.
Vol. 43 Myoclonus: *S. Fahn, C.D. Marsden, and M.H. Van Woert, editors*, 752 pp., 1986.
Vol. 42 Progress in Aphasiology: *F. Clifford Rose, editor*, 384 pp.,1984.
Vol. 41 The Olivopontocerebellar Atrophies: *R.C. Duvoisin and A. Plaitokis, editors*, 304 pp., 1984.
Vol. 40 Parkinson-Specific Motor and Mental Disorders, Role of Pallidum: Pathophysiological, Biochemical, and Therapeutic Aspects: *R.G. Hassler and J.F. Christ, editors*, 601 pp., 1984.
Vol. 38 The Dementias: *R. Mayeux and W.G. Rosen*, 288 pp., 1983.
Vol. 37 Experimental Therapeutics of Movement Disorders: *S. Fahn, D.B. Calne, and I. Shoulson, editors*, 339 pp., 1983.

Contents

Contributing Authors

Karrar H. Ali, M.P.H.
Abbott Laboratories
100 Abbott Park Road
Department 42J, Building AP6C-1
Abbott Park, Illinois 60064

David E. Blum, M.D.
Barrow Neurological Institute
SJHMC
350 West Thomas Road
Phoenix, Arizona 85013

Martin J. Brodie, M.B.Ch.B., M.R.C.P., M.D., F.R.C.P.
Professor of Medicine and Clinical Pharmacology
Epilepsy Research Unit
Department of Medicine and Therapeutics
Western Infirmary
Glasgow G11 6NT
Scotland

Jeffrey Buchhalter, M.D., Ph.D.
Section of Child Neurology
Mayo Clinic
Rochester, Minnesota 55905

Theresa L. Collins
Department of Neurology 701-LC1
Yale University School of Medicine
333 Cedar Street
New Haven, Connecticut 06510

Joyce A. Cramer, B.S.
Departments of Neurology and Psychiatry
Yale University School of Medicine
950 Campbell Avenue
West Haven, Connecticut 06516

Marc A. Dichter, M.D., Ph.D.
Professor of Neurology and Pharmacology
Department of Neurology
University of Pennsylvania
3 W. Gates
3400 Spruce Street
Philadelphia, Pennsylvania 19104

Sureyya S. Dikmen, Ph.D.
Professor
Departments of Rehabilitation Medicine, Neurological Surgery, Psychiatry, and Behavioral Sciences
University of Washington
Box 356490
1959 NE Pacific Street
Seattle, Washington 98195

Matthew J. During, M.D.
Professor
Department of Molecular Medicine
University of Auckland
School of Medicine
85 Park Road, Grafton
Aukland
New Zealand

Jacqueline French, M.D.
Associate Professor
Department of Neurology
University of Pennsylvania
3 W. Gates
3400 Spruce Street
Philadelphia, Pennsylvania 19104

Hal Galbraith, M.S. Pharm.
Hoechst Marion Roussel
10236 Marion Park Drive
Kansas City, Missouri 64137

Elizabeth Garofalo, M.D.
Senior Director
Department of Clinical Research, CNS
Parke-Davis Pharmaceutical Research
Warner-Lambert Co.
2800 Plymouth Road
Ann Arbor, Michigan 48105

Russel G. Katz, M.D.
Deputy Director
Division of Neuropharmacological Drug Products-HED-120
Food and Drug Administration
5600 Fishers Lane
Rockville, Maryland 20857

Harvey J. Kupferberg, Ph.D.
Chief Preclinical Pharmacology Section
Epilepsy Branch,
National Institute of Neurological Disorders and Stroke
National Institutes of Health
7550 Wisconsin Avenue
Federal Building, Room 516
Bethesda, Maryland 20892

Ilo Leppik, M.D.
MINCEP Epilepsy Care
5775 Wayzata Boulevard
Suite 255
Minneapolis, Minnesota 55416

René H. Levy
Department of Pharmaceutics
University of Washington
4165 Health Science Building BG-20
Seattle, Washington 98195

James L. Marks, Ph.D.
Department of Biochemistry
Parke-Davis Pharmaceutical Research Division
Warner-Lambert Co.
2800 Plymouth Road
Ann Arbor, Michigan 48105

Gary G. Mather, Ph.D.
Department of Pharmaceutics
University of Washington
H 165 Health Science Building BG-20
Seattle, Washington 98195

Richard H. Mattson, M.D.
Department of Neurology 701-LC 1
Yale University School of Medicine
333 Cedar Street
New Haven, Connecticut 06510

Kimford J. Meador, M.D.
Professor of Neurology and Pharmacology and Pediatrics Section of Neurophysiology
Department of Neurology
Medical College of Georgia
1120 15th Street
Augusta, Georgia 30912

Eli M. Mizrahi, M.D.
Associate Professor of Neurology and Pediatrics
Section of Neurophysiology
Baylor College of Medicine
1 Baylor Plaza
Houston, Texas 77039

Martha J. Morrell, M.D.
Associate Professor of Neurology and Neurological Sciences
Department of Neurology
Stanford University Medical School
300 Pasteur Drive
Stanford, California 94305

Azmi A. Nabulsi, M.D., M.P.H.
Medical Director
Abbott Laboratories
100 Abbott Park Road
Abbott Park, Illinois 60064

John M. Pellock, M.D.
Professor of Neurology, Pediatrics, Pharmacy, and Pharmaceutics
Division of Child Neurology
Medical College of Virginia
Virginia Commonwealth University
307 College Street
Randolph Minor Hall, 7th Floor
Richmond, Virginia 23213

Ognen A.C. Petroff, M.D.
Associate Professor of Neurology
Department of Neurology
Yale University School of Medicine
333 Cedar Street, LC1-701
New Haven, Connecticut 06520

Gordon W. Pledger, Ph.D.
Senior Research Fellow
Department of Biostatistics
R.W. Johnson Pharmaceutical Research Institute
920 Route 202
P.O. Box 300
Raritan, New Jersey 08869

Roger J. Porter, M.D.
Vice President Clinical Pharmacology
Wyeth-Ayerst Laboratories
145 King of Prussia Road
Radnor, Pennsylania 19101
Adjunct Professor of Pharmacology
Uniformed Services University of the Health Sciences
Bethesda, Maryland 20814

Ross A. Reife, M.D.
Senior Director
Global Clinical Research and Development
R. W. Johnson Pharmaceutical Research Institute
920 Route 202
Raritan, New Jersey 08861
Assistant Professor of Clinical Neurology
Thomas Jefferson University
11th and Walnut Street
Philadelphia, Pennsylvania 19107

Michael A. Rogawski, M.D., Ph.D.
Chief, Neuronal Excitability Section
Epilepsy Research Branch
National Institute of Neurological Disorders and Stroke
National Institutes of Health
10 Center Drive, MSC 1408
Bethesda, Maryland 20892

Todd Sahlroot, Ph.D.
Division of Biometrics
Food and Drug Administration
5600 Fisher Lane
Room 18845, HFD-173
Rockville, Maryland 20857

Richard D. Scheyer, M.D.
Associate Processor of Neurology,
Department of Neurology, 701-LC1
Yale University School of Medicine
333 Cedar Street
New Haven, Connecticut 06510

Brett E. Skolnick, Ph.D.
Department of Neurology
Pennsylvania Hospital
305 Spruce Street
Philadelphia, Pennsylvania 19146

Dennis D. Spencer, M.D.
Harvey and Kate Cushing Professor of Neurosurgery
Chairman
Department of Neurology
Yale University School of Medicine
333 Cedar Street
New Haven, Connecticut 06520

Neil M. Sussman, M.D.
Clinical Associate Professor
Department of Neurology
Yale University School of Medicine
333 Cedar Street
New Haven, Connecticut 06520

Charles P. Taylor, Ph.D.
Research Fellow
Department of Neuroscience Therapeutics
Parke-Davis Pharmaceutical Research Division
Warner-Lambert Co.
2800 Plymouth Road
Ann Arbor, Michigan 48105

Nancy R. Temkin, Ph.D.
Departments of Neurological Surgery and Biostatistics
University of Washington
Box 359924
700 9th Avenue
Seattle, Washington 98104

David M. Treiman, M.D.
Department of Neurology
UCLA School of Medicine
2905 Woodwardia Drive
Los Angeles, California 90095

Steven D. Walker
Parke-Davis Pharmaceutical Research Division
2800 Plymouth Road
Ann Arbor, Michigan 48105

H. Steve White, Ph.D.
Associate Professor
Department of Pharmacology and Toxicology
Anticonvulsant Screening Project
University of Utah
20 S 2030 E, Room 408
Salt Lake City, Utah 84112

H. Richard Winn, M.D.
Professor and Chairman
Department of Neurological Surgery
University of Washington
Harborview Medical Center
700 9th Avenue
Seattle, Washington 98104

Harold H. Wolf, Ph.D.
Professor of Pharmacology
Department of Pharmacology and Toxicology
Anticonvulsant Screening Project
University of Utah
408 Biomedical Polymers Research Building
Salt Lake City, Utah 84112

José H. Woodhead
Senior Research Specialist
Department of Pharmacology and Toxicology
Anticonvulsant Screening Project
University of Utah
20 S 2030 E, Room 408
Salt Lake City, Utah 84112

Preface

During the past ten years there has been a revolution in antiepileptic drug development. In 1993, there was a limited group of drugs in common use for the treatment of seizures. In the ensuing four years, four new Antiepileptic Drugs (AEDs) were approved for use in the United States and several others were approved in Europe and Asia. In addition, at least six other drugs were in various stages of clinical evaluation and others are moving from the laboratory to the clinical domain. It has been estimated that to bring a new AED from the laboratory to clinical approval may cost over $200,000,000 and take more than eight years.

Until recently, our concepts about new drug development were as stagnant as the list of available drugs for epilepsy. Clinical trials focused on add-on, placebo-controlled protocols that were performed in adults with partial seizures who had proved refractory to available AEDs. Although cumbersome, these types of trials were proven to be useful, as evidenced by their ability to demonstrate efficacy for gabapentin, lamictal, and topiramate. Yet even from the very beginning of modern AED testing, during the development of felbamate, there was an understanding that these trials alone would not be optimal for new drug testing, and new trial designs had to be created. The process of bringing new AEDs through development to ultimate approval has been a learning process for all involved. Trials with standard designs are now being performed more efficiently. In addition, we are becoming more innovative in creating novel designs to facilitate drug evaluation in different seizure types and in different patient populations.

Many of the concepts of antiepileptic drug development will be discussed in this book. The first section deals with the mechanisms by which promising new compounds are identified and evaluated for both efficacy and safety in preclinical trials. Issues related to standard and novel AED trial designs are also addressed. Trials in alternative populations such as women and children and for special seizure problems, such as status epilepticus, are discussed. The regulatory process, both in the United States and around the world, is explored, as are issues related to postmarketing surveillance. Finally, data from previous trials are reanalyzed so that past experience can serve as a template for future efforts.

The drug development process continues to evolve. The trial designs are cumbersome, lengthy, and may create ethical concerns about the safety of patients. In addition, clinical trials are designed for registration by the various regulatory bodies and frequently do not provide sufficient clinically relevant information. In other words, after $200 million and an extraordinary effort, clinicians may still not know in what settings a drug will be appropriate or how best to use it.

Epilepsy remains a major clinical problem. It has been estimated that as many as 40 percent of individuals with epilepsy do not have their seizures completely controlled by medication, despite all the new AEDs that have recently been developed. The antiepileptic development process must continue. By systematically examining our past efforts, the process can become more efficient and eventually more effective. The goal of eliminating all seizures without compromising quality of life is still far away, but at least we can be confident that there is progress.

Acknowledgments

The editors would like to thank the symposium organizing committee and the pharmaceutical industry advisory committee for their guidance and support for The Symposium on Antiepileptic Drug Development held in Charleston, South Carolina, in March 1996, which became the foundation for this book. We would also like to express our special gratitude to Ms. Mary Ann Brodie. Without her organizational skills and editorial assistance neither the symposium nor this book would have been possible. Her tireless efforts and dedication are greatly appreciated by the editors and the authors. In addition, we are very appreciative of the efforts of Shauna Williams during the editing process.

The Symposium on Antiepileptic Drug Development was supported by generous unrestricted educational grants from Bristol-Myers Squibb, Ciba Geneva, Dainippon, Digitrace, Glaxo Wellcome, Hoechst Marion Roussel, Ortho-McNeill, Parke-Davis, and SmithKline Beecham.

ADVANCES IN NEUROLOGY
Volume 76

Antiepileptic Drug Development.
Advances in Neurology, Vol. 76,
edited by J. French, I. Leppik, and M. A. Dichter.
Lippincott–Raven Publishers, Philadelphia © 1998.

1

Mechanisms of Action of New Antiepileptic Drugs

Marc A. Dichter

Department of Neurology, University of Pennsylvania, Philadelphia, Pennsylvania 19104.

INTRODUCTION

The epilepsies comprise a family of disorders having in common spontaneous, periodic disturbances in the normal electrical activity of the brain that are associated with changes in behavior. Each disturbance is called a seizure, and patients have epilepsy if they have recurrent spontaneous seizures. Both the electrical and behavioral aspects of seizures can be quite variable and complex, even in a given individual patient, and the classification of seizures has proved to be a complicated task. Seizures can be caused by a variety of pathologic conditions, including genetic abnormalities and acquired injuries. In addition, a wide variety of physiologic perturbations in brain function may produce seizures. Finally, the mechanisms by which seizures are generated and their behavioral manifestations are directly related to where in the brain the abnormality occurs. If antiepileptic drugs (AEDs) are designed to suppress seizures, it is clear that agents with quite different mechanisms of action could be effective against different types of epileptic seizures. Although it would be useful to be able to interrupt seizure activity at some "final common path" and treat patients with one, universally effective drug, it is not clear that such a goal will be possible, or that a strategy of having multiple drugs available to target multiple seizure mechanisms might not be almost as effective.

At the present time, some of the mechanisms that underlie different forms of seizures are moderately well understood, whereas other components of the epilepsy problem are much less well characterized. In addition, there is available a group of drugs known to be effective in suppressing seizures, and some of the mechanisms by which these drugs work have been characterized. New AEDs are being developed utilizing two complementary strategies. Animal models of human seizures can be created in the laboratory and used to screen new compounds for antiseizure activity. Alternatively, new drugs can be developed with specific cellular or molecular targets that are thought to be important in seizure generation. Both of these strategies have recently been successful and will be reviewed in this chapter from the perspective of drugs involved and in Chapters 2 and 3 from the perspective of future drug screening.

Mechanisms Underlying Focal Epileptiform Activity

Focal or partial seizures occur in an area of cortex that exhibits excess excitability. The interictal spike discharge in the electroencephalogram (EEG) is a manifestation of hyperexcitable brain and serves as a marker for an area of localized abnormal excitability. Interictal discharges (IDs) occur when a group of pyramidal neurons synchronously develop large depolarizing potentials, on which bursts of action potentials are superimposed. At the cellular level, this has been called the paroxysmal depolarizing shift (PDS) or depolarizing shift (DS). It is usually followed by a large, prolonged hyperpolarization (the post-DS HP), which is the cellular correlate of the slow wave that usually follows EEG spike discharges. Neurons are alternately excited during the DS and inhibited during the HP. The DS is generated by a combination of synaptic currents (mediated by the excitatory neurotransmitters glutamate and aspartate) and voltage-dependent depolarizing currents, especially calcium currents. The post-DS HP is also thought to be produced by a combination of synaptic events, especially those mediated by γ-aminobutyric acid (GABA) via both $GABA_A$ and $GABA_B$ receptors, voltage-dependent currents (mostly potassium currents), and calcium-dependent currents (potassium and possibly chloride).

IDs can convert to seizures when inhibitory mechanisms decrease in potency or when excitatory mechanisms become enhanced. This transition involves both an "escape" of the local discharge and spread of the discharge to nearby and distant areas of brain.

Mechanisms Underlying Primary Generalized Seizures

Many forms of primary generalized epilepsy are thought to be genetic. They are generally characterized by bilateral synchronous EEG spike-and-wave discharges. These discharges appear to be generated by thalamocortical rhythms. Under normal circumstances, the thalamocortical network generates relatively low-frequency oscillations, the nature of which depend on the arousal state of the individual (1). During epileptiform events, however, neurons become more synchronized, and larger, high-voltage waveforms emerge. It is likely that specific neurons in the thalamus that have large, voltage-dependent calcium (Ca^{2+}) currents (T currents) produce relatively large and long-lasting depolarizations that trigger bursts of action potentials. These same neurons seem to develop relatively long-lasting hyperpolarizations following their bursts, partially caused by voltage- and Ca^{2+}-dependent currents and partially caused by $GABA_B$-receptor-mediated inhibitory postsynaptic potentials (IPSPs). It has been hypothesized that either enhanced inhibitory inputs into the thalamic relay cells or T currents that are unusually large or have different activation/inactivation kinetics may foster the development of the 3- to 4-Hz spike-and-wave activity commonly seen in generalized epilepsy (2).

When the duration of the spike-and-wave discharges increases, more of the normal brain activity can be entrained, probably through mechanisms similar to those discussed above in regard to the transition to seizures in partial epilepsy; generalized tonic-clonic seizures then develop.

MECHANISMS OF ACTION OF "CONVENTIONAL" ANTIEPILEPTIC DRUGS

Based on the brief descriptions of epilepsy mechanisms presented above, several possible targets for AEDs can be identified. All forms of seizures are associated with bursting behavior in neurons, and dampening of repetitive action potential generation would therefore be a potentially useful target. This would need to be done carefully, as all the information transfer of the brain is coded by trains of action potentials, and it is important that any drug administered on a long-term basis not interfere with normal brain function. An additional target for AEDs would be other voltage-dependent currents involved in maintaining neuronal excitability. In addition, as synaptic inhibition plays a major role in all forms of epilepsy, drugs that enhance inhibition should be protective in most cases. Similarly, drugs that dampen synaptic excitation may be useful to suppress seizure generation and spread.

All the "conventional" AEDs currently available were developed without prior knowledge of drug mechanisms and were then studied in the laboratory to try to elucidate cellular mechanisms. They appear to exert their antiseizure activity via one of three mechanisms: inhibition of voltage-dependent sodium (Na^+) currents, enhancement of the actions of GABA on $GABA_A$ receptors, and suppression of voltage-dependent Ca^{2+} currents (3).

Inhibition of Voltage-Dependent Sodium Currents

All neurons in the central nervous system develop action potentials based on the opening and closing of Na^+ channels in response to membrane depolarization. Neurons may fire at relatively low frequency or may fire bursts or trains of higher-frequency action potentials in response to some stimuli. Several of the most potent AEDs in common use, including phenytoin (PHT) (4), carbamazepine (CBZ) (5), phenobarbital (PHB), and valproic acid (VPA) (6), appear to suppress these Na^+ currents in a voltage- and use-dependent manner. This means that the more the neuron is depolarized, and the more it fires, the more effective is the drug in suppressing the repetitive firing. Thus, these drugs appear to be effective against epileptic firing modes while interfering very little, if at all, with normal firing modes. This has been demonstrated by recording from neurons in the current clamp mode with sharp intracellular microelectrodes and showing that the drugs block the sustained repetitive firing (SRF) that occurs when a long depolarizing pulse is triggered (4). It can be demonstrated more quantitatively by performing voltage clamping on individual neurons and demonstrating a direct effect on Na^+ currents that is both voltage- and use-dependent (7).

Enhancement of GABA-Mediated Inhibition

All neurons within the mammalian central nervous system have GABA receptors that when activated produce hyperpolarizing inhibition. It has been well established that reduction of GABA-mediated inhibition results in seizures and that enhancement of inhibition is associated with a suppression of seizures. Several potent antiseizure drugs appear to work by enhancing the actions of GABA at $GABA_A$ receptors: the barbiturates act to prolong inhibition by keeping GABA-activated channels open longer, and the benzodiazepines act to increase the frequency of chloride (Cl^-) channel opening, thereby making inhibitory postsynaptic potentials larger (8). These two classes of drugs can have additive effects. These drugs both bind to specific sites on the GABA receptor complex (GRC) and act to alter the channel kinetics allosterically. The GRC consists of a pentameric unit made up of three different subunits, α, β, and γ, probably with the configuration $2\alpha{:}2\beta{:}1\gamma$. Multiple forms of each subunit exist, and GABA receptors in different brain regions and at different developmental times can be found to have various combinations of the subunits. This can confer subtle but important differences in the pharmacology of the GRC. At the present time, none of the currently available drugs appears to be significantly subunit-specific.

Reduction in Voltage-Dependent Calcium Currents (T Currents)

Ethosuximide and dimethadione are effective in absence epilepsy but are not effective in focal seizures or in suppressing the development of generalized tonic-clonic seizures. These drugs are uniquely capable of suppressing low-threshold, transient Ca^{2+} currents, which appear to be quite prominent in neurons within the intralaminar nuclei of the thalamus (9). It is thought that this is the mechanism by which these drugs suppress absence seizures. It must be pointed out, however, that absence seizures can also be suppressed by benzodiazepines working via enhancement of $GABA_A$ receptors; by VPA working via some other, unknown, mechanism; and, at least in experimental animals, by antagonists of the $GABA_B$ receptor.

MECHANISMS OF ACTION OF NEW ANTIEPILEPTIC DRUGS

Some of the new AEDs appear to act via mechanisms similar to those of older AEDs, whereas others appear to act via relatively novel mechanisms.

Inhibition of Voltage-Dependent Sodium Currents

Lamotrigine (LTG) has a clinical profile similar to, but perhaps broader than, those of PHT and CBZ. One of its principal mechanisms of action, analogous to that of PHT and CBZ, appears to be the suppression of voltage-dependent Na^+ currents in a voltage- and use-dependent fashion (10). LTG has been discussed as an agent that can suppress the release of glutamate from neurons, and speculation initially focused on whether this was a unique mechanism of action. However, it is likely that this effect is a consequence of blocking the Na^+ channels responsible for triggering the release of neurotransmitter from axonal endings.

Oxcarbazepine (OXC) (10,11-dihydro-10-oxo-carbamazepine) is a new AED that resembles CBZ and has a similar spectrum of antiseizure activity. OXC is really a prodrug, being quickly metabolized in the body to the 10-monohydroxyl compound (10,11-dihydro-10-hydroxycarbazepine, or MHD), which appears to be the active agent. OXC (MHD) can block SRF and therefore is likely to be acting on voltage-dependent Na^+ currents (11,12). The actions have not yet been described with voltage clamp techniques. Unlike its relative, CBZ, MHD has also been demonstrated to block glutamatergic excitatory postsynaptic potentials (EPSPs) in corticostriatal slice (13). This appeared to be the result of a presynaptic mechanism and was postulated to be related to a reduction in voltage-dependent Ca^{2+} currents. Additional work examining cortical and striatal neurons with both current clamp and voltage clamp recordings confirmed a blocking action on high-voltage-activated Ca^{2+} currents (14). The blocking action persisted in the presence of nifedipine, suggesting that L-type dihydropyridine-sensitive Ca^{2+} currents were *not* those affected by MHD. Interestingly, such an action has not been demonstrated for CBZ at comparable pharmacologic concentrations, although these experiments were performed by different investigators in different preparations (11). Thus, whether this action of MHD on voltage-dependent Ca^{2+} currents truly represents a significant difference for this drug's mechanism of action with regard to CBZ remains to be determined.

Zonisamide also appears to work via suppressing voltage-dependent Na^+ currents (15), although less has been published about the mechanism of action of this new AED. Similarly, topiramate (TPM) has been reported to suppress SRF, and it is therefore thought that suppression of Na^+ currents is one of its mechanisms of action (16).

Enhancement of GABA-Mediated Inhibition

Several of the new AEDs appear to act via enhancement of GABA-mediated inhibition, but by new mechanisms. In fact, two of the new drugs were specifically designed to enhance the effects of GABA by blocking its metabolism or blocking its uptake from the synaptic cleft. Vigabatrin (VGB) was designed as a GABA transaminase (GABA-T) inhibitor (17). The parent compound is activated once it binds to GABA-T and forms a reactive radical that covalently binds to the enzyme and inactivates it. Thus, VGB is called a suicide substrate inhibitor. GABA levels in the brain increase quickly after administration of VGB, and synaptic inhibition is also increased. Recent use of magnetic resonance spectroscopy has demonstrated that for many patients there is a ceiling effect, and doses of approximately 3 g/d produce maximal increases in GABA (18,19). Unlike the enhancement of GABA-mediated inhibition produced by PHB and benzodiazepines, which is restricted to synaptic function involving $GABA_A$ receptors, enhancement by VGB is *not* receptor-specific, and all effects of GABA are enhanced. This means that $GABA_B$ receptors can also be stimulated by the excess GABA released from nerve terminals. As $GABA_B$ receptors can be situated postsynaptically, where they mediate inhibition, or presynaptically, where they mediate reduction in synaptic neurotransmitter release, the net effect of VGB administration may be more variable than that of PHB or benzodiazepines. If the $GABA_B$ receptors on inhibitory terminals are preferentially activated, inhibition may actually be reduced by VGB.

In an analogous way, tiagabine (TGB) was also designed to enhance GABA-mediated inhibition, by blocking the reuptake of GABA released during synaptic activity (20). The effects of TGB effects are also not receptor subtype-specific. Prolongation of the actions of GABA is unlikely to prolong routine $GABA_A$ receptor-mediated IPSPs, as this is likely controlled by the channel kinetics. However, prolonged presence of GABA at synaptic clefts is more likely to activate $GABA_D$ receptors (21) and produce mixed net results, depending on the region of the brain involved and the state of the $GABA_B$ receptors. In fact, TGB can reduce IPSPs in some preparations (22) and cause increases in some kinds of seizures, but produce an antiseizure effect in other preparations.

Felbamate (FBM) has also been shown to enhance GABA-mediated IPSPs, in a manner appearing more similar to that of PHB and benzodiazepines (23). This is a receptor-specific stimulation, but its mechanism at the single-channel level has not yet been elucidated. The effects of FBM on GABA occur at relatively high concentrations compared with the serum concentrations at which the drug is active, so it is not known how much this action contributes to the antiseizure effects of FBM. However, other known mechanisms of action of FBM also occur at relatively high concentrations, and it has been speculated that FBM may work through several relatively low-affinity actions, the sum of which may be more important than each of the individual mechanisms.

Gabapentin (GBP) was designed as a GABA prodrug that would cross the blood-brain barrier and activate GABA receptors in the brain. This does not appear to be its mechanism, however, and it has been increasingly difficult to demonstrate any profound effect of GBP on GABA systems (24). GBP does not bind to any component of the GRC and does not activate Cl^- channels. GBP may, however, potentiate the release of GABA from neurons (25–27), and this could explain some of its antiseizure activity. GBP may also increase the concentration of GABA in the brain (28). GBP can also be shown to inhibit voltage-dependent Na^+ currents, but it is much more effective after cells have been exposed chronically to the drug than after acute exposure (29).

TPM, a drug just approved for release in the United States by the FDA (December 1996), is active against both partial and generalized seizures and has been postulated to have several cellular mechanisms of action, including an enhancement of GABAA-receptor-mediated inhibition. TPM does not bind to any known component of the GABA receptor complex, but in physiologic experiments TPM can be shown to enhance GABA-mediated Cl^- channel openings in a manner similar to that of the benzodiazepines (30). However, benzodiazepine antagonists do not block the effects of TPM. TPM alone does not appear capable of opening the Cl^- channels, even at high concentrations. TPM, as mentioned above, has also been demonstrated to block voltage-dependent Na^+ channels. TPM also has another unique cellular mechanism of action. At slightly higher concentrations, it is able to block the kainate subtype of glutamate receptors (16), although is appears ineffective at AMPA (α-amino-3-hydroxy-5-methyl-4-isoxazolepropionic acid) or NMDA (*N*-methyl-D-aspartate) receptors. How this action would translate into an antiseizure effect is not yet known, as the role of kainate receptors in the development of seizures remains unknown.

Reduction in Voltage-Dependent Calcium Currents

None of the new AEDs recently released in the United States or Europe or currently in clinical testing appear to have this as their primary mechanism of action, probably because of the relative lack of interest in drugs to treat primary generalized absence epilepsy and perhaps because of the fact that drugs with a number of different cellular mechanisms could be effective against these types of seizures, so that even screening with animal models might not pick up drugs with this specific mechanism. Part of the effect of zonisamide may be attributable to this mechanism (31). Experimental studies have suggested that drugs that work against other classes of voltage-dependent calcium currents might be useful in suppressing both interictal activity and the transition to seizures (32–37), but to date the clinical utility of drugs acting on voltage-dependent calcium currents has been relatively unimpressive.

Inhibition of Glutamate Receptors

In the last decade, much work has focused on the role of different glutamate receptors in the epileptic process and on the possibility of developing antagonists of these receptors as AEDs (38). Suffice it to say that to date, this has been a disappointing endeavor, and no drugs acting at either AMPA or NMDA receptors are clinically available. It has been proposed that one component of the action of FBM is to block NMDA receptors (23), but this occurs at relatively high concentrations, and its clinical significance remains to be determined. At least one other drug, MK801, acting specifically at the NMDA receptor proceeded to clinical trials, but at low doses it was ineffective and at higher doses too toxic for use. Remacemide is another new AED that appears to act at NMDA receptors and is currently in clinical trials (39). Interestingly, remacemide also acts at voltage-dependent Na^+ channels and therefore may have a mixed mechanism of action.

CONCLUSIONS AND FUTURE DIRECTIONS

In addition to the AEDs that have been available in the United States for more than 15 years, three new AEDs have been approved for use in the United States within the past 3 years, one new AED will be marketed in early 1997, and several new AEDs are available in Europe or Asia and are being clinically tested in the United States. Through many years, we have learned to classify the mechanisms of action of the conventional AEDs into three broad categories. Interestingly, these are the categories of mechanisms of action for most of the new AEDs as well. However, it is likely that these mechanisms of action are not capable of explaining all the antiseizure effects of many AEDs. For example, although VPA blocks voltage-dependent Na^+ currents, its broad spectrum of action indicates that it must also have other antiseizure effects that are not shared by PHT and CBZ. Similarly, LTG acts very much like PHT and CBZ on Na^+ currents, but also appears to have a broader spectrum of action and is likely to operate by other mechanisms.

In general, we examine newly discovered AEDs only with epilepsy model screening, using a set of pharmacologic and electrophysiologic tests that have been developed during the last two decades. There are many other possible mechanisms by which these drugs might work for which we have no test or for which we are not testing. The importance of this observation is underscored by recent advances in the analysis of some forms of inherited epilepsy. We now know that one form of epilepsy results from alterations in energy metabolism (40,41), another from an altered cysteine protease inhibitor (42), and a third from an altered nicotinic cholinergic receptor subunit (43). Drugs might be discovered that can operate on any of these systems, or compensate downstream from any of these defects. Such drugs might be effective AEDs, at least for these seizure types, and their mechanisms of action might never be uncovered because they would not be analyzed for the relevant processes. Thus, what we uncover as a mechanism of action for a given drug will depend critically on how the search is carried out.

Another component of AED mechanisms of action relates to the time course of most experiments. In general, drugs are examined in cellular or molecular preparations with acute application. Thus, if for a drug to work some form of chronic exposure is needed (even for hours), its action may be missed by routine experiments. This can be correlated with clinical data, in that most drugs appear to act by the time they reach equilibrium with brain levels, and so these drugs should act acutely in experimental preparations. Other drugs, especially those for which there is no parenteral route of administration, may not work so quickly.

A third caveat with regard to studies of the mechanisms of action of AEDs is the concept that a drug has only one mechanism of action or one main mechanism. This may be true for some drugs, but others may be effective because they have some unique combination of mechanisms that together produce the desired effect. In fact, one can make the case that for a number of complex neurologic diseases, such as epilepsy, Parkinson's disease, or depression, drugs with mixed mechanisms may be more effective clinically than highly targeted drugs with single, precise mechanisms of action. Certainly, each of the "conventional" AEDs—PHT, CBZ, and PHB—has multiple mechanisms that may be contributing to its final antiseizure effects. In this regard, even subtle differences may account for why some patients respond better to one Na^+-channel blocker than another. It is extremely important to recognize this issue, as current thinking about managed care in medicine tends to lump drugs together by their putative mechanism of action and allow pharmacists to substitute drugs arbitrarily within these categories. Our clinical experience would indicate that this is not going to be appropriate for epilepsy.

Finally, all AEDs have side effects, and it is often the side effect profile of a drug that determines how well it is accepted. Moreover, the nonneurologic side effects of most of the drugs differ significantly, again suggesting major differences in how drugs work in the body, even if they are thought to have common mechanisms of action. For example, the ability of PHT to produce gum hyperplasia and hirsutism, and its interaction with folic acid metabolism, are consequences of the "mechanisms of action" of PHT. These must be different from those associated with CBZ, because CBZ does not produce these effects. CBZ, on the other hand, suppresses the bone marrow, by another "mechanism of action" that is not shared by PHT. Thus, two "Na^+-channel blockers" also have multiple other "mechanisms of action." Side effects are caused by "mechanisms of action," and in general differ considerably from one AED to another.

AEDs can be discovered by screening new compounds against animal models of seizures (or epilepsy) or by screening against a discrete receptor, channel, transporter, neurotransmitter, or metabolic reaction. As we learn more about mechanisms underlying interictal discharges, the transition to seizures, the spread of seizure activity, and the development of the chronically hyperexcitable state that we call epilepsy, we may be in a position to develop drugs that can specifically interfere with one or another of these processes. The goal of modern pharmacology is to develop such drugs. Whether this goal will be reached for epilepsy in the near future remains to be determined. In the meanwhile, if we want to develop drugs with new and novel mechanisms of action, we may need to screen our compounds against different, and perhaps more representative, epilepsy models. Thus, we may need to use genetic models of different syndromes or models of chronic epilepsy rather than of acute seizures. Moreover, if we want to develop drugs to prevent the development of epilepsy, we may need to use models of epileptogenesis. In addition, we will need to refine the clinical evaluation of drugs that appear promising in the laboratory or preclinical stage, so as to be able detect drugs that may be very effective for a specific subpopulation of individuals with epilepsy. Finally, if we could learn more about the mechanisms of action by which drugs produce unwanted side effects, we might be able to develop strategies designed to make those drugs that are effective better tolerated.

REFERENCES

1. Steriade M, McCormick D, Sejnowski T. Thalamocortical oscillations in the sleeping and aroused brain. *Science* 1993;262:679–685.
2. Coulter DA, Huguenard JR, Prince DA. Calcium currents in rat thalamocortical relay neurones: kinetic properties of the transient, low-threshold current. *J Physiol (Lond)* 1989;414:587–604.
3. Macdonald R, Kelly K. Antiepileptic drug mechanisms of action. *Epilepsia* 1993;34:S1–S8.
4. McLean M, Macdonald R. Multiple actions of phenytoin on mouse spinal cord neurons in cell culture. *J Pharmacol Exp Ther* 1983;227:779–789.
5. McLean M, Macdonald R. Carbamazepine and 10,11-epoxycarbamazepine produce use- and voltage-dependent limitation of rapidly firing action potentials of mouse central neurons in cell culture. *J Pharmacol Exp Ther* 1986;238:727–738.
6. McLean M, Macdonald R. Sodium valproate, but not ethosuximide, produces use- and voltage-dependent limitation of high-frequency repetitive firing of action potentials of mouse central neurons in cell culture. *J Pharmacol Exp Ther* 1986;237:1001–1011.
7. Ragsdale D, Scheuer T, Catterall W. Frequency- and voltage-dependent inhibition of type IIA Na channels, expressed in a mammalian cell line, by local anesthetic, antiarrhythmic, and anticonvulsant drugs. *Mol Pharmacol* 1991;40:756–765.
8. Twyman R, Rogers C, Macdonald R. Differential regulation of gamma-aminobutyric acid receptor channels by diazepam and phenobarbital. *Ann Neurol* 1989;25: 213–220.
9. Coulter DA, Huguenard JR, Prince DA. Characterization of ethosuximide reduction of low-threshold calcium current in thalamic neurons. *Ann Neurol* 1989;25: 582–593.
10. Lang DG, Wang CM, Cooper BR. Lamotrigine, phenytoin, and carbamazepine interactions on the sodium current present in N4TG1 mouse neuroblastoma cells. *J Pharmacol Exp Ther* 1993;266:829–835.
11. Wamil A, Portet C, Jensen P, Schmutz M, McLean M. Oxcarbazepine and its monohydroxy metabolite limit action potential firing by mouse central neurons in cell culture. *Epilepsia* 1992;32:S65–S66.
12. McLean M, Schmutz M, Wamil A, Olpe H, Portet C, Feldmann K. Oxcarbazepine: mechanisms of action. *Epilepsia* 1994;35:S5–S9.
13. Calabresi P, De Murtas M, Stefani A, Pisani A, Sancesario G, Mercuri N, Bernardi G. Action of GP 47779, the active metabolite of oxcarbazepine, on the corticostriatal system. I. Modulation of corticostriatal synaptic transmission. *Epilepsia* 1995;36:990–996.
14. Stefani A, Pisani A, De Murtas M, Mercuri N, Marciani M, Bernardi G, Calabresi P. Action of GP 47779, the active metabolite of oxcarbazepine, on the corticostriatal system. II. Modulation of HVA calcium currents. *Epilepsia* 1995;36:997–1002.
15. Rock DM, Macdonald RL, Taylor CP. Blockade of sustained repetitive action potentials in cultured spinal cord neurons by zonisamide (AD 810, CI 912), a novel anticonvulsant. *Epilepsy Res* 1989;3:138–143.
16. Coulter D, Sombati S, Delorenzo R. Selective effects of topiramate on sustained repetitive firing and spontaneous bursting in cultured hippocampal neurons. *Epilepsia* 1993;34:123(abst).
17. Sabers A, Gram L. Pharmacology of vigabatrin. *Pharmacol Toxicol* 1992;70:237–243.
18. Petroff OA, Rothman DL, Behar KL, Mattson RH. Human brain GABA levels rise after initiation of vigabatrin therapy but fail to rise further with increasing dose. *Neurology* 1996;46:1459–1463.
19. Mattson RH, Petroff OA, Rothman D, Behar K. Vigabatrin: effect on brain GABA levels measured by nuclear magnetic resonance spectroscopy. *Acta Neurol Scand Suppl* 1995;162:27–30.
20. Nielsen EB, Suzdak PD, Andersen KE, Knutsen LJ, Sonnewald U, Braestrup C. Characterization of tiagabine (NO-328), a new potent and selective GABA uptake inhibitor. *Eur J Pharmacol* 1991;196:257–266.
21. Thompson SM, Gahwiler BH. Effects of the GABA uptake inhibitor tiagabine on inhibitory synaptic potentials in rat hippocampal slice cultures. *J Neurophysiol* 1992;67:1698–1701.
22. Oh DJ, Dichter MA. Effect of a gamma-aminobutyric acid uptake inhibitor, NNC-711, on spontaneous postsynaptic currents in cultured rat hippocampal neurons: implications for antiepileptic drug development. *Epilepsia* 1994;35:426–430.
23. Rho JM, Donevan SD, Rogawski MA. Mechanism of action of the anticonvulsant felbamate: opposing effects on *N*-methyl-D-aspartate and gamma-aminobutyric acid A receptors. *Ann Neurol* 1994;35:229–234.
24. Goa KL, Sorkin EM. Gabapentin. A review of its pharmacological properties and clinical potential in epilepsy. *Drugs* 1993;46:409–427.
25. Kocsis JD, Honmou O. Gabapentin increases GABA-induced depolarization in rat neonatal optic nerve. *Neurosci Lett* 1994;169:181–184.
26. Gotz E, Feuerstein TJ, Lais A, Meyer DK. Effects of gabapentin on release of gamma-aminobutyric acid from slices of rat neostriatum. *Arzneimittelforschung* 1993;43:636–638.
27. Honmou O, Oyelese AA, Kocsis JD. The anticonvulsant gabapentin enhances promoted release of GABA in hippocampus: a field potential analysis. *Brain Res* 1995; 692:273–277.
28. Petroff OA, Rothman DL, Behar KL, Lamoureux D, Mattson RH. The effect of gabapentin on brain gamma-aminobutyric acid in patients with epilepsy. *Ann Neurol* 1996;39:95–99.
29. Wamil AW, McLean MJ. Limitation by gabapentin of high-frequency action potential firing by mouse central neurons in cell culture. *Epilepsy Res* 1994;17:1–11.
30. Twyman R, Brown S, White S. The anticonvulsant topiramate potentiates GABA-evoked chloride currents. *Ann Neurol* (*in press*).

31. Suzuki S, Kawakami K, Nishimura S, et al. Zonisamide blocks T-type calcium channel in cultured neurons of rat cerebral cortex. *Exp Epilepsy Res* 1992;12:21–27.
32. De Sarro G, De Sarro A, Federico F, Meldrum BS. Anticonvulsant properties of some calcium antagonists on sound-induced seizures in genetically epilepsy-prone rats. *Gen Pharmacol* 1990;21:769–778.
33. Meyer FB, Anderson RE, Sundt TM Jr, Sharbrough FW. Selective central nervous system calcium channel blockers—a new class of anticonvulsant agents. *Mayo Clin Proc* 1986;61:239–247.
34. Walden J, Straub H, Speckmann EJ. Epileptogenesis: contributions of calcium ions and antiepileptic calcium antagonists. *Acta Neurol Scand Suppl* 1992;140:41–46.
35. Speckmann EJ, Walden J. Anticonvulsant effects of calcium channel blockers in partial and generalized model epilepsies. *Funct Neurol* 1986;1:521–527.
36. Delumeau JC, Bentue-Ferrer D, Saiag B, Allain H. Clinical neuropharmacology of calcium antagonists. *Fundam Clin Pharmacol* 1989;3(Suppl):89s–102s.
37. Walden J, Speckmann EJ, Witte OW. Suppression of focal epileptiform discharges by intraventricular perfusion of a calcium antagonist. *Electroencephalogr Clin Neurophysiol* 1985;61:299–309.
38. Rogawski M. The NMDA receptor, NMDA antagonists, and epilepsy therapy. *Drugs* 1992;44:279–292.
39. Muir E, Palmer G. Remacemide. In: Pisani F, Perucca G, Avanzini G, Richens A, eds. *New Antiepileptic Drugs*. Amsterdam: Elsevier Science Publishers; 1991: 147–152.
40. Rosing HS, Hopkins LC, Wallace DC, Epstein CM, Weidenheim K. Maternally inherited mitochondrial myopathy and myoclonic epilepsy. *Ann Neurol* 1985;17: 228–237.
41. Shoffner JM, Lott MT, Lezza AM, Seibel P, Ballinger SW, Wallace DC. Myoclonic epilepsy and ragged-red fiber disease (MERRF) is associated with a mitochondrial DNA tRNA(Lys) mutation. *Cell* 1990;61: 931–937.
42. Pennacchio L, Lehesjoki A, Stone N, et al. Mutations in the gene encoding cystatin B in progressive myoclonus epilepsy (*EPM1*). *Science* 1996;271: 1731–1734.
43. Steinlein O, Mulley J, Propiing P, Wallace R, Phillips H, Sutherland G, et al. A missense mutation in the neuronal nicotinic acetylcholine receptor a4 subunit is associated with autosomal dominant nocturnal frontal lobe epilepsy. *Nat Genet* 1995;11:1–5.

Antiepileptic Drug Development.
Advances in Neurology, Vol. 76,
edited by J. French, I. Leppik, and M. A. Dichter.
Lippincott–Raven Publishers, Philadelphia © 1998.

2

Mechanism-Specific Pathways for New Antiepileptic Drug Discovery

Michael A. Rogawski

Neuronal Excitability Section, Epilepsy Research Branch, National Institute of Neurological Disorders and Stroke, National Institutes of Health, Bethesda, Maryland 20892.

ANTIEPILEPTIC DRUG DISCOVERY: SCREENING VERSUS MECHANISM-SPECIFIC APPROACHES

How can more effective, better-tolerated antiepileptic drugs be identified? Most presently available antiepileptic drugs were discovered by drug screening using mechanism-neutral animal models. These animal models are used to identify potentially effective antiepileptic drugs based on their ability to protect against seizures (or a seizurelike behavioral response, such as tonic hindlimb extension) at doses that fail to induce generalized neurologic toxicity. Although none of the common screening models represent true models of epilepsy (characterized by spontaneous, recurrent seizures), activity in the models is an excellent predictor of efficacy in the treatment of human seizure disorders (1).

It can be argued that such mechanism-neutral screening methods have advantages over mechanism-based approaches, in that they allow for the identification of antiepileptic drugs that act by as yet unidentified molecular mechanisms or via complex actions on several targets. Thus, it is unlikely that mechanism-based approaches will eliminate the use of animal models. Nevertheless, in recent decades a number of specific molecular targets in the central nervous system have been identified where it is believed that anticonvulsant drugs act to produce their antiseizure effects. As in other therapeutic areas, there has been a movement on the part of the pharmaceutical industry to utilize this new knowledge in mechanism-based drug development. By targeting specific brain mechanisms, it is hoped that it will be possible to interfere with seizure-generating mechanisms in a highly selective fashion, so that seizures are prevented without the normal functioning of the brain being affected. However, if we consider that the molecular targets involved in seizure generation are also key mediators of neuronal excitability, vital to the normal functioning of the brain and spinal cord, it becomes evident that the problem of creating a drug that will prevent seizure activity while at the same time failing to cause significant impairment of normal neural activity is a major challenge. For example, it is well recognized that voltage-activated sodium (Na^+) channels are critically involved in seizure propagation by virtue of their role as mediators of the upstroke of fast action potentials. Indeed, the anticonvulsant activity of phenytoin is believed to reside in its ability to block Na^+ channels in a slow use-dependent and voltage-dependent fashion (2). Although the effect of phenytoin on Na^+ channels is similar to that of local anesthetics, the specific quantitative details of the blocking effects of phenytoin seem to endow it with just the right properties to be a minimally toxic anticonvulsant. Numerous other drugs are much more potent Na^+-channel blockers but are useless as anticonvulsants (3).

The mechanism of action of phenytoin was determined with in vitro electrophysiologic approaches using isolated cells. However, even with the availability of these tools and our present-day knowledge, it would have been difficult to select phenytoin from among the multitude of chemical compounds that can modify Na^+-channel activity. Rather, phenytoin was originally identified by a mechanism-neutral screening approach using the predecessor of today's maximal electroshock test (4). In fact, newer anticonvulsants that act on Na^+ channels (such as lamotrigine, zonisamide, and riluzole) were also identified in animal screening models, and only later were shown to interact with Na^+ channels in mechanism-based testing. To date, no Na^+-channel blocking anticonvulsant has been identified through the use of mechanism-based screening in a system designed to test activity on Na^+ channels. This is because the simplistic approach of maximizing activity on a specific drug target, which may be an appropriate strategy in other areas of pharmaceutical development, is not relevant in anticonvulsant drug discovery. In fact, as part of the drug development program of the Parke-Davis Pharmaceutical Research Division, Warner-Lambert Company, Roufos et al. (5) identified the phenylacetamide PD85,639 (*N*-[3-(2,6-dimethyl-1-piperidinyl)]-α-phenylbenzeneacetamide) as an extremely potent, use-dependent, centrally active Na^+ channel blocker (6). However, PD85,639 failed to exhibit anticonvulsant activity against tonic extensor seizures in the mouse, a model in which phenytoin is highly active. It would seem that the specific way in which phenytoin interacts with Na^+ channels is more important than the overall potency of its effect.

As indicated by this example, there are a number of key principals of drug discovery relevant to other therapeutic areas that require modification in antiepileptic drug discovery. First among these is the principal of maximization of receptor potency. As in the case of PD85,639, increasing receptor potency (at voltage-dependent Na^+ channels) does not necessarily lead to improved activity. Similarly, in the case of channel-blocking NMDA (*N*-methyl-D-aspartate) antagonists (discussed in more detail below), high-affinity dissociative anesthetic-like blockers, such as dizocilpine (MK-801) and phencyclidine are toxic, and not clinically useful anticonvulsants, whereas drugs that act at the same site on NMDA receptors but with lower affinity, such as memantine, remacemide and its metabolite ARL 12495, and ADCI, have promise. Possible explanations for this observation are discussed below (see also ref. 7).

In conventional drug discovery, a key goal is to maximize activity at the desired target site and reduce activity at other targets, with the aim of optimizing therapeutic activity and minimizing side effects. In some cases, this principal of optimization of target site selectivity may not be relevant in anticonvulsant drug discovery. Thus, it might be preferable for an anticonvulsant drug to interact simultaneously, but with modest activity, at several target sites (e.g., Na^+ channels, $GABA_A$ receptors, and excitatory amino acid receptors). The modest modifications of activity produced at each target might act synergistically to produce a robust protective effect against seizures. On the other hand, if the toxicities produced at each target site are different, it might be the case that the effect at each target (at an anticonvulsant dose) would be subthreshold for the differing toxicities. Thus, a drug that, for example, simultaneously affected Na^+ channels and $GABA_A$ receptors might exhibit enhanced anticonvulsant activity compared with the effect at each target site alone, because the effects at each target site would both lead to the final common effect of seizure protection. However, as the toxicities mediated at each target are different (symptoms of cerebellar impairment for Na^+-channel blockers and sedation for $GABA_A$ receptor potentiating agents), the toxicities would not be synergistic. If the effects at each target were modest and subthreshold, the drug might have good anticonvulsant activity with minimal toxicity. In fact, it is believed that several newly marketed and investigational anticonvulsant drugs may act in this way on several targets, including felbamate (8) and topiramate (9).

Finally, in conventional drug discovery, full agonist effects (high efficacy) are often the desired goal. For an antiepileptic drug, however, partial agonist effects may be preferable. For example, partial benzodiazepine receptor agonists may not have the side effects (sedation) and, most importantly, the tolerance liability of full agonists (10). At full receptor occupancy, partial agonists produce a biologic effect equivalent to that of partial receptor occupancy with a full agonist. If the anticonvulsant effects of a full agonist (e.g., diazepam) are produced with low receptor occupancy (as seems to be the case in some models; see ref. 11), whereas toxicity (such as sedation and muscle relaxation) requires high receptor occupancy, a partial agonist will have the ability to protect against seizures, but no dose of the partial agonist (even a very high one producing full receptor occupancy) will be sedative. Partial agonists also seem to be associated with less tolerance and physical dependence than do full agonists, but the reason for this is not well understood.

In sum, whereas in conventional drug discovery the goal is to identify molecules with high potency, high selectivity, and high efficacy, in anticonvulsant drug development compounds with modest potency that have activity at several relevant target sites and that are partial agonists may be preferred.

A final factor to consider in anticonvulsant drug discovery is the possibility that the epileptic brain may have unique drug sensitivities. Historically, anticonvulsant drugs were identified by testing in normal animals induced to have seizures. Moreover, current studies of the molecular bases of drug action typically utilize native or cloned receptors and channels from normal animals. However, there is emerging evidence that profound changes in excitability mechanisms occur in epilepsy. Thus, anticonvulsant drugs can have markedly different behavioral effects and toxicities in epileptic animals (12). This may be caused by alterations in neurotransmitter receptor expression accompanying the epileptic phenotype (13–15). Consideration of these receptor changes as well as the now well-established evidence of structural alterations in neural connectivity accompanying epilepsy (16) may lead to powerful new antiepileptic strategies.

With these general principles in mind, I will, in the remainder of this chapter, consider some of the molecular targets in the central nervous system that are of relevance for antiepileptic drug development. Despite the fact that most of these protein target molecules have been cloned, so that their primary amino acid structures are known, it is generally not possible to design *de novo* drugs that bind and modify the target in a desired way. Thus, the goal of "rational drug design" is not currently approachable. However, once an appropriate target has been selected, drug candidates can be identified in a process that perhaps can be referred to as "rational screening," in which a library of chemical compounds is randomly screened against the target site. Alternatively, if a prototype drug can be identified with at least some degree of desired activity at the target, analogues can be prepared and screened in an attempt to identify the pharmacophore for therapeutic activity or toxicity. This information can then be used to optimize target site activity or obtain other desirable characteristics (such as preferred pharmacokinetic properties or blood-brain barrier permeability). (In this chapter, the focus is on drugs for the treatment of generalized tonic-clonic and partial seizures; for new treatment strategies in absence epilepsy, see ref. 11.)

$GABA_A$ RECEPTOR, GABA TRANSAMINASE, AND GABA UPTAKE TRANSPORTER AS ANTICONVULSANT DRUG TARGETS

Of the approaches for the rational development of new anticonvulsant drugs, the most successful involve strategies to enhance synaptic inhibition, which is predominantly mediated by the inhibitory transmitter GABA (τ-aminobutyric acid) acting on $GABA_A$ receptors. It is possible to enhance GABA-mediated synaptic inhibition by a variety of approaches. The most direct is obviously the administration of a GABA agonist or prodrug (as GABA itself does not cross the blood-brain barrier). However, neither directly acting agonists such as THIP (4,5,6,7-tetrahydroisoxazolo-5,4-*C*-pyridine-3-ol) nor prodrugs such as progabide have demonstrated useful clinical anticonvulsant activity (17). An alternative strategy is to target enzymes involved in GABA synthesis so as to increase brain GABA levels. Although no anticonvulsant drug has been definitively linked to this mechanism, valproic acid has been demonstrated to enhance the activity of the GABA synthetic enzyme glutamic acid decarboxylase (GAD) in brain homogenates (18) and also to increase brain synthesis and levels of GABA (19,20). Recently, gabapentin has also been demonstrated to increase brain GABA levels (21), possibly by stimulation of GABA synthesis (22). However, it is yet to be established how significant the effects of valproate and gabapentin on GABA synthesis are in the overall anticonvulsant activity of the drugs.

Alternative approaches to increasing GABAergic tone include potentiation of the $GABA_A$ receptor (by drugs that bind to the receptor and allosterically modify its gating) or enhancement of synaptic GABA levels. The latter can be accomplished by inhibition of the GABA degradative enzyme GABA transaminase (GABA-T) or blockade of GABA uptake into neurons and/or glia.

Presently available drugs that potentiate $GABA_A$ receptors include the benzodiazepines and barbiturates. In addition, there are a variety of agents, including neuroactive steroids and loreclezole, that act similarly to barbiturates but probably interact with a distinct site on the $GABA_A$ receptor complex (11). Benzodiazepine receptor agonists, such as diazepam and lorazepam, have powerful anticonvulsant properties. Although such benzodiazepine agonists have an important role in the treatment of status epilepticus, two significant limitations largely preclude their use in long-term epilepsy therapy. The first limiting factor is that these benzodiazepines produce undesirable side effects, including sedation and muscle relaxation, at doses comparable with those that protect against seizures. The second and probably more important limitation is that tolerance develops to the anticonvulsant activity of benzodiazepine receptor agonists with long-term use. In recent years, considerable effort has been directed toward developing strategies for overcoming these limitations. A variety of benzodiazepines and drugs other than benzodiazepines have been identified that interact with the benzodiazepine binding site of the $GABA_A$ receptor complex in novel and potentially more favorable ways. In fact, partial benzodiazepine receptor agonists have been obtained with reduced liability for tolerance (10,23). In addition, subtype-selective benzodiazepine receptor agonists could theoretically overcome the disadvantageous side effects of nonselective drugs such as diazepam. Despite the potential of partial and subtype-selective benzodiazepine receptor agonists in epilepsy therapy, progress in this area has been limited, and there is no convincing evidence that any such benzodiazepine receptor ligands will have practical utility in the long-term treatment of epilepsy.

Like benzodiazepines, barbiturates are highly effective, broad-spectrum anticonvulsants. In addition to their ability to potentiate and also directly activate (24) $GABA_A$ receptors, barbiturates have effects on voltage-dependent calcium (Ca^{2+}) channels (25) (where it has been hypothesized that they may act to reduce glutamate release) and on AMPA (α-amino-3-hydroxy-5-methyl-4-isoxazolepropionic acid) receptors (26). The main impediment to the use of barbiturates in epilepsy therapy is their strong sedative activity. However, by optimizing the spectrum of effects on the various ion channel targets ($GABA_A$ receptors, Ca^{2+} channels, and AMPA receptors), it is conceivable that barbiturate-like compounds with improved side effect profiles could be obtained. In fact, felbamate, an anticonvulsant that more frequently causes agitation and insomnia than sedation, appears to act in part as a barbiturate-like modulator of $GABA_A$ receptors (27).

Another class of barbiturate-like allosteric $GABA_A$ receptor modulators comprises the neuroactive steroids (28). These steroids are devoid of traditional hormonal activity but instead produce a powerful potentiation of $GABA_A$ receptors (and, like barbiturates, also directly activate the receptors). A variety of synthetic steroids, including the steroid anesthetic alfaxalone, act in this fashion, as do certain endogenous ring A-reduced metabolites of progesterone and deoxycorticosterone, most notably epiallopregnanolone and allotetrahydrodeoxycorticosterone. Neuroactive steroids are protective against seizures induced by pentylenetetrazol and other GABA receptor antagonists (29), and in some cases they have also been found to be effective in the maximal electroshock test, albeit at higher (often nearly toxic) doses (30). Although tolerance to neuroactive steroids can occur at the receptor level (31), in an animal study tolerance to the anticonvulsant activity was not observed (32). Until recently, two significant problems have impeded the development of neuroactive steroids for use in epilepsy therapy. First, the therapeutic index (separation between the dose required for seizure protection and that producing motor impairment) of neuroactive steroids was relatively poor (29). Second, the steroids had poor bioavailability and were short-acting. Newer synthetic analogues, such as ganaxolone and Co 2-1068 (a prodrug; see ref. 33) appear to have reduced relative toxicity, are rapidly absorbed following oral administration, and have sufficiently prolonged actions to be administered on a thrice-daily schedule. In humans, ganaxolone was well tolerated with plasma concentrations (0.1 to 1 μM) in the range known from in vitro studies to modulate $GABA_A$ receptors (IC_{50} [concentration that inhibits 50%] for inhibition of [^{35}S]*t*-butylbicyclophosphorothionate binding of ~80 nM) (34). Adverse events observed most frequently in healthy volunteers included somnolence and dizziness. In an open-label, dose-escalation study in children refractory to conventional antiepileptic drugs, decreased seizure frequency was reported in 6 of 15 children and adolescents. Ganaxolone is currently undergoing controlled efficacy trials. Recently, neuroactive steroids that act as partial agonists at the putative neuroactive steroid site associated with $GABA_A$ receptors have been described (35). Whether such newer-generation neuroactive steroids will have anticonvulsant activity but produce less sedation (as is the case for partial benzodiazepine receptor agonists) remains to be determined. Preclinical studies indicate that the neuroactive steroids are highly effective in models of status epilepticus (36), indicating an additional potential use of this class of anticonvulsants.

In addition to the focus on targeting of postsynaptic $GABA_A$ receptors, there has been considerable interest and, indeed, success in the development of new antiepileptic drugs that modify GABA disposition in the brain. Vigabatrin (γ-vinyl-GABA), perhaps the most notable example, is an enzyme-activated irreversible inhibitor of GABA-T, the main degradative enzyme for GABA. The drug, which is a structural analogue of GABA, was synthesized specifically for the purpose of inhibiting the pyridoxal phosphate-dependent enzyme GABA-T, so it is indeed an example of rational drug design (37). Vigabatrin produces a twofold to threefold elevation of brain GABA levels (38), largely in intraneuronal pools that are available for release (39). Thus, it is believed that increased amounts of GABA are released in a use-dependent fashion as needed during seizures. There are now substantial clinical data supporting the efficacy of vigabatrin in the treatment of partial epilepsies (37,40). Although drowsiness and other side effects do occur with vigabatrin, these are often transient, and overall the drug is well tolerated in most subjects (41). In view of the critical importance of GABAergic neurotransmission in virtually all brain circuits, a drug that increases brain GABA levels might be expected to have substantial toxicity. However, the use-dependent action of vigabatrin may account for its selective protective action against seizures and good tolerability.

An alternative approach to enhancing synaptic GABA levels is blockade of GABA uptake into neurons and glia. Traditional GABA uptake blockers, such as nipecotic acid or guavacine, are polar compounds that do not penetrate the blood-brain barrier and are therefore unusable as anticonvulsants. In recent years, a variety of lipophilic analogues of nipecotic acid and guavacine have been described (42,43,44). These compounds, which include tiagabine, CI-966, NNC-711, and SKF 100330A, are highly potent and specific inhibitors of GABA uptake into glia and neurons, but they have essentially no activity on other uptake transporters. Using in vivo microdialysis, it has been possible to show that tiagabine increases extracellular GABA overflow in animals and awake human subjects (45; M. During, *unpublished observations*). Lipophilic GABA uptake inhibitors have a spectrum of anticonvulsant activity in animal seizure models similar to that of other drugs that act on brain GABA systems, such as the benzodiazepines (46). At doses higher than those required to protect against seizures, lipophilic GABA uptake inhibitors produce neurologic impairment, as do other drugs that enhance GABAergic neurotransmission. However, there is evidence that tolerance may develop to these side effects, but not to the anticonvulsant activity (47). In human clinical trials, tiagabine has shown efficacy in several monotherapy and add-on trials (48,49). Adverse events were not severe, and those that did occur (e.g., dizziness) were usually transient and did not require medical intervention (50). Importantly, there was no evidence of tolerance to the anticonvulsant activity of the drug with long-term dosing. GABA uptake blockers such as tiagabine are a promising new class of anticonvulsant drug with a well-defined mechanism of action.

EXCITATORY AMINO ACID RECEPTOR SYSTEMS AS ANTICONVULSANT DRUG TARGETS

The bulk of fast synaptic excitation in the central nervous system is mediated by the excitatory amino acid neurotransmitter glutamate acting on AMPA (α-amino-3-hydroxy-5-methyl-4-isoxazolepropionic acid) and NMDA (*N*-methyl-D-aspartic acid) receptors. A large body of evidence has been accumulated during the past 15 years supporting a role for NMDA and AMPA receptors in the expression of seizures in various in vivo and in vitro epilepsy models (51). Moreover, there is extensive evidence that NMDA (52) and AMPA (7) receptor antagonists have powerful anticonvulsant activity. Consequently, NMDA and AMPA receptors are important potential targets for the development of antiepileptic drugs. However, the early optimism regarding excitatory amino acid antagonists as antiepileptic drug candidates has been tempered by the recognition that such antagonists may have significant toxicities. Initially, most of the attention was focused on competitive NMDA recognition site antagonists. However, early clinical trials failed to provide much encouragement. For example, in a key open-label study of D-CPPene (an orally active cyclic phosphonate), all subjects withdrew prematurely because of side effects, including poor concentration, sedation, ataxia, depression, dysarthria, and amnesia (53). Given the critical role of NMDA receptors as mediators of central excitatory neurotransmission, this toxicity is not surprising. At present, the question of whether NMDA receptor antagonists can be developed that have sufficiently low toxicity to be clinically useful in epilepsy therapy remains unanswered.

Although development of competitive NMDA recognition site antagonists such as D-CPPene has largely been terminated, several other approaches to NMDA receptor blockade may have more promise, including competitive antagonism at the glycine site and low-affinity channel blockade. In addition, there is interest in subtype-selective NMDA receptor antagonists (i.e., those that target specific combinations of NMDA receptor subunits). At present, only NR2B selective antagonists are available. Thus, ifenprodil and eliprodil (SL 82.0715), potent allosteric (noncompetitive) inhibitors of the NMDA receptor, appear to antagonize selectively NMDA receptors composed of NR1A and NR2B subunits (54–57). Ifenprodil and eliprodil are effective neuroprotective agents with low toxicity. In addition, the two drugs have anticonvulsant activity in a broad spectrum of animal models (58,59). However, the anticonvulsant effects occur at high doses relative to the neuroprotection. Thus, it would appear that NR2B antagonists may not be optimally suited for seizure protection. Whether other subtype-selective antagonists will specifically target seizures remains to be determined.

Occupation of the glycine site is required for activation of the NMDA receptor (60,61). Consequently, agents that act as antagonists at this site produce as complete a functional block of the receptor as occurs with NMDA recognition site antagonists. However, evidence accumulated in recent years suggests that glycine site antagonists may have a more favorable side effect profile (62). In animals, glycine site antagonists may produce less neurobehavioral toxicity (63) and, indeed, may actually attenuate the adverse effects of channel-blocking NMDA receptor antagonists (64). In addition, glycine site antagonists may not induce neuronal vacuolization and necrosis as do high-affinity (dissociative anesthetic-like) channel blockers and competitive NMDA recognition site antagonists (65). Until recently, however, most selective glycine site antagonists were not of interest as drug candidates because they had poor blood-brain barrier penetrability. This situation has now changed with the identification of several related classes of glycine site antagonist that have good systemic bioavailability. For example, Kulagowski et al. (66) have described a series of 3′-substituted 3-phenyl-4-hydroxyquinolones (L-703,717; L-708,541; L-701,324; and L-705,022) that are highly potent glycine site antagonists in vitro and are effective anticonvulsants when administered either intraperitoneally or orally [ED_{50} (median effective dose) values for protection against reflex seizures in DBA/2 mice of <1 mg/kg]. More recently, a series of 1,4-dihydro-2,3-quinoxalinediones have been described that are similarly high-potency glycine site antagonists in vitro and have good systemic bioavailability. One such compound, 7-chloro-6-methyl-5-nitro-1,4-dihydro-2,3-quinoxalinedione (ACEA-1416), has particularly high anticonvulsant potency in the mouse maximal electroshock test (ED_{50} of ~1.5 mg/kg) (67). A related selective glycine site antagonist, licostinel (5-nitro-6,7-dichloro-1,4-dihydro-2,3-quinoxalinedione; ACEA-1021), which has only modestly reduced potency in the maximal electroshock test (see ref. 68), has been extensively studied in behavioral paradigms designed to assess whether the drug has liability for dissociative anesthetic-like side effects (69). In rats, ACEA-1021 was completely devoid of phencyclidine-like discriminative stimulus effects and it failed to disrupt prepulse inhibition of the acoustic startle reflex, suggesting that the drug may not produce the adverse neurobehavioral effects characteristic of other types of NMDA receptor antagonists. Although the glycine site-selective quinolones fail to block AMPA receptors, quinoxalinediones typically interact with the glutamate recognition site of AMPA receptors as well as the glycine site of NMDA receptors (70). Indeed, ACEA-1416 blocks AMPA receptor currents in cultured rat cortical neurons with a steady-state potency that is only 150 times less than its blocking potency against NMDA receptor currents, and there is evidence that its selectivity in vivo may be even lower (see ref. 67). As discussed below, AMPA receptor blockade can confer a powerful anticonvulsant effect, and the combined inhibition of NMDA and AMPA receptors may produce synergistic anticonvulsant effects (71). In fact, the quinoxalinedione AMPA receptor antagonist PNQX (1,4,7,8,9,10-hexahydro-9-methyl-6-nitropyrido[3,4-f]-quinoxaline-2,3-dione) has greater anticonvulsant activity than an analogue with similar potency, likely as a result of its additional NMDA receptor glycine site blocking activity (72). Thus, less selective antagonists such as ACEA-1416 and PNQX may in some situations be preferred to drugs with a single target of action. In any case, although animal studies suggest that glycine site antagonists may have lower toxicity than competitive NMDA recognition site antagonists, the proof of this concept awaits confirmation in clinical trials.

Another type of NMDA receptor antagonist that appears to have reduced toxicity are the low-affinity uncompetitive (channel-blocking) antagonists. Channel-blocking NMDA receptor antagonists are a group of structurally diverse compounds that have the common property of blocking NMDA receptor-mediated responses by binding to the cation channel of the NMDA receptor complex. As a result, their blocking action occurs in a use-dependent and often a voltage-dependent fashion (7,73). Like other types of NMDA receptor antagonists, channel-blocking NMDA receptor antagonists are potent, broad-spectrum anticonvulsants in a wide variety of animal seizure models. Theoretically, the use-dependent action (in which block occurs only when the channel is in the ligand-gated open state) may selectively target the overactive glutamate-mediated excitation postulated to occur during seizures (74). (This will be the case if stronger activation of the receptor leads to greater degrees of block, a property that must be verified experimentally for each antagonist.) Certain so-called dissociative anesthetic-like uncompetitive NMDA receptor antagonists, such as phencyclidine and dizocilpine, produce profound neurobehavioral side effects that limit their utility in epilepsy therapy. Others, however, are now recognized to have more favorable side effect profiles. These reduced-toxicity channel-blocking NMDA antagonists have been referred to as "low-affinity" uncompetitive antagonists. The reduced toxicity of these antagonists may, in part, relate to their faster apparent rates of block and unblock associated with their generally lower binding affinities (see refs. 7 and 75). However, this may not be the only factor that accounts for their more favorable toxicity characteristics. In addition, there may be regional differences between the blocking activities of dissociative anesthetic-like and low-affinity uncompetitive antagonists that could contribute to their distinct side effect profiles (76,77). The low-affinity antagonists include phenylcycloalkylamines, such as phenylcyclopentylamine (PPA), that are structurally related to phencyclidine, and also the cycloheptenimine ADCI, an analogue of dizocilpine. In addition, the antiparkinsonian drugs memantine (78), amantadine (75) and budipine (79); the antitussive dextromethorphan (80); and ARL 12495, the major metabolite of the anticonvulsant remacemide (81), are low-affinity uncompetitive NMDA antagonists with favorable toxicity characteristics. Indeed, all these latter compounds have been used clinically and rarely produce side effects at therapeutic doses (52,75). In fact, memantine is often administered to demented patients and reportedly improves cognitive performance. In animals, the low-affinity uncompetitive antagonists appear to produce less neurologic impairment and gross behavioral disruption than do high-affinity uncompetitive NMDA antagonists, and they have distinct discriminative stimulus properties from dissociative anesthetic-type uncompetitive NMDA antagonists (82). Several of these compounds are currently undergoing clinical trials in epilepsy.

Like NMDA receptor antagonists, selective AMPA receptor antagonists also have powerful anticonvulsant activity in animal seizure models. However, a key difference between NMDA and AMPA receptor antagonists is that NMDA receptor antagonists can prevent the development of kindled seizures in the amygdala kindling model, whereas AMPA receptor antagonists do not (83). On the other hand, AMPA receptor antagonists may be more effective in preventing the expression of kindled seizures in fully kindled animals. Thus, to the extent that kindling provides a model for some human epilepsies, NMDA receptor antagonists may be of utility in both prophylaxis and treatment, whereas AMPA receptor antagonists may be of particular value in treatment.

The availability of selective AMPA receptor antagonists dates to the discovery in the late 1980s that certain quinoxalinediones are relatively potent competitive AMPA recognition site antagonists (see ref. 84). Several such quinoxalinediones have been described with potent systemic anticonvulsant activity, including NBQX [2,3-dihydroxy-6-nitro-7-sulfamoylbenzo[F]quinoxaline; 85,86] and YM90K [6-(1*H*-imidazol-1-yl)-7-nitro-2,3-(1*H*,4*H*)-quinoxalinedione; 87]. In addition, several structurally novel selective competitive AMPA receptor antagonists with systemic anticonvulsant activity have been described, including a series of isatin oximes (88) and the decahydroisoquinoline-3-carboxylic acid LY293558 {(3*S*,4a*R*,6*R*,8a*R*)-6-(2-[1(2)*H*-tetrazole-5-yl]ethyl)decahydroisoquinoline-3-carboxylic acid} (89). Although these competitive AMPA recognition site antagonists are not typically orally active, this is not the case for the isatin oxime NS 229 and the structurally novel antagonist S 17625 [6,7-dichloro-2(1*H*)-oxoquinoline-3-phosphonic acid], which, although somewhat less potent than NBQX, has anticonvulsant activity on oral administration (90).

In addition to the diverse AMPA recognition site antagonists identified in recent years, a series of 2,3-benzodiazepines have been described that are highly selective, noncompetitive (allosteric) AMPA receptor antagonists. The first compound in this series was GYKI 52466 [1-(4-aminophenyl)-4-methyl-7,8-methylenedioxy-5*H*-2,3-benzodiazepine] (91,92). More recently, Tarnawa and colleagues (93) observed that certain 3*N*-substituted analogues of GYKI 52466 have enhanced potency, including the 3*N*-acetyl GYKI 53405 (94). Like competitive AMPA antagonists, the 2,3-benzodiazepine AMPA antagonists have anticonvulsant activity in various seizure models similar to that of the competitive antagonists (86,94–96). Nonetheless, there are modest differences in relative toxicity among the two types of antagonists that could be related to the difference in blocking mechanism (11) or to differences in kinetic properties of block (97) or subtype selectivity (98). Overall, however, in animals toxicity occurs at doses that are near those that protect against seizures, so that an assessment of the practical utility of these agents awaits the results of ongoing clinical trials. Studies in normal human volunteers with LY300164, the active (*R*)-enantiomer of GYKI, indicated that plasma concentrations (~2.5 μM) near the concentration that produces 50% block of AMPA receptors in vitro (94) were associated with toxic effects such as ataxia, diplopia, sedation, and euphoria. Whether lower plasma concentrations can confer therapeutic activity without toxicity remains to be determined. In animals, it has been demonstrated that low, nontoxic doses of AMPA receptor antagonists can potentiate the anticonvulsant activity of conventional antiepileptic agents (99) and NMDA antagonists (100,101). Thus, it may ultimately be the case that the most appropriate use of AMPA receptor antagonists is in combination therapy.

INHIBITION OF GLUTAMATE RELEASE

A particularly promising, but perhaps underappreciated, approach to reducing the presumed excessive glutamate-mediated excitation that underlies seizure activity is the suppression of glutamate release with drugs targeted at presynaptic release mechanisms. In fact, it has been proposed that the anticonvulsant activity of drugs that interact with voltage-activated Na^+ channels, such as phenytoin and lamotrigine, may to a greater or lesser extent involve this mechanism (102, 103). In addition, the anticonvulsant activity of barbiturates, such as phenobarbital, may in part be a consequence of their blocking effects on presynaptic Ca^{2+} channels mediating glutamate release (25). A variety of other agents that inhibit glutamate release have anticonvulsant activity, including Ca^{2+}-channel toxins such as ω-agatoxin IVA and ω-conotoxin MVIIC (which act predominantly at P- and Q-type Ca^{2+} channels) (104,105); κ-opioid agonists (which activate κ-opioid receptors—G protein-coupled receptors that inhibit Ca^{2+} channels and are powerful presynaptic inhibitors of glutamate release) (106–110); and metabotropic glutamate receptor agonists (111) (which may directly affect the release process by a mechanism independent of Ca^{2+} channels; 112). Indeed, the type 2/3 metabotropic glutamate receptor agonist (1S, 3S)-ACPD, a glutamate release inhibitor, not only protects against the expression of seizures, but, like postsynaptic NMDA receptor antagonists, also is highly effective in preventing the development of kindled seizures (113). Recently a series of *N,N'*-guanidines have been described that produce use-dependent inhibition of glutamate release, possibly by a nonselective action on voltage-activated Na^{+} and Ca^{2+} channels (114). One of these compounds, CNS 1237 [*N*-(5-acenaphthyl)-*N'*-(4-methoxynaphthyl)-guanidine], has systemically active neuroprotective and anticonvulsant activity (115,116). Although κ-opioid receptor agonists have dysphoric properties that may limit their potential utility in epilepsy therapy, the behavioral effects of other glutamate release antagonists are largely unexplored.

ADENOSINE BRAIN SYSTEMS AS ANTICONVULSANT DRUG TARGETS

Adenosine is a powerful inhibitory neuromodulator that may participate in the spontaneous arrest of seizures (117). This concept derives from several lines of experimental evidence. Among the most important is the observation that adenosine receptor antagonists such as caffeine and theophylline facilitate the spread and greatly extend the duration of seizures without affecting the threshold for seizure initiation. In fact, theophylline can produce potentially fatal status epilepticus in humans (118). Conversely, adenosine receptor agonists and adenosine uptake inhibitors reduce the severity and duration of seizures and prolong postictal refractoriness. In addition, it is now recognized that local brain adenosine levels rise dramatically during seizures in experimental animals and also in humans (119). Activation of excitatory amino acid receptors enhances adenosine release (120–122) and may be responsible for seizure-induced elevations in extracellular adenosine. Adenosine inhibits neuronal excitability by a variety of mechanisms, including direct (postsynaptic) hyperpolarization of neurons and inhibition of synaptic release, particularly of glutamate, via adenosine receptors on excitatory nerve terminals (123).

If adenosine normally functions to reduce the spread and duration of seizures, can drugs that interact with brain adenosine systems be of benefit in epilepsy therapy? Despite the effectiveness of adenosine A1 agonists in animal seizure models, it is unlikely that these compounds would be clinically useful anticonvulsants, because they have powerful cardiovascular effects as a result of their actions on peripheral adenosine receptors in the heart and vasculature. Even if these peripheral side effects could be overcome (e.g., by coadministration of a blood-brain barrier–impermeable adenosine antagonist such as 8-*p*-sulfophenyltheophylline), adenosine agonists may produce strong sedative and hypothermic effects at anticonvulsant doses that would limit their clinical utility (124). Consequently, alternative strategies will need to be developed. One approach is to utilize inhibitors of adenosine inactivation, which may specifically target epileptic brain regions by virtue of the fact that seizure activity is accompanied by local release of adenosine. Such agents would theoretically potentiate the protective effects of adenosine where needed without producing untoward side effects. There are multiple nucleoside transport (uptake) systems in brain that serve to inactivate released adenosine. Electrophysiologic studies in in vitro brain slice preparations have indicated that adenosine uptake inhibitors such as dipyridamole, dilazep, nitrobenzylthioguanosine, nitrobenzylthioinosine, hexobendine, and soluflazine, can potentiate the inhibitory effects of exogenous adenosine (125,126) and reduce epileptiform activity (127), although they generally have little effect on normal synaptic transmission. Moreover, microinjection of several adenosine uptake inhibitors into the rat prepiriform cortex reduced bicuculline-induced seizures (128). Thus, inhibition of adenosine uptake is a potentially promising anticonvulsant strategy. However, the available adenosine uptake inhibitors are generally of low potency or do not penetrate the blood-brain barrier.

Another approach to enhancing endogenous adenosine levels selectively is to inhibit adenosine metabolism (e.g., with adenosine kinase inhibitors, such as 5'-amino-5'-deoxyadenosine or 5'-iodotubercidin, or with adenosine deaminase inhibitors, such as 2'-deoxycoformycin). Although activation of excitatory amino acid receptors during seizures induces the release of adenosine, the protection afforded by this adenosine is obviously not optimal. Interestingly, adenosine kinase inhibitors appear to potentiate selectively the formation of extracellular adenosine in an activation-dependent fashion, so that basal adenosine release is enhanced to a much smaller extent than is excitatory amino acid receptor-evoked release (129). Although such enzyme inhibitors have been demonstrated to have anticonvulsant activity when injected locally (128), there is no evidence that they are effective with systemic administration.

Another class of adenosine-regulating agent is exemplified by acadesine (AICAr; 5-amino-1-[β-D-ribofuranosyl]imidazole-4-carboxamide), a purine nucleoside analogue that increases the availability of adenosine locally on depletion of adenosine triphosphate (as may occur in a seizure focus). Acadesine has been reported to have weak anticonvulsant activity that can be enhanced with the adenosine uptake blocker mioflazine (130). Acadesine has low blood-brain barrier permeability, and it will be necessary to develop analogues with improved bioavailability before the potential of this approach can be evaluated. In sum, enhancement of adenosine release, whether by adenosine uptake blockade, inhibition of adenosine metabolism, or promotion of adenosine release, would appear to be a promising investigational strategy for anticonvulsant drug development.

TABLE 1. *Mechanism-specific anticonvulsant drugs in preclinical and clinical development*

Target	Class	Examples	Stage of development
Na^+ channel	Voltage- and use-dependent inhibitor	Lamotrigine Riluzole	Marketed Marketed[a]
$GABA_A$ receptor	Neuroactive steroid	Ganaxolone	Clinical (early phase II)
$GABA_A$ receptor	Partial benzodiazepine receptor agonist	Abecarnil	Awaiting registration[b]
$GABA_A$ receptor	Subtype selective benzodiazepine receptor agonist	Zolpidem	Marketed[c]
GABA transporter (GAT-1)	Lipophilic GABA uptake inhibitor	Tiagabine	Clinical (phase III)
NMDA receptor	Glycine site antagonist	Licostinel (ACEA-1021)	Clinical (phase I)[d]
NMDA receptor	Low-affinity channel-blocking antagonist	Remacemide Memantine ADCI	Clinical (phase III) Marketed[e] Clinical (phase I)
AMPA receptor	Competitive AMPA recognition site antagonist	LY293558	Clinical (early phase I)[f]
AMPA receptor	Noncompetitive antagonist	LY300164	Clinical (late phase I)
κ-Opioid receptor	Agonist (glutamate release inhibitor)	Enadoline (CI-977)	Clinical (phase II)[g]
Na^+ and Ca^{2+} channels	Glutamate release inhibitor	CNS 1237	Preclinical

[a]Registered for amyotrophic lateral sclerosis.
[b]Submitted in Europe as anxiolytic.
[c]Registered as anxiolytic.
[d]Trials for stroke and traumatic brain injury suspended due to crystalluria.
[e]Utilized in dementia and Parkinson's disease.
[f]Under evaluation for amyotrophic lateral sclerosis and pain.
[g]Under evaluation for traumatic brain injury.

TABLE 2. *Anticonvulsant drugs with multiple sites of action*

Drug	Proposed mechanisms	References
Phenobarbital	1. Enhance (and directly activate) $GABA_A$ receptors 2. Inhibit glutamate release by blocking presynaptic voltage-activated Ca^{2+} channels 3. Inhibit AMPA receptors (subtype selective)	24–26
Gabapentin	1. Increase GABA synthesis and levels by activation of glutamic acid decarboxylase 2. Increase GABA levels by weak inactivation of GABA transaminase 3. Increase nonvesicular GABA release by competitive inhibition of L-amino acid transporter 4. Reduce glutamate synthesis and levels by competitive inhibition of branched-chain amino acid transporter	131,132
Remacemide[a]	1. Inhibit NMDA receptors (channel block and additional allosteric block) 2. Na^+ channel block	133,134
Felbamate	1. Barbiturate-like enhancement of $GABA_A$ receptors 2. Inhibit NMDA receptors (channel block and additional allosteric block)	8,27,135
Topiramate	1. Inhibit non-NMDA receptors (? selective for kainate subtype) 2. Enhance $GABA_A$ receptors 3. ? Na^+ channel block	9,136
D23129[b]	1. Enhance $GABA_A$ receptors 2. Open inwardly rectifying K^+ channels 3. Inhibit non-NMDA receptors (? selective for kainate subtype) 4. Stimulate GABA synthesis and turnover	137–140
ACEA-1416, PNQX	1. Inhibit NMDA receptors (competitive at glycine site) 2. Inhibit AMPA receptors (competitive at AMPA recognition site)	67,72

[a]Metabolized to ARL 12495.
[b]Desazoflupirtine (N-[2-amino-4-(4-fluorobenzylamino)phenyl]carbamic acid ethyl ester).

CONCLUSION

In recent years, a variety of mechanism-specific drugs with anticonvulsant properties have reached late-stage preclinical and clinical development (Table 1). Several of these are being evaluated specifically as antiepileptic agents, whereas others are under investigation for indications other than epilepsy. These mechanism-specific drugs may prove useful in epilepsy therapy. In addition, they provide the opportunity to test the potential of diverse anticonvulsant strategies in human epilepsies. Can a neuroactive steroid, partial benzodiazepine receptor agonist, GABA uptake inhibitor, NMDA receptor glycine site antagonist, low-affinity channel-blocking NMDA receptor antagonist, or AMPA receptor antagonist protect against seizures in humans without producing unacceptable side effects? It will be possible to find out with these new, relatively specific drugs. Ultimately, however, the most favorable results may be obtained by targeting multiple anticonvulsant sites with combinations of drugs or, even better, with a single drug that has multiple actions. Indeed, several marketed or promising anticonvulsant drugs appear to act at more than one site (Table 2). In the future, physicians will have an increasingly rich array of agents with which to tailor an optimal therapeutic regimen for their epileptic patients.

REFERENCES

1. White HS, Johnson M, Wolf HH, Kupferberg HJ. The early identification of anticonvulsant activity: role of the maximal electroshock and subcutaneous pentylenetetrazol seizure models. *Ital J Neurol Sci* 1995;16: 73–77.
2. Kuo CC, Bean BP. Slow binding of phenytoin to inactivated sodium channels in rat hippocampal neurons. *Mol Pharmacol* 1994;46:716–725.
3. McNeal ET, Lewandowski GA, Daly JW, Creveling CR. [^{3}H]Batrachotoxinin A 20α-benzoate binding to voltage-sensitive sodium channels: a rapid and quantitative assay for local anesthetic activity in a variety of drugs. *J Med Chem* 1985;28:381–388.
4. Friedlander WJ. Putnam, Merritt, and the discovery of Dilantin. *Epilepsia* 1986;27(Suppl 3):S1–S20.
5. Roufos I, Hays SJ, Dooley DJ, Schwarz RD, Campbell GW, Probert AW Jr. Synthesis and pharmacological evaluation of phenylacetamides as sodium-channel blockers. *J Med Chem* 1994;37:268–274.

6. Ragsdale DS, Numann R, Catterall WA, Scheuer T. Inhibition of Na^+ channels by the novel blocker PD85,639. *Mol Pharmacol* 1993;43:949–954.
7. Rogawski MA. Therapeutic potential of excitatory amino acid antagonists: channel blockers and 2,3-benzodiazepines. *Trends Pharmacol Sci* 1993;14:325–331.
8. Rho JM, Donevan SD, Rogawski MA. Mechanism of action of the anticonvulsant felbamate: opposing effects on *N*-methyl-D-aspartate and γ-aminobutyric $acid_A$ receptors. *Ann Neurol* 1994;35:229–234.
9. Severt L, Coulter DA, Sombati S, Delorenzo RJ. Topiramate selectively blocks kainate currents in cultured hippocampal neurons. *Epilepsia* 1995;36(Suppl 4):38.
10. Costa E, Auta J, Caruncho H, Guidotti A, Impagnatiello F, Pesold C, Thompson DM. A search for a new anticonvulsant and anxiolytic benzodiazepine devoid of side effects and tolerance liability. In: Biggio G, Sanna E, Costa E, eds. *$GABA_A$ Receptors and Anxiety: from Neurobiology to Treatment.* New York: Raven Press; 1995;75–92.
11. Rogawski MA. Epilepsy. In: Pullan L, Patel J, eds. *Neurotherapeutics: Emerging Strategies.* Totowa, NJ: Humana Press; 1996;193–273.
12. Hönack D, Löscher W. Kindling increases the sensitivity of rats to adverse effects of certain antiepileptic drugs. *Epilepsia* 1995;36:763–771.
13. Kohr G, De Koninck Y, Mody I. Properties of NMDA receptor channels in neurons acutely isolated from epileptic (kindled) rats. *J Neurosci* 1993;13:3612–3627.
14. Buhl EH, Otis TS, Mody I. Zinc-induced collapse of augmented inhibition by GABA in a temporal lobe epilepsy model. *Science* 1996;271:369–373.
15. Prince HK, Conn PJ, Blackstone CD, Huganir RL, Levey AI. Down-regulation of AMPA receptor subunit GluR2 in amygdaloid kindling. *J Neurochem* 1995;64:462–465.
16. Sloviter RS. The functional organization of the hippocampal dentate gyrus and its relevance to the pathogenesis of temporal lobe epilepsy. *Ann Neurol* 1994;35:640–654.
17. Gram L. Tiagabine: a novel drug with a GABAergic mechanism of action. *Epilepsia* 1994;35(Suppl 5):S85–S87.
18. Löscher W. Valproate-induced changes in GABA metabolism at the subcellular level. *Biochem Pharmacol* 1981;30:1364–1366.
19. Chapman A, Keane PE, Meldrum BS, Simiand J, Vernieres JC. Mechanism of anticonvulsant action of valproate. *Prog Neurobiol* 1982;19:315–359.
20. Löscher W. Valproate enhances GABA turnover in the substantia nigra. *Brain Res* 1989;501:198–203.
21. Petroff OA, Rothman DL, Behar KL, Lamoureux D, Mattson RH. The effect of gabapentin on brain γ-aminobutyric acid in patients with epilepsy. *Ann Neurol* 1996;39:95–99.
22. Löscher W, Hönack D, Taylor CP. Gabapentin increases aminooxyacetic acid-induced GABA accumulation in several regions of rat brain. *Neurosci Lett* 1991;128:150–154.
23. Rundfeldt C, Wla P, Hönack D, Löscher W. Anticonvulsant tolerance and withdrawal characteristics of benzodiazepine receptor ligands in different seizure models in mice. Comparison of diazepam, bretazenil, and abecarnil. *J Pharmacol Exp Ther* 1995;275:693–702.
24. Rho JM, Donevan SD, Rogawski MA. Direct activation of $GABA_A$ receptors by barbiturates in cultured rat hippocampal neurons. *J Physiol (Lond)* 1996;497 (Pt. 2):509–522.
25. french-Mullen JMH, Barker JL, Rogawski MA. Calcium current block by (–)-pentobarbital, phenobarbital, and CHEB but not (+)-pentobarbital in acutely isolated hippocampal CA1 neurons: comparison with effects on GABA-activated Cl^- current. *J Neurosci* 1993;13:3211–3221.
26. Taverna FA, Cameron BR, Hampson DL, Wang LY, MacDonald JF. Sensitivity of AMPA receptors to pentobarbital. *Eur J Pharmacol* 1994;267:R3–5.
27. Rho JM, Donevan SD, Rogawski MA. Barbiturate-like actions of the propanediol dicarbamates felbamate and meprobamate. *J Pharmacol Exper Ther* 1997;280:1383–1391.
28. Gee KW, McCauley LD, Lan NC. A putative receptor for neurosteroids on the $GABA_A$ receptor complex: the pharmacological properties and therapeutic potential of epalons. *Crit Rev Neurobiol* 1995;9:207–227.
29. Kokate TG, Svensson BE, Rogawski MA. Anticonvulsant activity of neurosteroids: correlation with γ-aminobutyric acid-evoked chloride current potentiation. *J Pharmacol Exp Ther* 1994;270:1223–1229.
30. Lambert JJ, Belelli D, Hill-Venning C, Peters JA. Neurosteroids and $GABA_A$ receptor function. *Trends Pharmacol Sci* 1995;16:295–303.
31. Yu R, Ticku MK. Chronic neurosteroid treatment decreases the efficacy of benzodiazepine ligands and neurosteroids at the γ-aminobutyric $acid_A$ receptor complex in mammalian cortical neurons. *J Pharmacol Exp Ther* 1995;275:784–789.
32. Kokate TG, Yamaguchi SI, Rogawski MA. Lack of tolerance to the anticonvulsant activity of the neuroactive steroid pregnanolone with chronic dosing in mice. *Epilepsia* 1995;36(Suppl 4):90.
33. Carter RB, Yang KC, Robledo S, Suruki M, White HS, Upasani RB. Characterization of the anticonvulsant properties of Co 2-1068, a novel neuroactive steroid modulator of the $GABA_A$ receptor. *Soc Neurosci Abst* 1996;22:2105.
34. Lechtenberg R, Lee DA, Villeneuve N, Dulac O, Densel MB, Monaghan EP. Initial human experience with ganaxolone, a neuroactive steroid with antiepileptic activity. *J Clin Pharmacol* 1996;36:858.
35. Hawkinson JE, Drewe JA, Kimbrough CL, Chen JS, Hogenkamp DJ, Lan NC, Gee KW, Shen KZ, Whittemore ER, Woodward RM. 3α-Hydroxy-3β-trifluoromethyl-5α-pregnan-20-one (Co 2-1970): a partial agonist at the neuroactive steroid site of the γ-aminobutyric $acid_A$ receptor. *Mol Pharmacol* 1996;49:897–906.
36. Kokate TG, Cohen AL, Karp E, Rogawski MA. Neuroactive steroids protect against pilocarpine- and kainic acid-induced limbic seizures and status epilepticus in mice. *Neuropharmacology* 1996;35:423–431.
37. Mumford JP, Cannon DJ. Vigabatrin. *Epilepsia* 1994;35(Suppl 5):S25–S28.
38. Petroff OA, Rothman DL, Behar KL, Mattson RH. Initial observations on effect of vigabatrin on in vivo ^1H spectroscopic measurements of γ-aminobutyric acid, glutamate, and glutamine in human brain. *Epilepsia* 1995;36:457–464.
39. Qume M, Whitton PS, Fowler LJ. The effect of chronic

treatment with the GABA transaminase inhibitors γ-vinyl-GABA and ethanolamine-*O*-sulphate on the in vivo release of GABA from rat hippocampus. *J Neurochem* 1995;64:2256–2261.
40. French JA, Mosier M, Walker S, Sommerville K, Sussman N. A double-blind, placebo-controlled study of vigabatrin three g/day in patients with uncontrolled complex partial seizures. Vigabatrin Protocol 024 Investigative Cohort. *Neurology* 1996;46:54–61.
41. Reynolds H. γ-Vinyl GABA (vigabatrin): clinical experience in adult and adolescent patients with intractable epilepsy. *Epilepsia* 1992;33(Suppl 5): S30–S35.
42. Braestrup C, Nielsen EB, Sonnewald U, Knutsen LJS, Andersen KE, Jansen JA, Frederiksen K, Andersen PH, Mortensen A, Suzdak PD. (*R*)-*N*-[4,4-Bis(3-methyl-2-thienyl)but-3-en-1-yl]nipecotic acid binds with high affinity to the brain τ-aminobutyric acid uptake carrier. *J Neurochem* 1990;54:639–747.
43. Suzdak PD. Lipophilic GABA uptake inhibitors: biochemistry, pharmacology and therapeutic potential. *Drugs of the Future* 1993;18:1129–1136.
44. Andersen KE, Braestrup C, Grønwald FC, Jørgensen AS, Bielsen EB, Sonnewald U, Sørensen PO, Suzdak PD, Knutsen LJS. The synthesis of novel GABA uptake inhibitors. 1. Elucidation of the structure-activity studies leading to the choice of (*R*)-1-[4,4-Bis(3-methyl-2-thienyl)-3-butenyl]-3-piperidinecarboxylic acid (tiagabine) as an anticonvulsant drug candidate. *J Med Chem* 1993;36:1716–1725.
45. Fink-Jensen A, Suzdak PD, Swedberg MDB, Judge ME, Hansen L, Nielsen PG. The γ-aminobutyric acid (GABA) uptake inhibitor, tiagabine, increases extracellular brain levels of GABA in awake rats. *Eur J Pharmacol* 1992;220:197–201.
46. Suzdak PD, Jansen JA. A review of the preclinical pharmacology of tiagabine: a potent and selective anticonvulsant GABA uptake inhibitor. *Epilepsia* 1995; 36:612–626.
47. Suzdak PD. Lack of tolerance to the anticonvulsant effects of tiagabine following chronic (21 day) treatment. *Epilepsy Res* 1994;19:205–213.
48. Schachter SC. Tiagabine monotherapy in the treatment of partial epilepsy. *Epilepsia* 1995;36(Suppl 6):S2–S6.
49. Ben-Menachem E. International experience with tiagabine add-on therapy. *Epilepsia* 1995;36(Suppl 6): S14–S21.
50. Leppik IE. Tiagabine: the safety landscape. *Epilepsia* 1995;36(Suppl 6):S10–S13.
51. Rogawski MA. Excitatory amino acids and seizures. In: Stone TW, ed. *CNS Neurotransmitters and Neuromodulators*; vol 2. *Glutamate*. Boca Raton, FL: CRC Press; 1995;219–237.
52. Rogawski MA. The NMDA receptor, NMDA antagonists, and epilepsy therapy. A status report. *Drugs* 1992;44:279–292.
53. Sveinbjornsdottir S, Sander JW, Upton D, Thompson PJ, Patsalos PN, Hirt D, Emre M, Lowe D, Duncan JS. The excitatory amino acid antagonist D-CPP-ene (SDZ EAA-494) in patients with epilepsy. *Epilepsy Res* 1993;16:165–174.
54. Williams K. Ifenprodil discriminates subtypes of the *N*-methyl-D-aspartate receptor: selectivity and mechanisms at recombinant heteromeric receptors. *Mol Pharmacol* 1993;44:851–859.
55. Cordon JJ, Coughenour LL. A comparison of the binding of ifenprodil, eliprodil, haloperidol, and trifluperidol to the NMDA receptor complex in rat brain: further evidence of selectivity for the NR2B receptor subtype. *Soc Neurosci Abst* 1995;21:84.
56. Gallagher MJ, Huang H, Pritchett DB, Lynch DR. Interactions between ifenprodil and the NR2B subunit of the *N*-methyl-D-aspartate receptor. *J Biol Chem* 1996; 271:9603–9611.
57. Priestley T, Laughton P, Myers J, Le Bourdelles B, Kerby J, Whiting PJ. Pharmacological properties of recombinant human *N*-methyl-D-aspartate receptors comprising NR1a/NR2A and NR1a/NR2B subunit assemblies expressed in permanently transfected mouse fibroblast cells. *Mol Pharmacol* 1995;48:841–848.
58. De Sarro GB, De Sarro A. Anticonvulsant properties of non-competitive antagonists of the *N*-methyl-D-aspartate receptor in genetically epilepsy-prone rats: comparison with CPPene. *Neuropharmacology* 1993; 32:51–58.
59. Scatton B, Avenet P, Benavides J, Carter C, Duverger D, Oblin A, Perrault G, Sanger DJ, Schoemaker H. Neuroprotective potential of the polyamine site-directed NMDA receptor antagonists—ifenprodil and eliprodil. In: Palfreyman MG, Reynolds IJ, Skolnick P, eds. *Direct and Allosteric Control of Glutamate Receptors*. Boca Raton, FL: CRC Press; 1994;139–154.
60. Johnson JW, Ascher P. Glycine potentiates the NMDA response in cultured mouse brain neurons. *Nature* 1987;325:529–531.
61. Kleckner NW, Dingledine R. Requirement for glycine in activation of NMDA-receptors expressed in *Xenopus* oocytes. *Science* 1988;241:835–837.
62. Kemp JA, Leeson PD. The glycine site of the NMDA receptor—five years on. *Trends Pharmacol Sci* 1993; 14:20–25.
63. Koek W, Colpaert FC. Selective blockade of *N*-methyl-D-aspartate (NMDA)-induced convulsions by NMDA antagonists and putative glycine antagonists: relationship with phencyclidine-like behavioral effects. *J Pharmacol Exp Ther* 1990;252:349–357.
64. Bristow LJ, Hutson PH, Thorn L, Tricklebank MD. The glycine/NMDA receptor antagonist, *R*-(+)-HA-966, blocks activation of the mesolimbic dopaminergic system induced by phencyclidine and dizocilpine (MK-801) in rodents. *Br J Pharmacol* 1993;108: 1156–1163.
65. Hargreaves RJ, Hill RG, Iversen LL. Neuroprotective NMDA antagonists: the controversy over their potential for adverse effects on cortical neuronal morphology. *Acta Neurochir Suppl (Wien)* 1994;60:15–19.
66. Kulagowski JJ, Baker R, Curtis NR, Leeson PD, Mawer IM, Moseley AM, Ridgill MP, Rowley M, Stansfield I, Foster AC, Grimwood S, Hill RG, Kemp JA, Marshall GR, Saywell KL, Tricklebank MD. 3′-(Arylmethyl)- and 3′-(aryloxy)-3-phenyl-4-hydroxyquinolin-2(1*H*)-ones: orally active antagonists of the glycine site on the NMDA receptor. *J Med Chem* 1994;37:1402–1405.
67. Ilyin VI, Whittemore ER, Tran M, Shen K-Z, Cai S-X, Kher SM, Keana JFW, Weber E, Woodward RM. Pharmacology of ACEA-1416: a potent, systemically active NMDA receptor glycine site antagonist. *Eur J Pharmacol (in press)*.
68. Woodward RM, Huettner JE, Guastella J, Keana JF, Weber E. In vitro pharmacology of ACEA-1021 and ACEA-1031: systemically active quinoxalinediones with high affinity and selectivity for *N*-methyl-D-as-

partate receptor glycine sites. *Mol Pharmacol* 1995; 47:568–581.

69. Balster RL, Mansbach RS, Shelton KL, Nicholson KL, Grech DM, Wiley JL, Li H, Weber E. Behavioral pharmacology of two novel substituted quinoxalinedione glutamate antagonists. *Behav Pharmacol* 1995; 6:577–589.
70. Randle JC, Guet T, Bobichon C, Moreau C, Curutchet P, Lambolez B, de Carvalho LP, Cordi A, Lepagnol JM. Quinoxaline derivatives: structure-activity relationships and physiological implications of inhibition of *N*-methyl-D-aspartate and non-*N*-methyl-D-aspartate receptor-mediated currents and synaptic potentials. *Mol Pharmacol* 1992;41:337–345.
71. Löscher W, Hönack D. Over-additive anticonvulsant effect of memantine and NBQX in kindled rats. *Eur J Pharmacol* 1994;259:R3–R5.
72. Bigge CF, Malone TC, Boxer PA, Nelson CB, Ortwine DF, Schelkun RM, Retz DM, Lescosky LJ, Borosky SA, Vartanian MG, Schwarz RD, Campbell GW, Robichaud LJ, Wätjen F. Synthesis of 1,4,7,8,9,10-hexahydro-9-methyl-6-nitropyrido[3,4-f]-quinoxaline-2,3-dione and related quinoxalinediones: characterization of α-amino-3-hydroxy-5-methyl-4-isoxazolepropionic acid (and *N*-methyl-D-aspartate) receptor and anticonvulsant activity. *J Med Chem* 1995;38:3720–3740.
73. MacDonald JF, Bartlett MC, Mody I, Pahapill P, Reynolds JN, Salter MW, Schneiderman JH, Pennefather PS. Actions of ketamine, phencyclidine, and MK-801 on NMDA receptor currents in cultured mouse hippocampal neurons. *J Physiol (Lond)* 1991;432: 483–508.
74. Kemp JA, Foster AC, Wong EHF. Non-competitive antagonists of excitatory amino acid receptors. *Trends Neurosci* 1987;10:294–299.
75. Parsons CG, Quack G, Bresink I, Baran L, Przegalinski E, Kostowski W, Krzascik P, Hartmann S, Danysz W. Comparison of the potency, kinetics, and voltage-dependency of a series of uncompetitive NMDA receptor antagonists in vitro with anticonvulsive and motor impairment activity in vivo. *Neuropharmacology* 1995;10:1239–1258.
76. Porter RHP, Greenamyre JT. Regional variations in the pharmacology of NMDA receptor channel blockers: implications for therapeutic potential. *J Neurochem* 1995;64:614–623.
77. Bresink I, Danysz W, Parsons CG, Mutschler E. Different binding affinities of NMDA receptor channel blockers in various brain regions—indication of NMDA receptor heterogeneity. *Neuropharmacology* 1995;34:533-540.
78. Frankiewicz T, Potier B, Bashir ZI, Collingridge GL, Parsons CG. Effects of memantine and MK-801 on NMDA-induced currents in cultured neurones and on synaptic transmission and LTP in area CA1 of rat hippocampal slices. *Br J Pharmacol* 1996;117: 689–697.
79. Jackisch R, Kruchen A, Sauermann W, Hertting G, Feuerstein TJ. The antiparkinsonian drugs budipine and biperiden are use-dependent (uncompetitive) NMDA receptor antagonists. *Eur J Pharmacol* 1994; 264:207–211.
80. Netzer R, Pflimlin P, Trube G. Dextromethorphan blocks *N*-methyl-D-aspartate-induced currents and voltage-operated inward currents in cultured cortical neurons. *Eur J Pharmacol* 1993;238:209–216.
81. Palmer GC, Murray RJ, Wilson TC, Eisman MS, Ray RK, Griffith RC, Napier JJ, Fedorchuk M, Stagnitto ML, Garske GE. Biological profile of the metabolites and potential metabolites of the anticonvulsant remacemide. *Epilepsy Res* 1992;12:9–20.
82. Grant KA, Colombo G, Grant J, Rogawski MA. Dizocilpine-like discriminative stimulus effects of low-affinity uncompetitive NMDA antagonists. *Neuropharmacology* 1996;35:1709–1719.
83. Dürmüller N, Craggs M, Meldrum BS. The effect of the non-NMDA receptor antagonist GYKI 52466 and NBQX and the competitive NMDA receptor antagonist D-CPPene on the development of amygdala kindling and on amygdala-kindled seizures. *Epilepsy Res* 1994;17:167–174.
84. Honoré T. Inhibitors of kainate and AMPA ionophore receptors. In: Meldrum BS, ed. *Excitatory Amino Acid Antagonists*. Oxford: Blackwell Scientific Publications; 1991;180–194.
85. Sheardown MJ, Nielsen EØ, Hansen AJ, Jacobsen P, Honoré T. 2,3-Dihydroxy-6-nitro-7-sulfamoyl-benzo[F]quinoxaline: a neuroprotectant for cerebral ischemia. *Science* 1990;247:571–574.
86. Yamaguchi S, Donevan SD, Rogawski MA. Anticonvulsant activity of AMPA/kainate antagonists: comparison of GYKI 52466 and NBQX in maximal electroshock and chemoconvulsant models. *Epilepsy Res* 1993;15:179–184.
87. Shimizu-Sasamata M, Kawasaki-Yatsugi S, Okada M, Sakamoto S, Yatsugi S, Togami J, Hatanaka K, Ohmori J, Koshiya K, Usuda S, Murase K. YM90K: pharmacological characterization as a selective and potent α-amino-3-hydroxy-5-methylisoxazole-4-propionate/kainate receptor antagonist. *J Pharmacol Exp Ther* 1996;276:84–92.
88. Wätjen F, Nielsen EØ, Drejer J, Jensen LH. Isatin oximes—a novel series of bioavailable non-NMDA antagonists. *Bioorg Med Chem Lett* 1993;3:105–106.
89. Schoepp DD, Lodge D, Bleakman D, Leander JD, Tizzano JP, Wright RA, Palmer AJ, Salhoff CR, Ornstein PL. In vitro and in vivo antagonism of AMPA receptor activation by (3*S*,4a*R*,6*R*,8a*R*)-6-[2-(1(2)*H*-tetrazole-5-yl) ethyl] decahydroisoquinoline-3-carboxylic acid. *Neuropharmacology* 1995;34:1159–1168.
90. Desos P, Lepagnol JM, Morain P, Lestage P, Cordi AA. Structure-activity relationships in a series of 2(1*H*)-quinolones bearing different acidic function in the 3-position: 6,7-dichloro-2(1*H*)-oxoquinoline-3-phosphonic acid, a potent and selective AMPA/kainate antagonist with neuroprotective properties. *J Med Chem* 1996;39:197–206.
91. Tarnawa I, Engberg I, Flatman JA. GYKI 52466, an inhibitor of spinal reflexes, is a potent quisqualate antagonist. In: Lubec G, Rosenthal GA, eds. *Amino Acids. Chemistry, Biology, and Medicine*. Leiden: ESCOM Scientific Publishers; 1990;538–546.
92. Donevan SD, Rogawski MA. GYKI 52466, a 2,3-benzodiazepine, is a highly selective, noncompetitive antagonist of AMPA/kainate receptor responses. *Neuron* 1993;10:51–59.
93. Tarnawa I, Berzsenyi P, Andrási F, Botka P, Hámori T, Ling I, Körösi J. Structure-activity relationships of 2,3-benzodiazepine compounds with glutamate antagonistic action. *Bioorg Med Chem Lett* 1993;3:99–104.
94. Donevan SD, Yamaguchi S, Rogawski MA. Non-*N*-methyl-D-aspartate receptor antagonism by 3-*N*-substi-

tuted 2,3-benzodiazepines: relationship to anticonvulsant activity. *J Pharmacol Exp Ther* 1994;271:25–29.
95. Chapman AG, Smith SE, Meldrum BS. The anticonvulsant effect of the non-NMDA antagonists, NBQX and GYKI 52466, in mice. *Epilepsy Res* 1991;9: 92–96.
96. Löscher W, Hönack D. Effects of the non-NMDA antagonists NBQX and the 2,3-benzodiazepine GYKI 52466 on different seizure types in mice: comparison with diazepam and interactions with flumazenil. *Br J Pharmacol* 1994;113:1349–1357.
97. Parsons CG, Gruner R, Rozental J. Comparative patch clamp studies on the kinetics and selectivity of glutamate receptor antagonism by 2,3-dihydroxy-6-nitro-7-sulfamoylbenzo[F]quinoxaline (NBQX) and 1-(4-amino-phenyl)-4-methyl-7,8-methyl-endioxyl-5*H*-2,3-benzodiazepine (GYKI 52466). *Neuropharmacology* 1994;33:589–604.
98. Rogawski MA, Donevan SD. Functional and pharmacological properties of AMPA receptors in type I and type II cultured rat hippocampal neurons. *Soc Neurosci Abst* 1996;1281.
99. Zarnowski T, Kleinrok Z, Turski WA, Czuczwar SJ. 2,3-Dihydroxy-6-nitro-7-sulfamoylbenzo[F]quinoxaline enhances the protective activity of common antiepileptic drugs against maximal electroshock-induced seizures in mice. *Neuropharmacology* 1993;32: 895–900.
100. Löscher W, Rundfeldt C, Hönack D. Low doses of NMDA receptor antagonists synergistically increase the anticonvulsant effect of the AMPA receptor antagonist NBQX in the kindling model of epilepsy. *Eur J Neurosci* 1993;5:1545–1550.
101. Czuczwar SJ, Borowicz KK, Kleinrok Z, Tutka P, Zarnowski T, Turski WA. Influence of combined treatment with NMDA and non-NMDA receptor antagonists on electroconvulsions in mice. *Eur J Pharmacol* 1995;281:327–333.
102. Taylor CP, Meldrum BS. Na^+ channels as targets for neuroprotective drugs. *Trends Pharmacol Sci* 1995;16:309–316.
103. Xie X, Lancaster B, Peakman T, Garthwaite J. Interaction of the antiepileptic drug lamotrigine with recombinant rat brain type IIA Na^+ channels and with native Na^+ channels in rat hippocampal neurones. *Pflügers Arch* 1995;430:437–446.
104. Robichaud LJ, Wurster S, Boxer PA. The voltage-sensitive Ca^{2+} channel (VSCC) antagonists ω-Aga-IVA and ω-CTX-MVIIC inhibit spontaneous epileptiform discharges in the rat cortical wedge. *Brain Res* 1994;643:352–356.
105. Jackson HC, Scheideler MA. Behavioural and anticonvulsant effects of Ca^{2+} channel toxins in DBA/2 mice. *Psychopharmacology* 1996;126:85–90.
106. Gross RA, Macdonald RL. Dynorphin A selectively reduces a large transient (N-type) calcium current of mouse dorsal root ganglion neurons in cell culture. *Proc Natl Acad Sci U S A* 1987;84:5469–5473.
107. Conner-Kerr TA, Terrian DM. Inhibition of glutamate release: a potential mechanism of action for the anticonvulsant U-54494A in the guinea pig hippocampus. *Brain Res Bull* 1993;31:573–580.
108. Brotchie JM. Modulation of glutamate release by a kappa-opioid receptor agonist in rodent and primate striatum. *Eur J Pharmacol* 1995;281:R1–R2.
109. Przewocka B, Machelska H, Lason W. Kappa-opioid receptor agonists inhibit the pilocarpine-induced seizures and toxicity in the mouse. *Eur Neuropsychopharmacol* 1994;4:527–533.
110. De Sarro G, Trimarchi GR, Sinopoli S, Masuda Y, De Sarro A. Anticonvulsant effects of U-54494A and U-50488H in genetically epilepsy-prone rats and DBA/2 mice: a possible involvement of glycine/NMDA receptor complex. *Gen Pharmacol* 1993;24:439–447.
111. Dalby NO, Thomsen C. Modulation of seizure activity in mice by metabotropic glutamate receptor ligands. *J Pharmacol Exp Ther* 1996;276:516–522.
112. Scanziani M, Gahwiler BH, Thompson SM. Presynaptic inhibition of excitatory synaptic transmission by muscarinic and metabotropic glutamate receptor activation in the hippocampus: are Ca^{2+} channels involved? *Neuropharmacology* 1995;34:1549–1557.
113. Attwell PJE, Kaura S, Sigala G, Bradford HF, Croucher MJ, Jane DE, Watkins JC. Blockade of both epileptogenesis and glutamate release by (1S,3S)-ACPD, a presynaptic glutamate receptor agonist. *Brain Res* 1995;698:155–162.
114. Reddy NL, Connaughton S, Daly D, Fischer JB, Goldin SM, Hu L-Y, Subbarao K, Durant GJ. Synthesis and characterization of *N*-(acenaphth-5-yl)-*N'*-(4-methoxynaphth-1-yl)-guanidine as a glutamate release inhibitor and potential anti-ischemic agent. *Bioorg Med Chem Lett* 1995;5:2259–2262.
115. Goldin SM, Subbarao K, Sharma R, Knapp AG, Fischer JB, Daly D, Durant GJ, Reddy NL, Hu L-Y, Magar S, Perlman ME, Chen J, Graham SH, Holt WF, Berlove D, Margolin LD. Neuroprotective use-dependent blockers of Na^+ and Ca^{2+} channels controlling presynaptic release of glutamate. *Ann N Y Acad Sci* 1995;765:210–229.
116. Reddy NL, Fan W, Magar SS, Yost E, Durant GJ. *N,N'*-diarylguanidines: synthesis and their anti-seizure activity in the audiogenic (DBA/2) mouse model. *Abst Am Chem Soc* 1996;211:MEDI 57.
117. Dragunow M. Adenosine: the brain's natural anticonvulsant? *Trends Pharmacol Sci* 1986;7:128–130.
118. Zwillich CW, Sutton FD, Neff TA, Cohn WM, Matthay RA, Weinberger MM. Theophylline-induced seizures in adults. Correlation with serum concentrations. *Ann Intern Med* 1975;82:784–787.
119. During MJ, Spencer DD. Adenosine: a potential mediator of seizure arrest and postictal refractoriness. *Ann Neurol* 1992;32:618–624.
120. Craig CG, White TD. *N*-methyl-D-aspartate- and non-*N*-methyl-D-aspartate-evoked adenosine release from rat cortical slices: distinct purinergic sources and mechanisms of release. *J Neurochem* 1993;60: 1073–1080.
121. Manzoni OJ, Manabe T, Nicoll RA. Release of adenosine by activation of NMDA receptors in the hippocampus. *Science* 1994;265:2098–2101.
122. Kaiser MG, During MJ. Combining laser Doppler flowmetry with microdialysis: a novel approach to investigate the coupling of regional cerebral blood flow to neuronal activity. *J Neurosci Methods* 1995;60: 165–173.
123. Proctor WR, Dunwiddie TV. Pre- and postsynaptic actions of adenosine in the in vitro hippocampus. *Brain Res* 1987;426:187–190.
124. Dunwiddie TV, Worth T. Sedative and anticonvulsant

effects of adenosine analogs in mouse and rat. *J Pharmacol Exp Ther* 1982;220:70–76.
125. Sanderson G, Scholfield CN. Effects of adenosine uptake blockers and adenosine on evoked potentials of guinea-pig olfactory cortex. *Pflugers Arch* 1986;406: 25–30.
126. Ashton D, Willems R, De Prins E, Van Belle H, Wauquier A. The nucleoside-transport inhibitor soluflazine (R 64 719) increases the effects of adenosine in the guinea-pig hippocampal slice and is antagonized by adenosine deaminase. *Eur J Pharmacol* 1987;142: 403–408.
127. Ashton D, De Prins E, Willems R, Van Belle H, Wauquier A. Anticonvulsant action of the nucleoside transport inhibitor, soluflazine, on synaptic and non-synaptic epileptogenesis in the guinea-pig hippocampus. *Epilepsy Res* 1988;2:65–71.
128. Zhang G, Franklin PH, Murray TF. Manipulation of endogenous adenosine in the rat prepiriform cortex modulates seizure susceptibility. *J Pharmacol Exp Ther* 1993;264:1415–1424.
129. White TD. Potentiation of excitatory amino acid-evoked adenosine release from rat cortex by inhibitors of adenosine kinase and adenosine deaminase and by acadesine. *Eur J Pharmacol* 1996;303:27–38.
130. Marangos PJ, Loftus T, Wiesner J, Lowe T, Rossi E, Browne CE, Gruber HE. Adenosinergic modulation of homocysteine-induced seizures in mice. *Epilepsia* 1990;31:239–246.
131. Goldlust A, Su TZ, Welty DF, Taylor CP, Oxender DL. Effects of anticonvulsant drug gabapentin on the enzymes in metabolic pathways of glutamate and GABA. *Epilepsy Res* 1995;22:1–11.
132. Honmou O, Oyelese AA, Kocsis JD. The anticonvulsant gabapentin enhances promoted release of GABA in hippocampus: a field potential analysis. *Brain Res* 1995;692:273–277.
133. Subramaniam S, Donevan SD, Rogawski MA. Block of the *N*-methyl-D-aspartate receptor by remacemide and its *de*-glycine metabolite. *J Pharmacol Exp Ther* 1996;276:161–168.
134. Srinivasan J, Richens A, Davies JA. The effect of the desglycinyl metabolite of remacemide hydrochloride (FPL 12495AA) and dizocilpine (MK-801) on endogenous amino acid release from mouse cortex. *Br J Pharmacol* 1995;116:3087–3092.
135. Subramaniam S, Rho JM, Penix L, Donevan SD, Fielding RP, Rogawski MA. Felbamate block of the *N*-methyl-D-aspartate receptor. *J Pharmacol Exp Ther* 1995;273:878–886.
136. White HS, Brown SD, Skeen GA, Twyman RE. The investigational anticonvulsant topiramate potentiates GABA-evoked currents in mouse cortical neurons. *Epilepsia* 1995;36(Suppl 4):34.
137. Rundfeldt C, Rohlfs A, Netzer R. Multiple actions of the new anticonvulsant D-23129 on voltage-gated inward currents and GABA-induced currents in cultured neuronal cells. *Naunyn Schmiedebergs Arch Pharmacol* 1995;351(Suppl):R160.
138. Rundfeldt C, Bartsch R. The new anticonvulsant D-23129 acts as a potent potassium channel opener in neuronal cells. *Naunyn Schmiedebergs Arch Pharmacol* 1996;353(Suppl 4):R97.
139. Skeen GA, Wolf HH, White HS. D-23129 attenuates glutamate-evoked whole-cell currents of mouse cortical neurons through an interaction with kainate-sensitive ion channels. *Soc Neurosci Abst* 1995;21: 353.131.
140. Kapetanovic IM, Yonekawa WD, Kupferberg HJ. The effects of D-23129, a new experimental anticonvulsant drug, on neurotransmitter amino acids in the hippocampus in vitro. *Epilepsy Res* 1995;22: 167–173.

Antiepileptic Drug Development.
Advances in Neurology, Vol. 76,
edited by J. French, I. Leppik, and M. A. Dichter.
Lippincott–Raven Publishers, Philadelphia © 1998.

3

The National Institutes of Health Anticonvulsant Drug Development Program: Screening for Efficacy

H. Steve White, Harold H. Wolf, José H. Woodhead, and Harvey J. Kupferberg

Department of Pharmacology and Toxicology, Anticonvulsant Screening Project, University of Utah, Salt Lake City, Utah 84112 and Epilepsy Branch, National Institute of Neurological Disorders and Stroke, National Institutes of Health, Bethesda, Maryland 20892.

INTRODUCTION

The current era of antiepileptic drug (AED) discovery was ushered in largely by the efforts of the National Institutes of Health-sponsored Antiepileptic Drug Development (ADD) Program. This program, which represents a collaborative effort between government, the pharmaceutical industry, and academia, was established in 1974 to foster the development of new and less toxic drugs for the treatment of seizure disorders. One important aspect of the ADD program has been the University of Utah Anticonvulsant Screening Project (ASP). Compounds submitted to the ADD Program for evaluation are tested at the ASP for their ability to prevent seizures in a number of well-defined animal seizure models. Indeed, the majority of the newer AEDs now available or under clinical evaluation have resulted from the wide-scale screening of thousands of chemically divergent structures in these animal models. Since its inception, the ASP has tested >18,000 compounds. The mission of the ASP is to identify and then characterize the anticonvulsant potential of those biologically active compounds that display a reasonable degree of separation between their anticonvulsant and behaviorally toxic doses. In addition, the ASP initiates pilot studies to identify the mechanism of action of interesting drugs and examines the potential of a candidate drug to produce tolerance and drug-drug interactions.

This chapter briefly describes the procedures employed by the ASP to identify and characterize the anticonvulsant profile of those compounds that may ultimately represent the next generation of new AEDs. The discussion focuses on the process through which a compound is evaluated and advanced to more extensive evaluation. It is beyond the scope of this review to provide extensive details of the technical procedures employed in each of the seizure models, and interested readers are referred to a detailed summary published in White et al. in 1995 (1) for more specific details.

MECHANISTIC VERSUS NONMECHANISTIC DISCOVERY OF ANTIEPILEPTIC DRUGS

The mechanistic approach to AED discovery assumes that a specific mechanism of action contributes to the initiation, propagation, and/or abatement of seizure activity. Indeed, the present era of AED development is driven largely by a greater understanding of the molecular mechanisms underlying seizure disorders. In recent years, the mechanistic approach has been directed at developing drugs that either enhance γ-aminobutyric acid (GABA)-mediated inhibition or reduce glutamate-mediated excitation. In the case of the inhibitory neurotransmitter GABA, this approach has led to the successful development of tiagabine and vigabatrin. By targeting the process whereby neuronally released GABA is removed from the synaptic cleft, scientists at Novo Nordisk provided the epilepsy community with tiagabine, a selective GABA uptake inhibitor (2). The principle mechanism of tiagabine appears to be related to its ability to inhibit neuronal and glial uptake of GABA. Vigabatrin, a close structural analogue of GABA, emerged from a mechanistically oriented drug-discovery program that targeted GABA γ-oxoglutarate transaminase (GABA-T; EC 2.6.1.19), the enzyme responsible for the metabolism of GABA.

Tiagabine and vigabatrin represent the best examples whereby the mechanistic approach has resulted in two clinically effective AEDs. However, it is important to note that their discovery relied entirely on a thorough understanding of the basic mechanisms through which GABA is removed from the synaptic cleft and metabolized. Thus, as the scientific community gains a greater understanding of the molecular biology underlying the pathophysiology of seizure disorders, there are likely to be more successful drugs that have been developed by the mechanistic approach. As discussed by Taylor and Marks in Chapter 4, great strides have been made in recent years, not only toward identifying new targets, but also toward identifying active drugs through high-volume screening techniques that target specific molecular mechanisms.

Regardless of the approach employed to synthesize a new chemical entity for the treatment of seizures, that chemical is not likely to be tested in humans unless it has demonstrated some degree of efficacy in preclinical animal models. Herein lies one of the most often discussed paradoxes associated with the current-day AED discovery process: What is the most appropriate animal model to employ when screening for efficacy?

With one exception, all the new drugs currently in clinical development have been found to be active in at least one of the two animal models routinely employed in most screening programs—the maximal electroshock (MES) seizure test and the subcutaneous pentylenetetrazol (sc PTZ) seizure test. It is often argued that these models identify only "me too"-type AEDs. However, it should be mentioned that all the newer drugs that have been derived from mechanistically based programs and presumably represent state-of-the-art attempts to design and synthesize novel chemical compounds have been shown to be active in at least one of these two animal models. The only known exception to this generalization is UCB LO59 (levetiracetam), synthesized by UCB Pharmaceuticals, which appears to represent a truly unique compound that is inactive against seizures induced by either MES or sc PTZ (3). It is active against audiogenic seizures in the genetically susceptible DBA/2 mouse and is also extremely active in several kindling models (3,4). More important is the finding that this compound is effective in controlled clinical trials (5–8). At the present time, the anticonvulsant mechanism of action of UCB LO59 has yet to be identified. Thus, UCB LO59 represents a good example of a novel AED that evolved from a nonmechanistic drug discovery program. The identification of the mechanism(s) of action of UCB LO59 will lead to a greater understanding of the pathophysiology underlying some drug-resistant seizure disorders and foster the development of a new series of AEDs.

The above discussion underscores some of the basic faults associated with any rigid program of drug development but does not address the basic question: Is there an appropriate animal model that can be employed in a high-throughput in vivo screening program that will lessen the likelihood that novel AEDs such as UCB LO59 will go undetected? Unfortunately, at the present time no one knows the answer to this question. However, compounds like UCB LO59 demonstrate the importance of maintaining a somewhat flexible approach to AED discovery.

ANTICONVULSTANT SCREENING PROJECT TESTING PROTOCOL

As discussed above, the choice of a particular animal model for the identification of potential AEDs can be based on either mechanistic or nonmechanistic principles. The nonmechanistic approach is best suited for the initial screening and identification of biologic activity, as it assumes that the pharmacodynamic effect of a drug is independent of its mechanism of action. The ASP and a number of drug discovery programs within the pharmaceutical industry employ a combination of nonmechanistic, mechanistic, and syndrome-specific animal models to identify and characterize the anticonvulsant profiles of potential AEDs. Furthermore, these animal models display well-defined seizure endpoints and require minimal technical expertise. This approach is ideally suited to the wide variety and large number of chemical entities that are evaluated annually by the ASP.

The current in vivo testing procedures employed by the ASP have evolved during the last 22 years to include a number of different animal seizure models that have historically proved to be extremely useful in identifying clinically effective AEDs (see White et al., ref. 9, for further discussion). The flow chart shown in Fig. 1 summarizes the path that a candidate substance is likely to take once it is added to the ADD Program and sent to the ASP for testing. As shown in this figure, there are four distinct phases to the testing protocol of the ASP: identification, quantification, differentiation, and advanced testing. The remainder of this chapter is devoted to a discussion of the rationale of this approach and briefly describes the attendant criteria that lead to the advancement of a candidate substance.

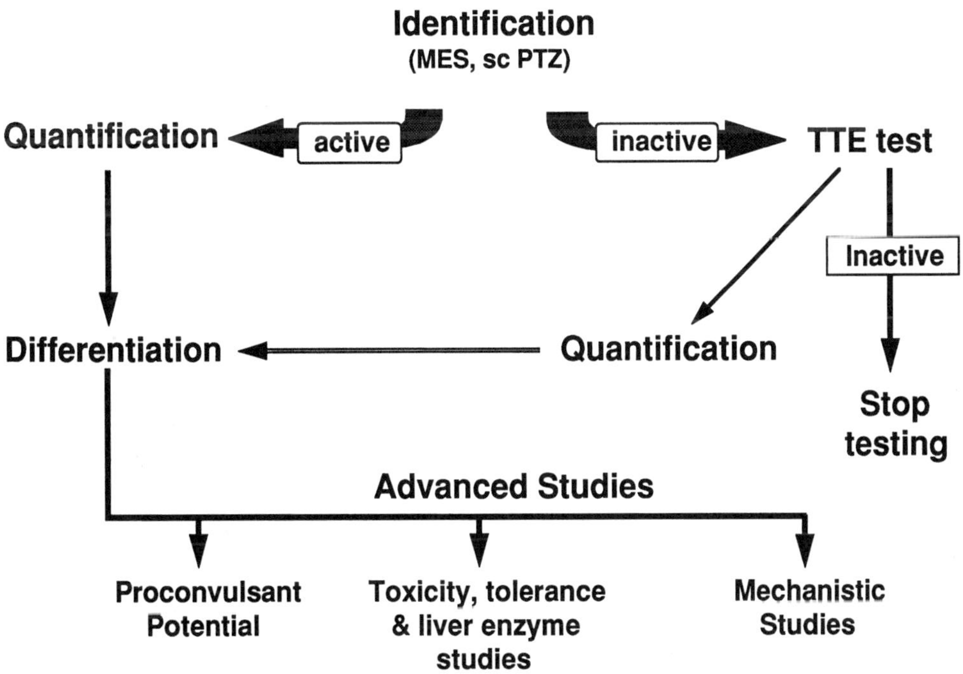

FIG. 1. ASP testing protocol.

Identification

The ASP uses both electrically and chemically (sc PTZ) induced seizures for its initial nonmechanistic identification tests. Anticonvulsant activity is determined following intraperitoneal administration in CF#1 mice and oral administration in Sprague Dawley rats. The effect of a test substance on minimal motor impairment is also assessed in the early testing phases. This helps to differentiate promising candidate substances that display good anticonvulsant activity with minimal to no toxicity from those substances that display little or no separation between efficacy and toxicity.

Maximal Electroshock Seizure Pattern Test

The MES test is an excellent animal model for the identification of new AEDs that block seizure spread and as such are likely to be effective for the management of generalized tonic-clonic seizures in humans (see White et al., ref. 9, for historical review and references.) This particular test has been used extensively in the search for new AEDs since Putnam and Merritt (10) successfully identified phenytoin in a systematic screening program. Their demonstration that it was feasible to discover a clinically effective AED using an experimental animal model provided the rationale for the introduction of the MES test into the routine screening protocol of numerous laboratories.

The induction of an MES seizure with a supramaximal current (i.e., usually three to four times the threshold current required to induce a tonic extension seizure) delivered via corneal or pineal electrodes results in a behavioral seizure in mice and rats that is characterized by tonic extension of both forelimbs and hindlimbs. The tonic extension phase is followed by brief episodes of clonic activity of the forelimbs and hindlimbs that lead to a prolonged postictal period lasting several minutes. The associated electroencephalogram (EEG) displays high-frequency, high-amplitude spiking activity that correlates with the behavioral seizure. Efficacy in this test is based on the ability of a drug to block the tonic hindlimb extension component of the MES seizure. Thus, it is not necessary for a candidate AED to block the secondary clonic activity that follows the tonic extension component.

One particular disadvantage associated with the use of rats in the MES test, as opposed to mice, is that not all rats display a full hindlimb tonic extension seizure in response to a supramaximal stimulation. The incidence of nonresponders in Sprague Dawley-derived rats is approximately 10% to 15% but can increase markedly with increasing age and seasonal variations (11). For this reason, it becomes necessary to prescreen all rats the day before a drug trial to identify and eliminate nonresponders from the experimental group. In doing this, the potential for false-positives is reduced.

Subcutaneous Pentylenetetrazol Seizure Test

When used appropriately, the sc PTZ test is an effective animal model that identifies those compounds that raise seizure threshold. The early observation that PTZ-induced seizures could be blocked by trimethadione (12), coupled with the clinical finding that trimethadione was effective in reducing *petit mal* seizures (13), provided the clinical correlation suggesting that this test would be useful for identifying drugs effective in the treatment of absence seizures (see White et al., ref. 9, for references and additional discussion). The behavioral seizure that results from the administration of sc PTZ is markedly different from an MES-induced seizure. Depending on the dose administered, PTZ can produce myoclonic jerks; repeated clonic seizures of the vibrissae, forelimbs, and hindlimbs without loss of righting reflex; clonic seizures of the limbs with loss of righting reflex; and loss of righting reflex followed by tonic extension of the forelimbs and hindlimbs (14). The importance of this point relies on the observation that the pharmacologic profile of the PTZ test differs depending on the endpoint selected. In this respect, it is possible to convert a rather discriminating threshold model into a nondiscriminating seizure test by simply choosing an inappropriate endpoint (15).

Threshold Tonic Extension Seizure Test

As discussed above, UCB LO59 represents the only example of a drug that was inactive in both the MES and sc PTZ tests but active against audiogenic seizures and kindled seizures. As a result of this observation, the ASP modified its initial identification procedures in 1994 to include a nondiscriminating threshold tonic extension (TTE) seizure test. The TTE test is a nonselective, electroconvulsive seizure model that, as shown in Fig. 1, is used only with those compounds found to be inactive in both the MES and sc PTZ tests. For the most part, MES- and sc PTZ-active compounds are active in this test. In this respect, the pharmacologic profile of the TTE test is similar to that associated with the audiogenic seizure-susceptible mouse model (see below).

Initial Testing for Minimal Motor Impairment

All mice and rats used in the initial identification tests are tested for minimal motor impairment before being subjected to the anticonvulsant tests. Minimal motor impairment in mice is established by the rotorod procedure of Dunham and Miya (16). When a mouse is placed on a rod that rotates at a speed of 6 rpm, the animal can maintain its equilibrium for long periods of time. Inability of a treated mouse to maintain its equilibrium in three trials during 1 minute is taken as the endpoint. In rats, motor deficit is indicated by ataxia, which may include a circular or zigzag gait, abnormal body posture and spread of the legs, tremors, hyperactivity, lack of exploratory behavior, somnolence, stupor, catalepsy, loss of placing response, and changes in muscle tone.

Identification Testing Protocol

In the initial identification tests, a minimal number of mice are tested for MES and sc PTZ protection at 0.5 and 4 hours after an intraperitoneal dose of 30, 100, or 300 mg of the test substance per kilogram. If this preliminary testing in mice suggests that a candidate substance possesses satisfactory anticonvulsant activity, the compound is then screened in rats following an oral dose of 30 mg/kg. Rats are tested at five-time intervals between 0.25 and 4 hours. For the MES test, a 60-Hz alternating current electrical stimulus of 50 mA (mice) and 150 mA (rats) is delivered to the anesthetized cornea (0.5% tetracaine HCl in 0.9% saline solution) for a duration of 0.2 second. For the sc PTZ test, the ASP routinely administers a subcutaneous dose of PTZ to mice (85 mg/kg) and rats (70 mg/kg) to produce a minimal clonic seizure of the vibrissae and/or forelimbs that persists for at least 5 seconds. Animals are observed during a 30-minute period for the presence or absence of a clonic seizure.

The primary technical difference between the TTE test and the MES test is the current employed. The TTE test uses sufficient current to elicit threshold hindlimb tonic extension in 97% of the animals challenged, whereas the MES test uses a supramaximal current (four to five times threshold). For this test, 20 CF#1 mice are pretreated intraperitoneally with 100 mg of the test substance per kilogram. At varying times (0.25, 0.5, 1, 2, and 4 hours) after treatment, individual mice (four at each time point) are challenged with sufficient current (12 to 15 mA for 0.2 second) delivered through corneal electrodes to elicit a threshold tonic extension seizure (17). Animals not displaying hindlimb tonic extension are considered protected. Active compounds are then screened again at the same dose and time points in the MES test to verify that they were truly inactive against MES seizures. No further testing is conducted on compounds found inactive in this test (Fig. 1).

The results obtained from these three initial identification tests and the motor impairment tests provide useful information regarding the overall potential of an investigational AED. For example, the results obtained from the MES and sc PTZ tests (mice and rats), the TTE test (mice), and neurologic deficit tests (mice and rats) provide information concerning the oral bioavailability, species variation, duration of action, toxicity, efficacy, and clinical utility of a test substance. Those compounds displaying a favorable anticonvulsant profile without substantial neurotoxicity or death are then subjected to further testing to quantify and define their anticonvulsant potential.

Finally, it is important to note that all testing and dosing protocols should remain flexible so that they can be modified when additional appropriate information regarding pharmacokinetics and mechanism of action supports such a modification. Vigabatrin represents one example for which such a change was warranted. In most animal models, vigabatrin displays a time to peak effect that is between 24 and 48 hours. This long time to peak effect reflects the slow yet irreversible inhibition of GABA-T and subsequent increase in brain GABA concentrations following vigabatrin administration. Thus, the anticonvulsant activity of vigabatrin went undetected when it was originally tested in the standard protocol, but was observed at 24 hours when consideration was given to these factors.

Quantification of Anticonvulsant Activity and Behavioral Toxicity

These studies are designed to provide in-depth information pertaining to the time of peak effect (TPE) and median effective (ED_{50}) and median toxic (TD_{50}) doses of a candidate substance. Information obtained from the quantification studies conducted at the TPE can be used to estimate the protective index (PI) of a test substance. The PI is defined as the ratio between the TD_{50} and the ED_{50} and is an indicator useful for differentiating and advancing one analogue of a chemical series for further testing.

For the dose-response studies, groups of at least eight mice or rats are treated with various doses of the test substance until at least two points have been established between the limits of 0 and 100% protection or toxicity. The 95% confidence interval is then calculated for each quantitative determination by probit analysis (18).

Candidate substances that display a reasonable level of separation between activity and toxicity and represent a novel chemical series are advanced to more in-depth characterization.

Anticonvulsant Differentiation

Once the efficacy of a test substance against MES-, sc PTZ-, or TTE-induced seizures has been quantitated, a battery of tests are employed to characterize further the anticonvulsant profile of the substance. In this phase of testing, a substance is evaluated for its ability to block clonic seizures induced in mice by the GABA antagonists bicuculline (BIC) and picrotoxin (PIC) and non-convulsant spike-and-wave seizures induced in rats by γ-hydroxybutyrate (GHB). Efficacy against sound-induced seizures is also assessed in the Frings audiogenic seizure-susceptible mouse. In addition, a candidate substance is evaluated for its ability to modify both the behavioral and electrographic seizure in the fully hippocampal-kindled rat. The results from these tests provide useful information regarding the overall anticonvulsant profile of the most interesting and novel compounds identified earlier.

Subcutaneous Bicuculline and Subcutaneous Picrotoxin Tests

Seizures produced by the $GABA_A$ receptor antagonist BIC and the chloride-channel blocker PIC depend in part on the dose administered and the route of administration. In both cases, seizures can progress from clonus to tonic extension. Benzodiazepines and other $GABA_A$ receptor agonists are very effective against clonic seizures induced by these two GABA antagonists. However, like the sc PTZ test, the sc BIC and sc PIC tests become somewhat nondiscriminatory when tonic extension is employed as the endpoint.

Although it is tempting, one should not speculate about the mechanism of action of a drug based solely on its ability to prevent seizures induced by a chemoconvulsant with a known mechanism of action. For this reason, these two tests are employed only to provide additional efficacy data that may be useful for differentiating a candidate substance from the established and new AEDs.

Following the administration of BIC (2.7 mg/kg), mice are observed for 30 minutes for the presence of a minimal clonic seizure. Mice given PIC (2.5 mg/kg) are observed for 45 minutes. BIC and PIC seizures typically consist of an episode of clonic spasms of the forelimbs and hindlimbs, jaws, or vibrissae. BIC-induced clonic seizures are frequently followed by tonic extension of the hindlimbs and death. For those active compounds, activity is quantitated and the ED_{50} and 95% confidence interval determined.

γ-Hydroxybutyrate Spike-and-Wave Model of Absence

GHB-induced spike-and-wave seizures represent an excellent pharmacologic model for the initial identification of AEDs that may be useful in the treatment of generalized absence seizures (19). Shortly after systemic administration of a convulsant dose of GHB, the EEG of a treated animal is characterized by abnormal 6- to 7-Hz spike-and-wave discharges that persist for 2 to 4 hours. Ethosuximide and other antiabsence drugs are effective in reducing the severity and duration of GHB-induced spike-and-wave discharges. In addition, phenytoin and $GABA_A$ receptor agonists prolong GHB seizures (19). Thus, this represents a useful model not only to confirm the potential antiabsence activity of drugs found to be active in the sc PTZ test, but also to assess whether a drug with a phenytoin-like anticonvulsant profile or a known GABAmimetic will worsen GHB seizures. Such information is particularly useful when a candidate substance makes the transition from preclinical to clinical investigations.

For the studies conducted by the ASP, eight rats are treated orally with the dose of candidate substance that provides 97% protection against MES or sc PTZ seizures. At the TPE, 150 mg of GHB is administered per kilogram intraperitoneally and the EEG of individual rats is monitored for 2 hours; the severity of spike-and-wave seizures is evaluated by computer analysis of the EEG. Results obtained from a group of treated animals are compared with those obtained from a group of vehicle-treated rats.

Kindled Rat Model of Focal Seizures

None of the tests described thus far is very useful for identifying new drugs likely to be beneficial for the treatment of difficult-to-control seizure types and epilepsy syndromes such as complex partial seizures or Lennox-Gastaut syndrome. Of the numerous animal seizure models available, the kindling model provides useful information regarding the potential ability of an investigational drug to limit focal seizures originating from discrete limbic brain regions (e.g., amygdala, hippocampus) and is thought to represent a model of complex partial seizures (20,21). This conclusion is supported in part by the pharmacologic profile of the kindling model. For example, drugs effective against human partial seizures are also effective against fully kindled seizures in animals. This model not only provides an experimental model of focal seizures, but also provides a means of studying complex brain networks that may contribute to seizure spread and generalization from a focus (22,23). Furthermore, the kindling model probably represents the most suitable model available for evaluating the ability of an investigational substance to prevent the acquisition of a seizure focus (i.e., antiepileptic versus anticonvulsant potential). Because of the labor-intensive nature of these studies, only a few (approximately 20) of the most promising compounds are evaluated annually by the ASP.

Of the various kindling paradigms described in the literature for identifying the potential utility of a substance for treating complex partial seizures, the rapid hippocampal kindling model of Lothman et al. (22,23) appears to offer some distinct advantages for the routine screening and evaluation of new anticonvulsant substances. For example, this particular model is unique in that it provides a framework for assessing drug efficacy against focal seizures in a temporal fashion in each individual rat.

For these studies, the candidate substance is evaluated for its ability to block the kindled motor seizure (seizure scores of 4 and 5) and limbic behavioral seizure (seizure score between 1 and 3) and to effect changes in the afterdischarge duration. The procedures for surgical implantation of a bipolar electrode have been described previously (22). After a 1-week recovery period, animals are kindled to a stage 5 behavioral seizure (24) with a stimulus consisting of a 50-Hz, 10-second train of 1-ms biphasic 200-A pulses delivered every 30 minutes for 6 hours (12 stimulations per day) on alternating days, for a total of 60 stimulations (5 stimulus days). Drug testing is usually initiated after a 1-week, stimulus-free period. On each day of a drug trial, animals receive two to three suprathreshold stimulations delivered every 30 minutes before drug treatment. During these control blocks, the stability of the behavioral seizure stage and afterdischarge duration is assessed. Fifteen minutes after the last control block, a single dose of the test substance is administered intraperitoneally. After 15 minutes, each rat is then stimulated every 30 minutes for 3 to 4 hours. After each stimulation, individual seizure scores and afterdischarge durations are recorded. The group mean and standard error of the mean are calculated for each parameter. After the last stimulation, animals are allowed 4 to 5 drug- and stimulus-free days between subsequent drug tests.

With this approach, a drug that reduces the seizure score from 5 to 3 without any effect on afterdischarge duration would be presumed useful against secondary generalized seizures and would not likely be useful against focal seizures. In contrast, those drugs that reduce the seizure score from 5 to <1, in addition to reducing the electrographic afterdischarge, would be anticipated to be quite effective against focal seizures.

Audiogenic Seizures

Mice susceptible to audiogenic seizures (AGS) are commonly employed in the initial screening protocols of many laboratories. They are particularly useful for pharmacologic studies because they are nondiscriminating with respect to a wide variety of drugs active in the central nervous system (25). Thus, it is not likely that drugs with any anticonvulsant potential will be missed using this model. However, the main advantage of this model can also become a disadvantage for high-volume laboratories wherein several hundred compounds are evaluated annually. The ASP employs this model as an end-stage screen for a select number of the most promising candidate substances identified and characterized by more discriminating seizure models.

The DBA/2 mouse is the most commonly used strain of audiogenic mice. It is commercially available around the world and has been well characterized. Seizures that are evoked by a high-intensity sound stimulus are characterized by wild running followed by forelimb and hindlimb tonic extension that lasts for 15 to 25 seconds. The ASP employs male and female Frings AGS-susceptible mice (18 to 25 g body weight) that are obtained from an inhouse colony at the University of Utah (26). The behavioral seizure and pharmacologic profile of the Frings mouse is identical to that of the DBA/2 AGS-susceptible mouse. The major difference between these two strains is their developmental susceptibility to sound-induced seizures. For example, DBA/2 mice display a relatively narrow window of susceptibility (18 to 24 days), whereas the Frings strain retain their susceptibility well into adult life. This makes this particular strain extremely useful for long-term studies.

Typically, a dose-response study is conducted to determine the ED_{50} for a limited number of candidate substances. For these studies, groups of eight mice each are treated with varying doses of the test substance. At the predetermined TPE, individual mice are placed into a sound chamber and exposed to a sound stimulus of 110 decibels (11 kHz). Mice are observed for 25 seconds for the presence or absence of hindlimb tonic extension. Animals not displaying hindlimb tonic extension are considered protected. The severity of the seizure is also quantitated by assigning a numeric score to the observed response (e.g., no response, 0; wild running for <10 seconds, 1; wild running for >10 seconds, 2; clonic seizure, 3; forelimb extension/hindlimb flexion, 4; tonic seizure, 5). The anticonvulsant ED_{50} and 95% confidence interval are calculated by probit analysis (18).

Advanced Studies

Advanced pharmacologic and hepatic drug-metabolizing enzyme studies are used to help elucidate the proconvulsant potential, mechanism of action, potential for drug-drug interactions, and tolerance of the most promising candidate substances (Fig. 1).

Intravenous Pentylenetetrazol Seizure Threshold Test (Proconvulsant Potential)

A compound that prevents seizure spread (active in the MES test) may also lower seizure threshold (27). Such a compound may have proconvulsant activity and at the same time prevent generalized tonic seizures. For example, the cardiac antiarrhythmic drug mexiletine is a potent anti-MES compound, yet it lowers seizure threshold at doses slightly above the MES ED_{50} in mice. The ASP employs the timed intravenous PTZ seizure threshold test in mice to identify those MES compounds with proconvulsant potential (28).

The candidate substance is administered to mice intraperitoneally in doses representing the ED_{50} and TD_{50}. At the TPE by the MES test, an intravenous infusion of a 0.5% heparinized solution of PTZ (0.34 mL/min) is started. The time to the appearance of the first myoclonic jerk and the subsequent sustained clonic seizure is determined. Results obtained from groups of 10 treated and 10 vehicle-control mice are converted to the dose of PTZ in milligrams per kilogram necessary to produce the two endpoints. Proconvulsant drugs, such as lidocaine and mexiletine, lower the dose of PTZ required to produce the endpoint, whereas anticonvulsant drugs, such as valproic acid, ethosuximide, and phenobarbital, increase the required dose of PTZ.

In Vitro Mechanism-of-Action Studies

The mechanisms of action of currently marketed anticonvulsant drugs are not fully understood. Although numerous molecular targets exist wherein anticonvulsant drugs may exert an effect, the final common pathway appears to be through modulation of voltage-gated and/or neurotransmitter-gated ion channels (29,30,31). The common link among the various proposed mechanisms involves the ability of an anticonvulsant to modulate ion-channel function. For this reason, the mechanistic studies conducted by the ASP are directed at identifying a potential interaction of the candidate substance with voltage-sensitive (Na^+ and Ca^{2+}) and receptor-gated (glutamate and GABA) ion channels (1). With this approach, it would not be too surprising to find that a compound with a phenytoin-like anticonvulsant profile also inhibits voltage-sensitive Na^+ channels. In contrast, it would be particularly interesting to find that such a compound was without any effect on the Na^+ channel. The ASP employs this approach to assess how an investigational drug might differ mechanistically from the established AEDs. It is hoped that this procedure will result in the identification of mechanistically novel compounds.

Tolerance and Toxicity Studies

When a test substance demonstrates intrinsic anticonvulsant activity, a favorable PI relative to overall neurotoxicity, and an adequate duration of action, consideration must be given to the fact that in the clinical setting the drug will be administered during long time periods and often in conjunction with other drugs. These factors require consideration of self- and/or cross-tolerance as well as other drug-drug interactions. Tolerance can be metabolic (pharmacokinetic) or central (pharmacodynamic). Pharmacokinetic changes derive most often from effects on hepatic drug-metabolizing enzymes. Changes in the metabolism reactions can result in increased or decreased pharmacologic effects of the candidate substance and can also lead to alterations in toxicity and activity of concurrently administered drugs. The tolerance and liver microsomal enzyme studies conducted by the ASP have been designed to address this particular issue (1).

SUMMARY

The procedures employed by the ASP provide detailed information pertaining to the anticonvulsant profile of new candidate substances. In addition, the results obtained from tolerance and liver microsomal studies furnish critical information for predicting whether tolerance and/or serious drug-drug interactions are likely to develop following long-term administration of a candidate substance. Finally, in vitro mechanism-of-action studies supply preliminary information regarding the site of action of promising new anticonvulsant drdugs. It is anticipated that the testing protocol outlined above will identify safer and mechanistically novel substances to enhance significantly the quality of life of those epilepsy patients still suffering from uncontrolled seizure disorders and/or experiencing significant adverse drug effects.

REFERENCES

1. White HS, Woodhead JH, Franklin MR, Swinyard EA, Wolf HH. General principles: experimental selection, quantification, and evaluation of antiepileptic drugs. In: Levy RH, Mattson RH, Meldrum BS, eds. *Antiepileptic Drugs*. 4th ed. New York: Raven Press; 1995:99–110.
2. Suzdak PD, Jansen JA. A review of the preclinical pharmacology of tiagabine, a potent and selective anticonvulsant GABA uptake inhibitor. *Epilepsia* 1995;36: 612–626.
3. Löscher W, Hönack D. Profile of UCB L059, a novel anticonvulsant drug, in models of partial and generalized epilepsy in mice and rats. *Eur J Pharmacol* 1993; 232:147–158.
4. Klitgaard H, Matagne A, Gobert J, Wulfert E. Levetiracetam (UCB LO59) prevents limbic seizures induced by pilocarpine and kainic acid in rats. *Epilepsia* 1996;37(Suppl 5):118.
5. Abou-Khalil B, Nasreddine W, Fakhoury T, Atkinson D, Beydoun A. Efficacy and safety of UCB L059 as an adjunctive treatment in refractory partial epilepsy: results of open-label treatment at two centers. *Epilepsia* 1996; 37(Suppl 5):169.
6. Cameron N, Penovich PE, Ritter FJ, Espe-Lillo J. Open-label study of UCB L059 as add-on therapy in refractory partial epilepsy. *Epilepsia* 1996;37(Suppl 5):169.
7. Shorvon S, Janz D, Loiseau P, Lowenthal A, Bielen E, Johnscher G. Efficacy and tolerability of UCB L059 add-on treatment in refractory patients with partial-onset epileptic seizures. *Epilepsia* 1996;37(Suppl 5):170.
8. van Rijckevorsel K, Debrabandere L, Deberdt W. Evaluation of the efficacy and tolerability of UCB L059 in refractory epileptic patients with complex partial seizures: a 12-week, single-blind, add-on, rising-dose study. *Epilepsia* 1996;37(Suppl 5):169.
9. White HS, Johnson M, Wolf HH, Kupferberg HJ. The early identification of anticonvulsant activity: role of the maximal electroshock and subcutaneous pentylenetetrazol seizure models. *Ital J Neurol Sci* 1995;16: 73–77.
10. Putnam TJ, Merritt HH. Experimental determination of the anticonvulsant properties of some phenyl derivatives. *Science* 1937;85:525–526.
11. Swinyard EA, Woodhead JH, White HS, Franklin MR. General principles: experimental selection, quantification, and evaluation of anticonvulsants. In: Levy R, Mattson R, Meldrum B, Penry JK, Dreifuss FE, eds. *Antiepileptic Drugs*. 3rd ed. New York: Raven Press; 1989;85–102.
12. Everett GM, Richards RK. Comparative anticonvulsive action of 3,5,5-trimethyloxazolidine-2,4-dione (Tridione), Dilantin, and phenobarbital. *J Pharmacol Exp Ther* 1944;81:402–407.
13. Lennox WG. The *petit mal* epilepsies. Their treatment with Tridione. *JAMA* 1945;129:1069–1074.
14. Löscher W, Hönack D, Fassbender CP, Nolting B. The role of technical, biological, and pharmacological factors in the laboratory evaluation of anticonvulsant drugs. 3. Pentylenetetrazole seizure models. *Epilepsy Res* 1991;8:171–189.
15. Piredda SG, Woodhead JH, Swinyard EA. Effect of stimulus intensity on the profile of anticonvulsant activity of phenytoin, ethosuximide, and valproate. *J Pharmacol Exp Ther* 1985;232:741–745.
16. Dunham MS, Miya TA. A note on a simple apparatus for detecting neurological deficit in rats and mice. *J Am Pharm Assoc Sci Ed* 1957;46:208–209.
17. Woodbury LA, Davenport VD. Design and use of a new electroshock seizure apparatus, and analysis of factors altering seizure threshold and pattern. *Arch Int Pharmacodyn Ther* 1952;92:97–104.
18. Finney DJ. *Probit Analysis*. 3rd ed. London: Cambridge University Press; 1971.
19. Snead OC. Pharmacological models of generalized absence seizures in rodents. *J Neural Transm* 1992;35: 7–19.
20. McNamara JO, Byrne MC, Dasheiff RM, Fitz JG. The kindling model of epilepsy: a review. *Prog Neurobiol* 1980;15:139–159.
21. McNamara JO. Development of new pharmacological

agents for epilepsy: lessons from the kindling model. *Epilepsia* 1989;30:513–518.
22. Lothman EW, Salerno RA, Perlin JB, Kaiser DL. Screening and characterization of antiepileptic drugs with rapidly recurring hippocampal seizures in rats. *Epilepsy Res* 1988;2:366–379.
23. Lothman EW, Williamson JM. Closely spaced recurrent hippocampal seizures elicit two types of heightened epileptogenesis: a rapidly developing, transient kindling and a slowly developing, enduring kindling. *Brain Res* 1994;649:71–84.
24. Racine RJ. Modification of seizure activity by electrical stimulation: II. Motor seizure. *Electroencephalogr Clin Neurophysiol* 1972;32:281–294.
25. Chapman AA, Croucher MJ, Meldrum BS. Evaluation of anticonvulsant drugs in DBA/2 mice with sound-induced seizures. *Arzneimittelforschung/Drug Res* 1984; 34(II, No 10):1261–1264.
26. White HS, Patel S, Meldrum BS. Anticonvulsant profile of MDL 27,266, an orally active, broad-spectrum anticonvulsant agent. *Epilepsy Res* 1992;12:217–226.
27. Kupferberg HJ. Antiepileptic drug development program: a cooperative effort of government and industry. *Epilepsia* 1989;30(Suppl 1):S51–S56.
28. Orlof MJ, Williams HL, Pfeiffer CC. Timed intravenous infusion of Metrazol and strychnine for testing anticonvulsant drugs. *Proc Soc Exp Biol Med* 1949;70: 254–257.
29. Macdonald RL. Antiepileptic drug actions. *Epilepsia* 1989;30:S19–S28.
30. Rogawski MA, Porter RJ. Antiepileptic drugs: pharmacological mechanisms and clinical efficacy, with consideration of promising developmental-stage compounds. *Pharmacol Rev* 1990;42:223–286.
31. Macdonald RL, Kelly KM. Antiepileptic drug mechanisms of action. *Epilepsia* 1993;34:S1–S8.

Antiepileptic Drug Development.
Advances in Neurology, Vol. 76,
edited by J. French, I. Leppik, and M. A. Dichter.
Lippincott–Raven Publishers, Philadelphia © 1998.

4

Pharmaceutical Industry Screening for New Antiepileptic Drugs

Charles P. Taylor and James L. Marks

Department of Neuroscience Therapeutics and Department of Biochemistry, Parke-Davis Pharmaceutical Research Division, Warner-Lambert Co., Ann Arbor, Michigan 48105.

INTRODUCTION

The recent introduction of four new antiepileptic drugs (AEDs) to the marketplace in the United States, with several others nearing approval, has altered the economic and medical outlook for new anticonvulsants for the next 10 years. It is now less likely that novel anticonvulsant compounds with unknown mechanisms of action will be developed. The present trend is to investigate known molecular drug targets and develop therapeutic targets later in the development process. In addition, several new technologies have greatly altered the methods used for drug discovery in the pharmaceutical industry. Mass screening of large databases of compounds has become routine, with molecular techniques used to isolate single drug targets for pharmacologic testing. Combinatorial chemistry has recently emerged as a way to generate large numbers of related compounds for pharmacologic testing. This brief review highlight those trends of drug discovery within the pharmaceutical industry.

STRUCTURE-ACTIVITY RELATIONSHIPS

New drugs are usually discovered by testing in a standardized pharmacologic model (e.g., maximal electroshock following intraperitoneal administration of test compounds to a group of intact mice; alternatively, in vitro displacement of radioligands from a known drug binding site or inhibition of neurotransmitter uptake or enzyme activity). Typically, a single, well-known compound is used as a chemical template, and systematic chemical modifications are made to this chemical lead in an effort to improve potency or selectivity. Often, trends emerge that associate certain types of chemical modifications with increased potency or effectiveness. This type of work is called structure-activity analysis. Following optimization of potency or selectivity, typically another round of structural modifications is made to enhance physical or pharmacokinetic properties, such as oral absorption, elimination half-life, and aqueous solubility. The same basic approach has been used for at least the past 50 years to develop new drugs. However, methods of pharmacology and synthetic chemistry have evolved considerably during that time.

NEW ANTIEPILEPTIC DRUGS INTRODUCED IN THE 1990S

Table 1 lists several new AEDs that have recently reached the marketplace, or that will likely be introduced within the next few years. It is clear that the 1990s are a unique period in the discovery of AEDs; previously, there was never a decade in which so many new med-

TABLE 1. *Discovery methods of recent antiepileptic drugs*

Drug (year first published)	Discovery screen method	Mechanism	Indication	Market approval
Gabapentin (1975)	Semicarbazide seizures	Δ GABA metabolism (?)	Partial seizures	UK, 1992; US, 1993
Vigabatrin (1977)	GABA-T inhibition	GABA-T inhibition	Partial seizures	UK, 1990; US (?)
Zonisamide (1980)	Electroshock	Na^+ channel	Partial seizures	Japan, 1995
Felbamate (1984)	Electroshock (NINDS)	Na^+ channel (NMDA antagonist)	Partial seizures, Lennox-Gastaut syndrome	US, 1993; Europe, 1995
Lamotrigine (1984)	Electroshock (veratridine)	Na^+ channel	Partial seizures (absence?)	UK, 1991; US, 1996
Topiramate (1987)	Electroshock (NINDS)	Na^+ channel (AMPA antagonist, GABA modulator)	Partial seizures	UK, 1996; 1997
Tiagabine (1987)	[^{3}H]GABA uptake	GABA uptake inhibitor	Partial seizures	1997 (?)
Remacemide (1990)	Electroshock	Na^+ channel (NMDA antagonist metabolite)	Partial seizures (stroke?)	(?)

NINDS, National Institute of Neurological Diseases and Stroke, Antiepileptic Drug Discovery Project, aided in this discovery.

ications for epilepsy were introduced. As Table 1 shows, these drugs may be "novel," but they are not really new. Initial synthetic chemistry and pharmacology of most of these compounds was completed as long ago as the late 1970s. The tools used for the pharmacologic selection process varied somewhat, but in most cases, the primary test system was maximal electroshock in mice (1), a method adapted from technology available 60 years ago (2,3). Exceptions include drugs that selectively inhibit the GABA (τ-aminobutyric acid) transaminase enzyme (GABA-T), such as vigabatrin (4,5), or inhibit the synaptic reuptake of GABA, such as tiagabine (6) and gabapentin, which was designed as a structural analogue of GABA (7).

In recent years, the trend within the pharmaceutical industry has been toward mechanistically based drug screening. Therefore, it may be anticipated that new substances will have increasingly well-defined molecular sites of action. It will be the job of pharmaceutical and medical researchers not only to test known anticonvulsant drugs in epilepsy, but also to determine which of the various mechanistically defined drugs that become available might benefit from animal pharmacology or clinical studies for epilepsy. In many cases, the initial indication for new drugs might not be for epilepsy, but instead might be for cerebral ischemia, neurodegenerative diseases, pain, or some other problem.

NEW TECHNOLOGIES

Mass Screening of Chemical Databases

This section briefly reviews several new technologies that have become available within the past 10 years. The first is mass screening of large databases of known chemicals through highly automated pharmaceutical tests (8,9). As an example, Fig. 1 shows the typical screening capacity of a single radioligand binding assay at various times in the past 10 years at the Parke-Davis Pharmaceutical Research Division in Ann Arbor, Michigan. It is easy to appreciate that even a large library of >160,000 compounds can now be tested in the course of a few months.

The technologies enabling this drastic increase in screening capacity are based on the invention of miniaturized and mechanized methods carried out by computer-controlled

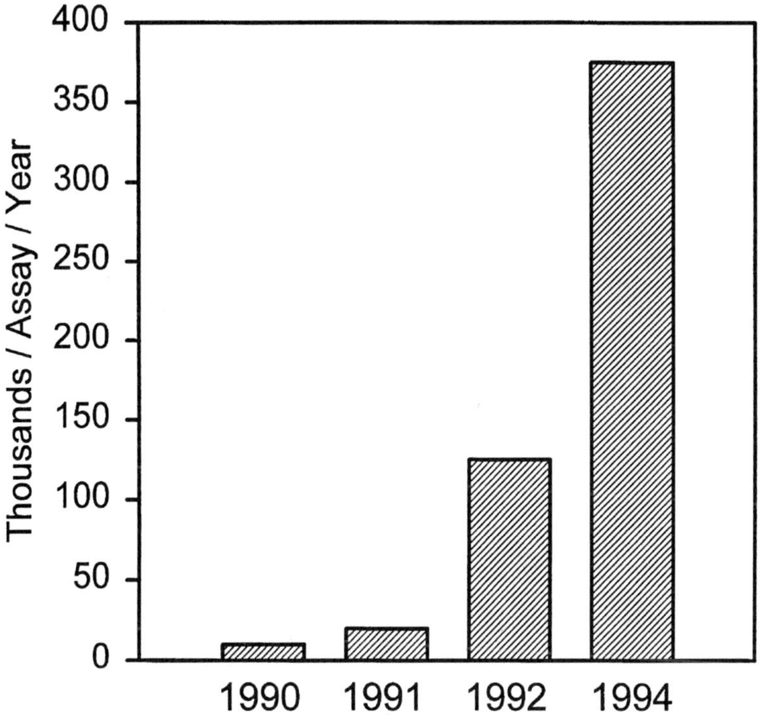

FIG. 1. Graph depicts the volume of mass screening (number of compounds from the Parke-Davis database tested in receptor binding assays) during a single month. Note the logarithmic growth in the number of compounds tested, illustrating the utility of new methods for mass screening.

robotics. The basics behind this method are shown in Fig. 2. Small quantities of individual chemical samples are weighed into small test tubes and then transferred to plastic 96-well microtiter plates. Each sample is dissolved in dimethylsulfoxide (DMSO) at an approximate concentration of 10 mg/mL. To speed up the screening process, and on the assumption that only a small fraction of experimental compounds will be active in any one pharmacologic test, 10 individual compounds are combined in each test well (each at a concentration of 1 mg/mL). Following this step, solutions in each well are diluted in physiologic salt solution to 1:1000 in a second 96-well plate used for the pharmaceutical test procedure, to an approximate final concentration of 10 μg/mL (roughly 20 to 50 μM) for each compound. The original plate with compounds in DMSO is retained for future use with different screen procedures.

A robotic device performs the test (e.g., by adding appropriate radioligands to a brain membrane preparation, or by performing a colorimetric enzyme reaction). If any of the 96 wells show significant inhibition of activity, the code numbers for the compounds in the "active" well are retrieved, and additional tests are done with separately weighed samples of the 10 compounds from the active well to determine which compound caused the activity. Finally, activity is confirmed by additional testing with a wide range of concentrations to determine an IC_{50} value (concentration that inhibits 50%). In this way, it is possible to screen rapidly through vast numbers of randomly chosen compounds, selecting only those with a given level of inhibitory potency. This mass screening approach is increasingly used to discover chemical leads for a wide variety of pharmacologic targets amenable to radioligand bind-

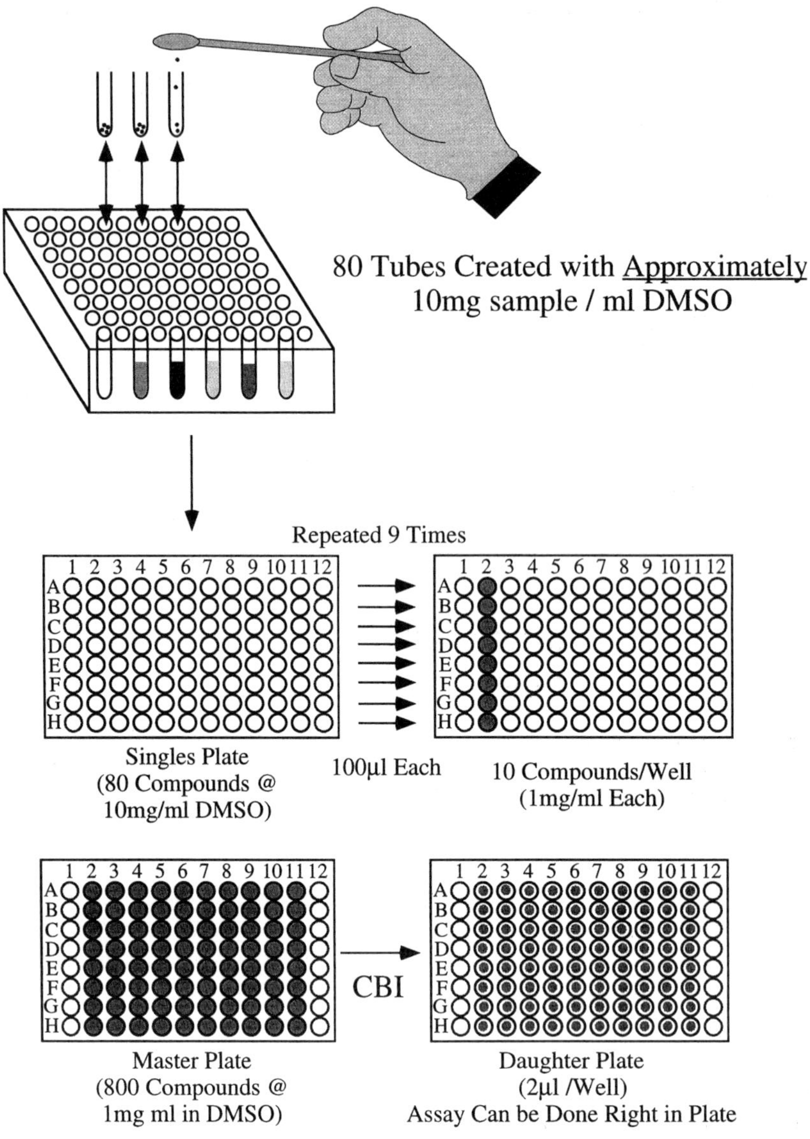

FIG. 2. Method for mass screening of compounds with 96-well format. Eighty compounds are weighed into 80 individual test tubes, with approximately 10 mg of each sample dissolved in 1.0 mL of DMSO, a universal solvent. One hundred microliters from each tube is pipetted into a 96-well microtiter plate; this is repeated until 80 compounds (each at 1 mg/mL DMSO) are pipetted, producing a "singles plate." From each of 10 singles plates, 2 μL is removed from each well with an automated pipettor and placed into a "master plate"; the master plate contains 10 individual compounds in each of 80 wells. The master plate is then diluted into a "daughter plate," which is used to complete the assay procedure. Each well on the daughter plate contains approximately 2 μg of each of 10 experimental compounds. Appropriate physiologic salt solutions, radiolabeled tracers, and enzymes are added to the daughter plate, and the assay is processed. Additional tests with other assay procedures can be performed with compounds from the same master plate, which is retained and stored at low temperature.

ing or colorimetric enzyme activity assays. Physiologic functional tests are also beginning to be performed with similar methods (see below).

Molecular Biologically Defined Targets

The recent availability of cloned neurotransmitter receptors, ion channels, and neurotransmitter transporters has enabled pharmacologic testing to be carried out in cell systems expressing only a single type of drug target (receptor), rather than the many related targets present in most mammalian neurons. This offers obvious advantages for the discovery and optimization of drugs that are selective for a particular receptor subtype and are inactive at other, related receptor subtypes.

Examples include the expression of single subtypes of voltage-gated calcium channels in stable cell lines (10,11), and the expression of defined NMDA-type (*N*-methyl-D-aspartate) and AMPA-type (α-amino-3-hydroxy-5-methyl-4-isoxazolepropionic acid) glutamate receptors in oocytes (12–14). Similar approaches have been used in many other areas that are less immediately relevant for epilepsy, including the cloning and expression of multiple subtypes of cholinergic, dopamine, or serotonin receptors and a wide variety of cellular enzymes.

The simplest technique for expressing cloned receptors or ion channels is to inject artificially produced mRNA coding for the desired protein with a micropipette directly through the cell membrane of a large oocyte taken from the South American clawed toad, *Xenopus laevis*. Within 3 days in vitro, the oocyte translates mRNA into proteins, which are expressed at the cell membrane and act functionally very much like a native mammalian ion channel or receptor. The oocyte then can be used for electrophysiologic experiments using the voltage-clamp technique to study agonist-induced responses (e.g., NMDA receptors) or voltage-gated ion-channel responses (e.g., Na^+ or Ca^{2+} channels).

However, because oocytes must be injected with mRNA individually, they are not suitable for producing large numbers of cells needed for biochemical experiments with radioligand binding or neurotransmitter release or uptake. For these experiments, usually it is necessary to transfect cloned DNA into a stable cell line that can be grown for many generations in vitro. This technique takes considerably more work, as the mammalian gene must be incorporated into a viral particle that is used to transfect mammalian cells, stably incorporating the cloned gene into the genome of the cell line. Once produced, however, quantities of the cell line can be stored in liquid nitrogen for future use, and the cells can be grown in vitro through many cell divisions to produce large numbers of cells for receptor binding, ion-flux experiments, or other biochemical experiments. Cell lines are also very useful for electrophysiology experiments using the voltage-clamp technique.

Examples of anticonvulsant targets that have already been studied with molecular biologic techniques include voltage-gated Na^+ channels (15), voltage-gated Ca^{2+} channels (16,17), voltage-gated K^+ channels (18), and subtypes of glutamate receptors (12–14,19), GABA receptors (20), and glutamate and GABA uptake carriers (21,22).

Physiologic Monitoring of Mass Screen Targets

Although adaptation to 96-well formats is more difficult, it is often desirable to study voltage-dependent ion channels and certain other targets by a functional biochemical assay rather than with radioligand binding techniques. Functional assays have the advantage of detecting potential inhibitor compounds that interact with more than a single type of receptor site on the protein. Examples of modulatory binding sites that would not be detected with radioligand assays using labeled receptor agonists or competitive antagonists include the benzodiazepine modulatory site of $GABA_A$ receptors (20), the GYKI

52466 site of AMPA-type glutamate receptors (23), and the blocker sites of voltage-gated cation channels. Usually, functional assays require living (cultured) cells or synaptosomes acutely purified from brain tissue that can be stimulated to cause an easily detectible physiologic response in vitro. Examples include cellular influx of radiolabeled cations through voltage-gated ion channels detected by scintillation counting, and increases in cytosolic Ca^{2+} concentration from cell excitation measured with Ca^{2+}-sensitive fluorometric dyes.

Two recently designed instruments allow fluorescent dye experiments to be carried out in a 96-well format, with simultaneous quantitative measurements of fluorescent activity in each of the wells updated several times each second (18,24). One potential disadvantage of these instruments is their expense, which can reach a very significant fraction of U.S.$1,000,000. Although these fluorescent detector devices do not allow quite the same high volume of screening that radioligand binding techniques do, they still provide a vast improvement in throughput over traditional electropysiologic or cuvette-based fluorimetric methods for studying voltage-gated ion channels and other targets.

Combinatorial Chemistry Techniques

In the past few years, new methods of chemical synthesis have become available. These methods allow the rapid synthesis of many chemically related compounds by solid-phase chemistry, similar to that sometimes used to make polypeptide molecules of up to 20 or 30 amino acids. Solid-phase chemistry utilizes a compound that is temporarily bonded chemically to the surface of a tiny pin in an array of many pins. Each pin is then submerged into various reaction mixtures, allowing derivatives to be made without the time-consuming filtration and purification typically required between each synthetic step with traditional methods. Furthermore, solid-phase chemistry is amenable to being performed using a miniaturized format, with many different compounds all made in parallel processes in miniaturized reaction chambers similar to the wells of a multi-well culture dish. This adaptation has been called combinatorial chemistry (9,25–28). The technique has the advantage of quickly generating large numbers of novel compounds. However, only very small quantities of each compound are usually obtained (40 mg or less), and these may be less pure than compounds made by traditional methods. However, subsequent to screening, additional quantities of particularly interesting compounds are usually synthesized by traditional methods to allow more extensive pharmacologic characterization and testing in animal models.

SUMMARY

It is clear that in coming years, many interesting new compounds will emerge from these and other strategies for drug discovery. In previous strategies of anticonvulsant discovery, whole-animal models of seizures were utilized from the initial stages; however, with the newer strategies, it will become necessary to select promising drug targets for clinical trials in epilepsy that have well-defined molecular targets of action but poorly defined actions in various animal seizure models. The new pharmaceutical discovery technologies of mass screening, cloned drug targets, and combinatorial chemistry will assist in the efficient discovery of novel drug candidates. Incidentally, these techniques also will minimize the use of large numbers of living laboratory animals for anticonvulsant drug screening.

REFERENCES

1. Swinyard EA. Electrically induced convulsions. In: Purpura DP, Penry JK, Tower DB, Walter RD, Woodbury DM, eds. *Experimental Models of Epilepsy*. New York: Raven Press; 1972:433–458.
2. Toman JEP, Swinyard EA, Goodman LS. Properties of maximal seizures and their alteration by anticonvulsant drugs and other agents. *J Neurophysiol* 1946;9:231–240.
3. Putnam TJ, Merritt HH. Experimental determination of the anticonvusant properties of some phenyl derivatives. *Science* 1937;85:525–526.
4. Gram L, Larsson OM, Johnsen A, Schousboe A. Experimental studies of the influence of vigabatrin on the GABA system. *Br J Clin Pharmacol* 1989;27:13S–18S.
5. Lippert B, Metcalf BW, Jung MJ, Casara P. 4-Amino-hex-5-enoic acid, a selective catalytic inhibitor of 4-

aminobutyric-acid aminotransferase in mammalian brain. *Eur J Biochem* 1977;74:441–445.
6. Suzdak PD, Jansen JA. A review of the preclinical pharmacology of tiagabine, a potent and selective anticonvulsant GABA uptake inhibitor. *Epilepsia* 1995;36:612–626.
7. Satzinger G. Antiepileptics from gamma-aminobutyric acid. *Drug Res* 1994;44:261–266.
8. Bevan P, Ryder H, Shaw I. Identifying small-molecule lead compounds: the screening approach to drug discovery. *Trends Biotechnol* 1995;13:115–121.
9. Kubinyi H. Strategies and recent technologies in drug discovery. *Pharmazie* 1995;50:647–662.
10. Williams ME, Marubio LM, Deal CR, Hans M, Brust PF, Philipson LH, Miller RJ, Johnson EC, Harpold MM, Ellis SB. Structure and functional characterization of neuronal alpha 1E calcium-channel subtypes. *Nature* 1994;269:22347–22357.
11. Williams ME, Brust PF, Feldman DH, Patthi S, Simerson S, Maroufi A, McCue AF, Velicelebi G, Ellis SB, Harpold MM. Structure and functional expression of an omega-conotoxin-sensitive human N-type calcium channel. *Science* 1992;257:389–395.
12. Cordi AA, Desos P, Randle JC, Lepagnol J. Structure-activity relationships in a series of 3-sulfonylamino-2-(1*H*)-quinolones, as new. *Bioorg Med Chem* 1995;3:129–141.
13. Earley WG, Kumar V, Mallamo JP, Subramanyam C, Dority JA, Jr, Miller MS, DeHaven Hudkins DL, Aimone LD, Kelly MD, Ault B. Novel benzo[*b*]quinolizinium cations as uncompetitive *N*-methyl-D-aspartic acid (NMDA) antagonists: the relationship between log D and agonist independent (closed) NMDA channel block. *J Med Chem* 1995;38:3586–3592.
14. Woodward RM, Huettner JE, Guastella J, Keana JF, Weber E. In vitro pharmacology of ACEA-1021 and ACEA-1031, systemically active quinoxalinediones with high affinity and selectivity for *N*-methyl-D-aspartate receptor glycine sites. *Annu Rev Neurosci* 1995;47:568–581.
15. Ragsdale DS, Scheuer T, Catterall WA. Frequency and voltage-dependent inhibition of type IIA Na^+ channels, expressed in a mammalian cell line, by local anesthetic, antiarrhythmic, and anticonvulsant drugs. *Mol Pharmacol* 1991;40:756–765.
16. Simerson S, Brust P, Zahl N, Gillespie A, Sionit P, Ellis S, Urrutia A, Deal C, Hans M, Velicelebi G, Stauderman K, Harpold MM. Pharmacological characterization of recombinant cell lines stably expressing human voltage-gated calcium-channel subunits alpha1A, alpha1B, and alpha1E. *Soc Neurosci Abst* 1995;21:339.
17. Rock DM, Stoehr SJ, Offord J, Palma A. Biophysical and pharmacological characterization of stably expressed class B and class E Ca^{2+} channels in HEK 293 cells. *Soc Neurosci Abst* 1995;21:1282.
18. Groppi VE. Development of a functional high-volume screen for K^+ channel modulators. Ion Channels and Drug Discovery, presentation at the IBC Conference, Philadelphia, PA, Dec. 1995.
19. Daggett LP, Sacaan AI, Akong M, Rao SP, Hess SD, Liaw C, Urrutia A, Jachec C, Ellis SB, Dreessen J, et al. Molecular and functional characterization of recombinant human metabotropic glutamate receptor subtype 5. *Neuropharmacol* 1995;34:871–886.
20. Macdonald RL, Olsen RW. $GABA_A$ receptor channels. *Annu Rev Neurosci* 1994;17:569–602.
21. Clark JA, Amara SG. Amino acid neurotransmitter transporters: structure, function, and molecular diversity. *Bioessays* 1993;15:323–332.
22. Amara SG, Kuhar MJ. Neurotransmitter transporters: recent progress. *Annu Rev Neurosci* 1993;16:73–93.
23. Donevan SD, Rogawski MA. GYKI 52466, a 2,3-benzodiazepine, is a highly selective, noncompetitive antagonist of AMPA/kainate receptor responses. *Neuron* 1993;10:51–59.
24. Akong M, Siegel R, Vasserman E, Rowe B, Karlton D, McNiel J, Varney M, Stauderman K, Velicelebi G. High-throughput measurement of intracellular Ca^{2+} by fluorescence imaging of a 96-well microtiter plate. *Soc Neurosci Abst* 1995;21:577.
25. Doyle PM. Combinatorial chemistry in the discovery and development of drugs. *J Chem Technol Biotechnol* 1995;64:317–324.
26. Jiracek J, Yiotakis A, Vincent B, Lecoq A, Nicolaou A, Checler F, Dive V. Development of highly potent and selective phosphinic peptide inhibitors of zinc endopeptidase 24-15 using combinatorial chemistry. *J Biol Chem* 1995;270:21701–21706.
27. Martin EJ, Blaney JM, Siani MA, Spellmeyer DC, Wong AK, Moos WH. Measuring diversity: experimental design of combinatorial libraries for drug discovery. *J Med Chem* 1995;38:1431–1436.
28. Chabala JC. Solid-phase combinatorial chemistry and novel tagging methods for identifying leads. *Curr Opin Biotechnol* 1995;6:632–639.

Antiepileptic Drug Development.
Advances in Neurology, Vol. 76,
edited by J. French, I. Leppik, and M. A. Dichter.
Lippincott–Raven Publishers, Philadelphia © 1998.

5

Metabolic Enzymes and Antiepileptic Drug Interactions

René H. Levy and Gary G. Mather

Department of Pharmaceutics, University of Washington, Seattle, Washington 98195.

INTRODUCTION

Numerous studies have shown that the identification of metabolic enzymes aids in the rational understanding of drug-drug interactions (1–4). A detailed knowledge of metabolic pathways and the enzymes involved in the metabolism of a drug is essential to avoid potential interactions, as it has been determined that the different human cytochromes P_{450} exhibit substrate specificity. This substrate specificity provides a framework to address both types of drug interactions—inhibitory interactions, which lead to toxicity, or inductive interactions, manifested as loss of efficacy. Recently, the number of studies relating to CYP_{450} isoforms and their interactions has expanded at a geometric pace. These studies can be categorized into three basic types: (a) those identifying the isoform(s) responsible for a drug's metabolism, (b) those reporting the inhibition of specific isozymes by a drug, and (c) studies suggesting induction or increased expression of a certain isozyme following exposure to a drug.

In the case of the antiepileptic drugs (AEDs), identification of the isoforms responsible for their metabolism has been limited to phenytoin (PHT) and carbamazepine (CBZ). In a previous review (5), this information was used to demonstrate the application of metabolic isozymes in inhibition-based interactions. For CBZ, 30% to 50% of the dose is eliminated by epoxidation at the 10-11 position, and CYP3A4 plays a dominant role in the formation of this metabolite (6). Thus, various inhibitors of CYP3A4 (erythromycin, troleandomycin and other macrolide antibiotics, propoxyphene, and stiripentol) produce elevations in CBZ levels (7). In the case of PHT, both CYP2C9 and CYP2C19 contribute to the formation of *p*-HPPH (*p*-hydroxyphenylphenylhydantoin), the primary metabolite of PHT in humans (8,9). Quantitatively, CYP2C9 is the major enzyme catalyzing *p*-HPPH formation, with CYP2C19 providing a smaller contribution, especially at low concentrations. Therefore, it can be predicted that any drug that inhibits CYP2C9 or CYP2C19 at therapeutic concentrations will decrease PHT clearance. Indeed, drugs that inhibit CYP2C9 result in major interactions with PHT (sulfaphenazole, phenylbutazone), whereas drugs inhibiting CYP2C19 are associated with minor interactions (fluoxetine, cimetidine, omeprazole, felbamate, topiramate) (9).

No analysis has been published to date that addresses induction-based interactions on the basis of metabolic isozymes. The relationship between enzyme induction and metabolic isozymes is particularly relevant for AEDs, as this therapeutic class includes some of the most potent inducing drugs. The induction spectra of various AEDs have not been characterized. The objective of this review is to provide an update of current information on metabolic enzymes involved in anticonvulsant metabolism and to evaluate how this isozyme information relates to metabolic induction by AEDs.

ENZYME IDENTIFICATION

As previously mentioned, the key to understanding a drug's interaction potential lies with identification of the enzymes responsible for its clearance in humans. When the major metabolites of a drug are known, studies designed to identify the enzymes responsible for their formation can be conducted. Indeed, this information is now required by the Food and Drug Administration before final approval can be granted for new drugs, and it has begun to appear in Physicians' Desk Reference and pharmacology reference texts.

The biotransformation of a drug is generally analyzed using a number of in vitro tests conducted in human tissues, cell fractions, or cDNA-expressed enzymes. These tests include the following:

1. Addition of isozyme selective inhibitors. When the metabolite of interest is formed in detectable amounts in suspensions of subcellular fractions (i.e., human liver microsomes), the rate of its formation can be determined. Reduction in the rate of metabolite formation in the presence of an isozyme selective inhibitor in vitro suggests a contribution by that isozyme.
2. Antibody studies. Similarly, addition to incubations in vitro of antibodies directed against the active site of a specific isozyme results in decreased metabolite formation if that isozyme is involved.
3. Correlation analyses. A high degree of correlation between the rate of metabolite formation and the expression level of a specific isozyme as determined by Western blot analysis is indicative of contribution by that isozyme. Correlation between the rate of metabolite formation and other prototypic enzyme activities also provides corroborative evidence.
4. cDNA-expressed enzymes. The cDNA-expressed enzymes, most of which are commercially available, are used to measure metabolite formation and thus confirm the involvement of a particular enzyme.

A definite conclusion regarding the role of an enzyme requires that several (if not all) of these tests have similar outcomes. Experience to date has shown that the concentration of the drug (substrate) must be kept at or close to therapeutic concentrations even though the tests are conducted in vitro. This ensures that the therapeutically relevant enzyme is identified (10). If the drug is studied at unrealistically high concentrations, a second enzyme may be identified as a participant in metabolite formation but have limited clinical relevance.

The isozymes identified as contributing to the metabolic elimination of many AEDs are listed in Table 1. The contribution by each isozyme is indicated as either major or minor. CYP3A4 plays a major role in the clearance of CBZ, midazolam, remacemide, tiagabine, and zonisamide, and a smaller role in the case of diazepam. CYP2C9 plays a major role in PHT clearance, whereas CYP2C19 contributes to the metabolism of diazepam, one enantiomer of mephenytoin, and PHT. Lamotrigine clearance has been shown to depend on UDPGT. Those drugs for which a single enzyme controls the major route of metabolic elimination are most prone to involvement in clinically significant interactions; examples are CBZ (CYP3A4), PHT (CYP2C9), and midazolam (CYP3A4).

ENZYME INDUCTION

Exposure to some environmental agents, cigarette smoke, and several different drugs has been shown to induce metabolic enzyme activity and shorten the plasma half-lives of other drugs in humans. Induction can alter a second drug's efficacy by reducing plasma levels or increase its toxicity if that drug is metabolically activated. Indeed, induction of mono-oxygenase and UDPGT activities is of clinical relevance to epileptologists, as the

TABLE 1. *Enzymes responsible for the metabolic elimination of antiepileptic drugs*

	2C9	2C19	2D6	2E1	3A4	UDPGT	References
Carbamazepine	+(2C8)				++		6
Diazepam		+			+		10
Lamotrigine						++	11,12
S-Mephenytoin		++					13,14
Midazolam					++		15,16
Phenytoin	++	+					8,9
Remacemide					++		17
Tiagabine					++		18
Zonisamide					++		19

AEDs CBZ, PHT, and phenobarbital are among the most potent inducing agents known. Although the exact mechanisms responsible for induction are not fully understood, it is clear that induction results in an increased amount or increased expression of enzyme. This may occur through increased production of mRNA or prolonged mRNA half-life (20). Regardless of the mechanism, enzyme induction can be demonstrated through *de novo* synthesis of proteins and occurs with some delay following exposure to the inducing agent. Thus, induction requires the study of intact cells and cannot be studied in subcellular fractions.

To predict how administration of a new drug will affect other medications when added to an existing treatment regimen requires the characterization of an induction spectrum for the new drug (and its metabolites, if they accumulate to significant circulating levels). Both in vivo and in vitro approaches have been used. To date, the most reliable information regarding induction comes from in vivo human studies.

1. In vitro systems. It has been shown that primary cultures of human hepatocytes retain the expression of several liver functions, including drug-metabolizing activities. Donato et al. (21) used 24-hour isolated hepatocytes to characterize the induction resulting from inclusion of phenobarbital, ethanol, and four other test compounds. After 48 hours of exposure, the inducing agent was removed and mono-oxygenase activity was assessed using compounds known to be metabolized by CYP1A2, CYP2E1, and CYP3A4. In this system, phenobarbital induced the activity of CYP3A4 but had little or no effect on CYP1A2 or CYP2E1. Conversely, exposure of hepatocytes to ethanol induced activity of CYP2E1, with marginal induction of CYP3A4 and no change in CYP1A2. The study also revealed a great interindividual variability in mono-oxygenase activity levels obtained from different liver donors. Until cryopreservation methods become perfected, the use of human tissues will require the culture of freshly isolated hepatocytes, thus limiting the usefulness of this approach for large-scale screening of potential inducers. Others have shown that phenobarbital induction in rat hepatocytes can be modulated by culture conditions (22), suggesting that culture conditions may also influence P_{450} expression in human hepatocytes. However, the use of primary cell cultures prepared from frozen human hepatocytes should provide useful information in the future (23).

2. In vivo studies. Typical studies measure the clearance of a drug in the absence and in the presence of the potential inducing agent. Increased clearance following several days' administration of the test compound implies induction. Identification of the isozymes that are induced relies on increased clearance of a drug (probe) whose metabolism has been characterized with respect to one metabolic isozyme. These tests require administration of a standard dose of a probe compound and some measure of its rate of metabolic disposition. The rate of metabolism in the control state is then compared with the rate following

a second administration of the probe compound after the subject has been treated with the potential inducer. Increases in the rate of the probe reaction suggest induction of the isozyme catalyzing the reaction.

Little information is available on specific isozyme induction, so it is worthwhile to examine the potential for induction of CYP3A4 and the CYP2C group of enzymes, as these isozymes catalyze the metabolic elimination of the majority of AEDs. The inductive effects of selected AEDs on CYP3A4 and CYP2C are summarized in Table 2.

Induction of CYP3A4

Induction of CYP3A4 by PHT is apparent from its effects on cyclosporine metabolism. Freeman et al. (24) reported that the AUC (area under the curve) for cyclosporine was reduced from 10.4±1.7 to 5.5±2.1 mg/L per hour and that half-life was reduced from 5.1±1.1 to 3.7±1.1 hours after 9 days of treatment with 300 to 400 mg PHT. Similar differences have been noted in the AUC of the CYP3A4 probe midazolam when healthy volunteers are compared with epileptic patients (25). The enzyme-inducing effect of PHT on CBZ metabolism has also been identified during the withdrawal of PHT from patients to whom the two drugs were coadministered (26).

CYP3A induction by CBZ has been studied extensively. The clearances of cyclosporine (27–29), oral contraceptives (30,31), and midazolam (25) are increased when CBZ is coadministered. CBZ is also known to induce its own metabolism, probably through increased expression of CYP3A4 (32,33).

TABLE 2. *Inductive effects of selected antiepileptic drugs*

	2C9	2C19	3A4	References
Phenytoin			++	24–26
Carbamazepine	++	?	+++	27–33,46
Phenobarbital	?		++	34–38,47, 51–54
Felbamate			+	39–41

Phenobarbital also appears to induce the expression of CYP3A4. Several cases have been reported demonstrating reduced plasma levels of cyclosporine and loss of efficacy in patients to whom phenobarbital was coadministered and a decrease in cyclosporine clearance when phenobarbital treatment ceased (34). Additionally, CBZ plasma clearance decreased after discontinuation of phenobarbital in patients to whom CBZ, PHT, and phenobarbital were coadministered (35). These studies are consistent with deinduction of CYP3A4 following discontinuation of phenobarbital. Other studies have shown that the plasma level-to-dose ratio of CBZ is reduced when phenobarbital is coadministered with CBZ (36–38).

In the case of felbamate, Albani et al. (39) found reductions in CBZ plasma levels when felbamate was added to treatment regimens. Subsequently, CBZ kinetics were determined in nine patients treated with CBZ monotherapy and again after coadministration of felbamate up to a maximum daily dose of 3000 mg. The apparent total body clearance of CBZ increased from a mean of 229.4 ± 68.7 to 324.3 ± 109.2 mL/h per kilogram (41). These studies suggest induction of CYP3A4 by felbamate.

Induction of CYP2C

The effects of AEDs on CYP2C isozymes are less well documented than their effects on CYP3A4. This is not surprising, as the question of inducibility of CYP2C enzymes has not been resolved. To evaluate the potential for induction of these enzymes, we have first examined the effects of the potent inducer rifampin on probe compounds. The inducibility of CYP2C9 can be inferred from two studies. Zilly et al. (42) reported that tolbutamide clearance was increased more than twofold following treatment with 1.2 g of rifampin daily for 8 days. Likewise, the clearance of 7-hydroxy-(*S*)-warfarin, a metabolite of (*S*)-warfarin, was increased from 0.41 to 1.18 mL/h per kilogram after 4 days of treatment with 600 mg of rifampin per day (43). Induction of CYP2C19 is also supported by two sets of findings. The study by Heimark et al. (43) showed increased clearance (0.14 to 0.56 mL/h per kilogram) of the 8-hydroxyl metabolite of (*R*)-wayfarin, formed by a CYP2C19-mediated reaction (2), following refampin treatment. Subsequently, Zhou et al. (44) noted increased excretion of 4'-hydroxymephenytoin in the urine of extensive metabolizers of (*S*)-mephenytoin with rifampin treatment but saw no effect in poor metabolizers.

The effects of PHT on the level of expression of CYP2C enzymes are unclear. As therapeutic levels of PHT are often higher than its K_m (which is also its K_i) for CYP2C9, inhibition is the predominant effect observed clinically (9), thus masking any inductive effect on the metabolism of other CYP2C9 substrates. To study the possibility of autoinduction, Browne et al. (45) followed the kinetics of PHT during continuous administration using isotopically labeled drug. However, the results of the study could not distinguish the phenomenon of autoinduction because of the nonlinear kinetics of PHT.

Addition of CBZ to treatment regimens with PHT decreased PHT half-lives from 10.6 hours to 6.4 hours after at least 9 days of CBZ treatment at a dosage of 600 mg/d (46). Although specific pathways of warfarin metabolism were not measured in this same study, warfarin half-lives and prothrombin times were decreased when CBZ was added. These findings suggest that CBZ induces CYP2C9, the major enzyme involved in the metabolism of PHT and of the active (*S*)-warfarin enantiomer, although CYP2C19 induction also may have contributed to the changes.

For phenobarbital, MacDonald et al. (47) reported lowered warfarin plasma levels, decreased prothrombin times, and nearly a 50% reduction in half-life following 3 weeks of treatment. Mungall et al. (48) used a population kinetics approach with patients taking racemic warfarin and observed almost a 50% increase in warfarin clearance when phenobarbital was coadministered. These studies are not conclusive, as the specific metabolic pathways of warfarin enantiomers were not measured, but decreases in prothrombin times suggest an effect on CYP2C9. Schellens et al. (49) found that the 8-hour recovery of urinary 4'-hydroxymephenytoin was not influenced by phenobarbital treatment of volunteers. Thus, phenobarbital appears to induce CYP2C9 but not CYP2C19. According to these findings, an increase in PHT clearance would be expected when PHT and phenobarbital are coadministered. However, Browne et al. (50) studied the interaction between phenobarbital and labeled PHT and found no significant changes after addition of phenobarbital. In clinical studies of groups of patients taking PHT alone or PHT combined with phenobarbital, the maintenance plasma PHT levels tended to be somewhat lower in the group with combined treatment (51–54). When individual patients were studied before and after the addition of phenobarbital to PHT, the plasma PHT levels declined in some, rose in others, and remained unchanged in still others.

The potential for felbamate to induce CYP2C enzymes has not been adequately investigated.

CONCLUSION

It is expected that the effects of enzyme induction will behave in a substrate-independent manner, enabling prediction of increased clearance (caused by enzyme induction) based on metabolic isozymes before the actual coadministration of two drugs. Thus, based on the inducibility of CYP3A4 by PHT, CBZ, phenobarbital, and felbamate, it can be inferred that these drugs will increase the clearances of other CYP3A4 substrates, such as the new protease inhibitors indinavir, saquinovir, and ritonavir. Whether the associated decrease in plasma level results in underdosage and loss of efficacy will depend on a number of factors: (a) the extent to which CYP3A4 contributes to the overall elimination of the substrate, (b) the potency and dose of the inducer, and (c) the initial concentration of substrate in relation to its therapeutic range.

ACKNOWLEDGMENT

Supported in part by National Institutes of Health Grant P01 GM32165-11.

REFERENCES

1. Pichard L, Fabre I, Fabre G, Domergue J, Saint Aubert B, Mourad G, Maurel P. Cyclosporin A drug interactions. *Drug Metab Dispos* 1990;18:595–606.
2. Kunze KL, Wienkers LC, Thummel KE, Trager WF. Warfarin-fluconazole I. Inhibition of the human cytochrome P_{450}-dependent metabolism of warfarin by fluconazole: in vitro studies. *Drug Metab Dispos* 1996; 24:414–421.
3. Black DJ, Kunze KL, Wienkers LC, Gidal BE, Seaton TL, McDonnell ND, Evans JS, Bauwens E, Trager WF. Warfarin-fluconazole II. A metabolically based drug interaction: in vivo studies. *Drug Metab Dispos* 1996;24: 422–428.
4. Mather GG, Levy RH. Pharmacokinetics of polypharmacy: prediction of drug interactions. In: Leppik IE, ed. *Rational Polypharmacy*. New York: Elsevier; 1996: 113–122.
5. Levy RH. Cytochrome P_{450} isozymes and antiepileptic drug interactions. *Epilepsia* 1995;36(Suppl 5):S8–S13.
6. Kerr BM, Thummel KE, Wurden CJ, Klein SM, Kroetz DL, Gonzalez FJ, Levy RH. Human liver carbamazepine metabolism: role of CYP3A4 and CYP2C8 in 10,11-epoxide formation. *Biochem Pharmacol* 1994; 47:1969–1979.
7. Levy RH, Wurden CJ. Carbamazepine: interactions with other drugs. In: Levy RH, Mattson RH, Meldrum BS, eds. *Antiepileptic Drugs*. 4th ed. New York: Raven Press; 1995:543–554.
8. Veronese ME, Mackenzie PI, Doecke CJ, McManus ME, Minors JO, Birkett DJ. Tolbutamide and phenytoin hydroxylations by cDNA-expressed human liver cytochrome P_{450} 2C9. *Biochem Biophys Res Commun* 1991;175:1112–1118.
9. Levy RH, Bajpai M. Phenytoin: interactions with other drugs. Mechanistic aspects. In: Levy RH, Mattson RH, Meldrum BS, eds. *Antiepileptic Drugs*. 4th ed. New York: Raven Press; 1995:329–338.
10. Yasumori, Nagata TK, Yang SK, Chen LS, Murayama N, Yamazoe Y, Kato R. Cytochrome P_{450}-mediated metabolism of diazepam in human and rat: involvement of human CYP2C in *N*-demethylation in the substrate concentration-dependent manner. *Pharmacogenetics* 1993; 3:291–301.
11. Dickins M, Sawyer DA, Morley TJ, Parsons DN. Lamotrigine: chemistry and biotransformation. In: Levy RH, Mattson RH, Meldrum BS, eds. *Antiepileptic Drugs*. 4th ed. New York: Raven Press; 1995:871–876.
12. Doig MV, Clare RA. Use of thermospray liquid chromatography-mass spectrometry to aid in the identification of urinary metabolites of a novel antiepilepitc drug, lamotrigine. *J Chromatogr* 1991;554:181–189.
13. Goldstein JA, Faletto MB, Romkes-Sparks R, Sullivan T, Kitareewan S, Raucy JL, Lasker JM, Ghanayem BI. Evidence that CYP2C19 is the major (*S*)-mephenytoin 4'-hydroxylase in humans. *Biochemistry* 1994;33: 1743–1752.
14. Wrighton SA, Stevens JC, Becker JW, VandenBranden M. Isolation and characterization of human liver cytochrome P_{450} 2C19: correlation between 2C19 and *S*-mephenytoin 4'-hydroxylation. *Arch Biochem Biophys* 1993;306:1–6.
15. Wrighton SA, Ring BJ. Inhibition of human CYP3A-catalyzed 1'-hydroxymidazolam formation by ketoconazole, nifedipine, erythromycin, cimetidine, and nizatidine. *Pharm Res* 1994;11:921–924.
16. Chaudhary AK, Belas FJ, Saleh SA, Wandel C, Wood AJJ, Blair IA. Quantitation of midazolam and its CYP3A4 metabolites from human plasma using liquid chromatography/tandem mass spectrometry (LC/MS/MS). *ISSX Proc* 1996;10:130.
17. Leach JP, Blacklaw J, Jamieson V, Jones T, Richens A, Brodie MJ. Mutual interaction between remacemide hydrochloride and carbamazepine: two drugs with active metabolites. *Epilepsia* 1996;37:1100–1106.
18. Bopp BA, Nequist GE, Rodrigues AD. Role of the cytochrome P_{450} 3A subfamily in the metabolism of [^{14}C]tiagabine by human hepatic microsomes. *Epilepsia* 1995;36(Suppl 3):S159.
19. Nakasa H, Komiya M, Ohmori S, Rikihisa T, Kiuchi M, Kitada M. Characterization of human liver microsomal cytochrome P_{450} involved in the reductive metabolism of zonisamide. *Mol Pharmacol* 1993;44:216–221.
20. Okey AB, Roberts EA, Harper PA, Denison MS. Induction of drug-metabolizing enzymes: mechanisms and consequences. *Clin Biochem* 1986;19:132–141.
21. Donato MT, Castell JV, Gomez-Lechon MJ. Effect of model inducers on cytochrome P_{450} activities of human hepatocytes in primary culture. *Drug Metab Dispos* 1995;23:553–558.
22. Sidhu JS, Farin FM, Omiecinski CJ. Influence of extracellular matrix overlay on phenobarbital-mediated induction of *CYP2B1*, *2B2*, and *3A1* genes in primary adult rat hepatocyte culture. *Arch Biochem Biophys* 1993;301:103–113.
23. Ruegg CE, Silber PM, Mughal RA, Ismail AJ, Li AP. P_{450} induction in primary human hepatocytes after cryopreservation. *ISSX Proc* 1996;10:200.
24. Freeman DJ, Laupacis A, Keown PA, Stiller CR, Carruthers SG. Evaluation of cyclosporin-phenytoin interaction with observations on cyclosporin metabolites. *Br J Clin Pharmacol* 1984;18:887–893.
25. Backman JT, Olkkola KT, Ojala M, Laaksovirta H, Neuvonen PJ. Concentrations and effects of oral midazolam are greatly reduced in patients treated with carbamazepine or phenytoin. *Epilepsia* 1996;37:253–257.
26. Chapron DJ, LaPierre BA, Abou-Elkair M. Unmasking the significant enzyme-induceing effects of phenytoin on serum carbamazepine concentrations during phenytoin withdrawal. *Ann Pharmacother* 1993;27:708–711.
27. Christians U, Sewing KF. Cyclosporin metabolism in transplant patients. *Pharmacol Ther* 1993;57:291–345.
28. Alvarez JS, Del Castillo JAS, Ortiz MJA. Effect of carbamazepine on ciclosporin blood level. *Nephron* 1991; 58:235–236.
29. Yee GC, McGuire TR. Pharmacokinetic drug interactions with cyclosporin (part 1). *Clin Pharmacokinet* 1990;19:319–332.
30. Back DJ, Orme ML. Pharmacokinetic drug interactions with oral contraceptives. *Clin Pharmacokinet* 1990;18: 472–484.
31. Crawford P, Chadwick DJ, Martin C, Tjia J, Back DJ,

Orme M. The interaction of phenytoin and carbamazepine with combined oral contraceptive steroids. *Br J Pharmacol* 1990;30:892–896.
32. Pitlick WH, Levy RH, Troupin AS, Green JR. Pharmacokinetic model to describe self-induced decreases in steady-state concentrations of carbamazepine. *J Pharm Sci* 1976;65:462.
33. Schäffler L, Bourgeois BFD, Lüders HO. Pharmacokinetics of carbamazepine: rapid reversibility of autoinduction of carbamazepine after temporary discontinuation. *Epilepsia* 1994;35:195–198.
34. Carstensen H, Jacobsen, Dieperink H. Interaction between cyclosporin A and phenobarbitone. *Br J Clin Pharmacol* 1986;21:550–551.
35. Tomson T, Spina E, Wedlund JE. Minor additive inducing effects of phenobarbital on carbamazepine clearance in patients on combined carbamazepine-phenytoin therapy. *Ther Drug Monit* 1987;9:117–119.
36. Christiansen J, Dam M. Influence of phenobarbital and diphenylhydantoin on plasma carbamazepine levels in patients with epilepsy. *Acta Neurol Scand* 1973;49: 543–546.
37. Schneider H. Carbamazepine: the influence of other antiepileptic drugs on its serum level. In: Schneider H, Janz D, Gardner-Thorpe C, Meinardi H, Sherwin AL, eds. *Clinical Pharmacology of Antiepileptic Drugs*. Berlin: Springer-Verlag; 1975:189–196.
38. Johannssen SI, Strandjord RE. The influence of phenobarbitone and phenytoin on carbamazepine serum levels. In: Schneider H, Janz D, Gardner-Thorpe C, Meinardi H, Sherwin AL, eds. *Clinical Pharmacology of Antiepileptic Drugs*. Berlin: Springer-Verlag; 1975: 201–205.
39. Albani F, Theodore WH, Washington P, Devinsky O, Bromfield E, Porter RJ, Nice FJ. Effect of felbamate on plasma levels of carbamazepine and its metabolites. *Epilepsia* 1991;32:130–132.
40. Wagner ML, Remmel RP, Graves NM, Leppik IE. Effect of felbamate on carbamazepine and its major metabolites. *Clin Pharmacol Ther* 1993;53:536–543.
41. Howard JR, Dix RK, Shumaker RC, Wichmann JK, Gilchrist J, Kucharczyk N, Perhach JL. Effect of felbamate on carbamazepine pharmacokinetics. *Epilepsia* 1992;33(Suppl):84–85.
42. Zilly W, Breimer DD, Richter E. Pharmacokinetic interactions with rifampicin. *Clin Pharmacokinet* 1977;2: 61–70.
43. Heimark LD, Gibaldi M, Trager WF, O'Reilly RA, Goulart DA. The mechanism of the warfarin-rifampin drug interaction in humans. *Clin Pharm Ther* 1987;42: 388–394.
44. Zhou HH, Anthony LB, Wood AJJ, Wilkinson GR. Induction of polymorphic 4'-hydroxylation of *S*-mephenytoin by rifampin. *Br J Clin Pharmacol* 1990; 30:471–475.
45. Browne TR, Evans JE, Szabo GK, Evans BA, Greenblatt DJ, Schumacher GE. Studies with stable isotopes I: changes in phenytoin pharmacokinetics and biotransformation during monotherapy. *J Clin Pharmacol* 1985; 25:43–50.
46. Hansen JM, Sierbak-Nielsen K, Skovsted L. Carbamazepine-induced acceleration of diphenylhydantoin and warfarin metabolism in man. *Clin Pharmacol Ther* 1971;12:539–543.
47. MacDonald MG, Robinson DS, Sylwester D, Jaffe JJ. The effects of phenobarbital, chloral betaine, and glutethimide administration on warfarin plasma levels and hypoprothrombinemic responses in man. *Clin Pharmacol Ther* 1968;10:80–84.
48. Mungall DR, Ludden TM, Marshall J, Hawkins DW, Talbert RL, Crawford MH. Population pharmacokinetics of racemic warfarin in adult patients. *J Pharmacokinet Biopharm* 1985;13:213–227.
49. Schellens JHM, vanderWart JHF, Brugman M, Breimer DD. Influence of enzyme induction and inhibition on the oxidation of nifedipine, sparteine, mephenytoin, and antipyrine in humans as assessed by a "cocktail" study design. *J Pharmacol Exp Ther* 1989;249:638–645.
50. Browne TR, Evans JE, Szabo GK, Evans BA, Greenblatt DJ, Schumacher DE. Studies with stable isotopes I: changes in phenytoin pharmacokinetics and biotransformation during monotherapy. *J Clin Pharmacol* 1985; 25:43–50.
51. Kutt H, Haynes J, Verebely K, McDowell F. The effect of phenobarbital on plasma dephenylhydantoin level and metabolism in man and in rat liver microsomes. *Neurology (Minneapolis)* 1969;19:611–616.
52. Sontaniemi E, Arvela P, Hakkarainen H, Huhti E. The clinical significance of microsomal enzyme induction in the therapy of epileptic patients. *Ann Clin Res* 1970; 2:223–227.
53. Booker HE, Tormey A, Toussaint J. Concurrent administration of phenobarbital and diphenylhydantoin: lack of interference effect. *Neurology (Minneapolis)* 1971; 21:383–385.
54. Morselli PL, Rizzo M, Garattini S. Interaction between phenobarbital and diphenylhydantoin in animals and in epileptic patients. *Ann N Y Acad Sci* 179:88–107

Antiepileptic Drug Development.
Advances in Neurology, Vol. 76,
edited by J. French, I. Leppik, and M. A. Dichter.
Lippincott–Raven Publishers, Philadelphia © 1998.

6

New Drugs for Persons with Epilepsy

David E. Blum

Barrow Neurological Institute, Phoenix, Arizona 85013.

INTRODUCTION

Epilepsy afflicts between .5% and 1% of the population. Drug treatment is the mainstay of therapy. The first modern pharmacologic treatment, bromide salt, was introduced more than 100 years ago; that drug was modestly effective and produced intolerable side effects. To greater or lesser degrees, the same issues face the currently available and newly developed drugs. These are summarized in Tables 1, 2, and 3.

Efficacy is the ability to control seizures. New drugs are tested for efficacy by determining their ability to reduce mean seizure frequency, or the fraction of patients in whom seizures are reduced by 50%. This is not enough. Adequacy of control depends on point of view. Many patients and clinicians settle for adequate control. In the Veterans Administration Cooperative Study, between 60% and 70% of patients were sufficiently pleased with their medication to stay on it, but in even the best group, only 47% of patients achieved a seizure-free state (1). Increasingly, studies have emphasized the importance of a seizure-free state in enabling patients to maintain their quality of life (2). Despite this, most drug trials do not focus on seizure-free outcomes, but rather use measures such as percentage of seizure reduction or percentage of patients who improve by 50%. For patients with more than four complex partial seizures per month (typical entry criteria for phase II and III studies), a 50% seizure reduction is not an adequate milestone. Patients who have three or four seizures a year cannot drive, generally lose their jobs, and live in fear of having seizures when in public, out on dates, or in athletic contests. There is reason to believe that continued seizures may lead to hippocampal sclerosis (3) and long-term memory dysfunction (4). Patients desperately need more effective treatments.

The most important side effects of anticonvulsants are related to central nervous system function. Barbiturate drugs, although still widely used, produce insidious side effects of sedation, depression, and personality change. Phenytoin, carbamazepine, and valproate all produce similar levels of mild, but still unsatisfactory, sedation and cognitive difficulties. Many patients did not realize how sedated they were by their drugs until they switched to felbamate monotherapy, and many patients are now reluctant to go back to their former medications despite the high risks associated with felbamate.

Another key failing is pharmacologic; no other class of drugs is plagued by as many oddities of pharmacology and drug interactions as the anticonvulsants. Narrow therapeutic ranges and unreliable pharmacology make accurate dosing difficult for many patients. Phenytoin exhibits nonlinear kinetics. Carbamazepine has a very narrow range and a short half-life. In addition, it causes many drug-drug interactions and autoinduction, and a metabolic degradation product of carbamazepine causes clinical toxicity. Valproate is

TABLE 1. *Shortcomings of current seizure drugs*

	Phenobarbital	Phenytoin	Carbamazepine	Valproate
Protein binding		90%	30%–50%	90+%
Metabolism		Nonlinear	Autoinduction	
Enzyme induction	+++	+++	++++++	
Therapeutic range ratio[a]	2	2	1.5	2
Doses per day	1	1 or 2	3	3
Toxicity	Connective tissue (long-term use)	Liver, cosmetic, dental, bones	Marrow, weight gain, hyponatremia	Liver, pancreas, platelets, weight gain, alopecia
Pregnancy	Decreased IQ	Hydantoin syndrome	Neural tube defects	Neural tube defects
Sedation or depression	Severe	Modest	Modest	Modest
Seizure-free rate[b]	36%	38%	47%	23%
Primary epilepsy	Fair	Sometimes	Sometimes	Good

[a]Therapeutic range ratio is the ratio of upper limit to lower limit of therapeutic range and indicates the narrow band required for appropriate dosing.
[b]One-year seizure-free rates for all seizure types, taken from the two VA collaborative studies (290).

heavily protein-bound and interacts with other anticonvulsants. Most anticonvulsants are enzyme inducers and alter metabolism of other drugs.

Finally, the drugs used for epilepsy cause side effects on a day-in, day-out basis that are a burden to patients' quality of life. Drowsiness, ataxia, and nausea are common side effects of all anticonvulsants—new and old. Phenytoin causes hirsutism and gingivitis. Carbamazepine causes blurred vision or diplopia. Valproate causes hair loss, weight gain, and tremor. Add to this a female patient's constant fear of birth defects and it is no wonder that patients resent, and often do not take, their medications.

New drugs for epilepsy have come from four avenues. Phenytoin, the most successful anticonvulsant of all time, was developed by systematic screening of candidate compounds in an animal model. This strategy continues today in the Anticonvulsant Drug Development Program. Some drugs have been acquired through mistakes. Bromides were first used in the mistaken belief that suppression of sexuality would suppress epilepsy. Lamotrigine was developed as a folate antagonist on the theory that phenytoin acts via an antifolate effect.

TABLE 2. *Comparative pharmacology of new drugs or drugs near release*

	Mechanism	Metabolism	Protein binding, %	t 1/2, h	Daily dose, mg/kg	Therapeutic range, µg/mL	Enzyme induction
Felbamate	–glycine +GABA	hepatic	30	16	40–60	50–100	inhibits
Gabapentin	+GABA	renal	0	6	30	?	no effect
Lamotrigine	$-Na^+$ channels	hepatic	55	20[a]	5–7	1–4	mixed
Topiramate	–EAA GABA	renal	0	16–20	6–10	?	no effect
Vigabatrin	–GABA breakdown	renal	0	100+[b]	50	N/A	no effect
Oxcarbazepine	$-Na^+$ channels	hepatic, 30% renal[c]	10	18[d]	40–50	?10–15	limited induction
Tiagabine	–GABA reuptake	hepatic	0	6	0.5–1	?	no effect
Zonisamide	$-Ca^{2+}$ T channels	hepatic	0	12–20	6–8	10–20	minimal

t 1/2, half-life; EAA, Excitatory Amino Acid.
[a]Half-life doubled in combination with valproic acid; reduced with enzyme-inducing drugs.
[b]Biologic half-life of GABA-T inhibition.
[c]Monohydroxyl derivative is partly renally excreted.
[d]Half-life of active metabolite.

TABLE 3. *Author's subjective summary of efficacy in various epilepsy syndromes, and toxicity summary*

	Partial seizures			Primary generalized seizures				
	Responder rate, %	Seizure-free, %	Subjective rating	T-C	Absence	L-G and IS	CNS toxicity	Organ damage and systemic toxicity
Felbamate	[a]	[a]	++++	+++	++	+++	insomnia, agitation, headache	marrow, hepatic, weight loss
Gabapentin	25–35	<1	+	N/A	N/A	N/A	mild sedation	weight gain
Lamotrigine	25–35	<3	+	++	++	++		rash
Topiramate	40–50	5–10	+++	+++	+++	+++	sedation (can be severe)	renal stones, mild weight loss
Vigabatrin	45–55	5–10	+++	?	?–	+++	depression, psychosis (rare), irritability	weight gain
Oxcarbazepine	?[b]	?	+++	?+	N/A	N/A	minimal	hyponatremia, leukopenia
Tiagabine	25–30[c]	?	+				minimal	none
Zonisamide	30–40	5	++	+	+	++	minimal	renal stones

CNS, central nervous system; L-G, Lennox-Gastaut syndrome; IS, infantile spasms; T-C, tonic-clonic seizures.
[a]Pivotal studies did not use standard, add-on strategy; appropriate numbers unknown.
[b]Efficacy is comparable with or better than that of carbamazepine. Not well tested in add-on trials.
[c]Responder rating in trials using enrichment design.

Some drugs were discovered by accident; valproate was being used as a vehicle for testing other compounds when its activity was noticed. Now we are entering an era of deliberate, rational drug development based on an understanding of basic mechanisms of the epilepsies. Vigabatrin and tiagabine are examples of the new wave of drug development. The choice of models dictates the drugs that will be discovered. There are no good models of infantile spasms or Lennox-Gastaut syndrome. There are no truly useful models of human temporal lobe or frontal lobe epilepsy. There is no active screening of compounds to inhibit development of mesial sclerosis, so the new drugs are "anticonvulsant" rather than "antiepileptic."

Despite all these difficulties, these are promising times for patients and exciting times for physicians treating epilepsy. Three new drugs have been released in the last 2 years, and new drug applications have been filed for three or four additional drugs. They are reviewed below in their estimated order of release in the United States. Although none of the new drugs is a panacea, each drug has unique advantages. Some have reduced side effect profiles, some have untroubling pharmacology, and some are effective for either common refractory epilepsies or for less common epilepsies that were not well treated with older drugs.

NEW FORMS OF OLD DRUGS

Intravenous formulations of carbamazepine and valproate are both under development. Tegretol is a novel, osmotically driven, sustained-release preparation (5). When used on a twice-daily dosing schedule, the sustained-release preparation is bioequivalent to dosing three or four times daily with conventional carbamazepine. Fosphenytoin is a phosphorylated prodrug that is rapidly converted to phenytoin (6). Conversion is by serum phosphoesterases, with a half-life of 15 minutes (7). The addition of a phosphate group leads to a molar conversion of 1.5, so that 3 mg of fosphenytoin is converted into 2 mg of phenytoin. With an infusion rate of 225 mg/min, fosphenytoin is bioequivalent to phenytoin infused at 50 mg/min. Local tissue reactions are markedly reduced, and the prodrug is safe to use by intramuscular injection. Release for general use in the United States is imminent for both preparations.

FELBAMATE

Felbamate was released for use in the United States 1993 as the first of the new drugs; it is marketed by Wallace Laboratories (8,9).

Mechanism

Felbamate seems to have a dual mechanism. It blocks the strychnine-insensitive glycine receptor (10), modulating NMDA (*N*-methyl-D-aspartate) receptor activity. Glycine blocked the anticonvulsant action of felbamate in electroshock models and in NMDA-induced seizure models (11). Felbamate reduces burst firing induced by kainate or quisqualate in neurons bathed in low-magnesium medium (12). In the same models, glycine showed no blocking effect on other anticonvulsants. Modulation of the strychnine-insensitive glycine receptor can be visualized in mouse cerebellar granule cells using a calcium-sensitive fluorescent dye (indo-1/AM) (13). A potential additional action at the NMDA receptor complex may involve a slowing of dissociation of dizocilpine (MK801) from the receptor complex. This altered dissociation is not affected by increased glycine levels, suggesting that this particular effect may not be mediated by actions directly at the glycine site (14).

Felbamate blockade of excitatory amino acid channels suggests a neuroprotective role. In rat hippocampal slice, glycine induced neurotoxicity resembling NMDA neurotoxicity (15). Felbamate was found to be neuroprotective in a kainic acid-induced model of status epilepticus in rats. Administration of relatively high doses of 100 to 300 mg of felbamate per kilogram led to preservation of performance on several behavioral tests and also to increased seizure latency with flurothyl inhalation in comparison with controls (16). Neuroprotection against hypoxia in a rat hippocampal slice preparation was seen with felbamate concentrations similar to those used in treatment of epilepsy in humans (17). Felbamate pretreatment was neuroprotective in 7-day-old rat pups subjected to carotid artery ligation. Infarct size was reduced by >40% (18). Glycine reverses hypoxic protection of felbamate (19,20).

A second mechanism is potentiation of chloride currents mediated by GABA (τ-aminobutyric acid). Rho et al. showed that in addition to actions on the glycine/NMDA system, felbamate potentiates the action of GABA in rat hippocampal voltage clamp models (21), possibly by binding to a unique, nonbarbiturate, nonbenzodiazepine site (22). Felbamate blocks isoniazid-induced seizures in mice (23). It also facilitates the effect of diazepam in that model and alters binding of TBPS, a benzodiazepine receptor inverse agonist. These findings also support an effect of felbamate on $GABA_A$ receptor function (23).

Pharmacology

Felbamate is 90% absorbed following an oral dose, with peak absorption in 3 to 6 hours. The half-life is approximately 20 hours (9). Felbamate is only modestly protein-bound. Clearance is hepatic through multiple pathways. Felbamate levels can be determined by high-performance liquid chromatography (24) or by isothermal gas chromatography (25). Typical doses are 30 to 60 mg/kg per day. The drug is supplied as an elixir and as 400- and 600-mg tablets.

Drug Interactions

Drug interactions are a major drawback of felbamate. It inhibits hepatic metabolism of most other anticonvulsants. Felbamate leads to 30% to 50% increases in levels of phenytoin (26), phenobarbital (27), and valproate (28). One of the most bothersome drug interactions is seen when felbamate is added to carbamazepine. Addition of felbamate leads to reductions in carbamazepine levels of 10% to 30%, with increases in levels of carbamazepine epoxide of up to 50% of pretreatment levels (29). This can lead to increases in both seizure frequency and toxic symptoms. Overall, doses of most other anticonvulsants need to be reduced by at least 30% when felbamate is added. Felbamate also interacts with warfarin (30,31), theophylline, and other drugs.

Efficacy

The efficacy of felbamate is high. One of the pivotal studies demonstrating efficacy of felbamate was a double-blind, active-control study comparing monotherapy with 3600 mg of felbamate per day against 15 mg of valproic acid per kilogram per day (32). The valproic acid dose was selected to lie at the lower end of the therapeutic range. Forty-four patients were randomized. The study continued for 112 days, or until "escape criteria" of predefined increases above baseline seizure frequency were reached. Escape criteria were met (treatment failure) by 19 patients on valproic acid and by three patients on felbamate. The felbamate group demonstrated a 50% to 65% reduction in seizure frequency compared with baseline. Felbamate was well tolerated and there were few adverse events (32). Another pivotal study for felbamate was a unique design, testing monotherapy against placebo in patients admitted to epilepsy telemetry units and taken off all other drugs (33). Eligible patients had one to two seizures per day. The endpoints of the study were time to fourth seizure and number of patients completing 10 days of therapy. The felbamate-treated patients had a lower mean seizure frequency and were more likely to complete 10 days of therapy than were controls. An interesting aspect of the study is that felbamate was well tolerated despite a rapid, 2-day dose escalation to 3600 mg (33). More traditional add-on trials have also been performed. Leppick et al. tested felbamate as add-on therapy in partial epilepsy in patients previously treated with either phenytoin or carbamazepine (34). The felbamate dose used was considerably lower than doses typically used in monotherapy (averaging 2300 mg/d in this trial), presumably to lessen drug interactions. Nevertheless, the drug was effective at lowering seizure counts to a modest degree. Side effects were nausea, sedation, and dizziness (34).

Impressive efficacy in pediatric epilepsy is an important advantage of felbamate. Felbamate was given to 73 patients with Lennox-Gastaut syndrome. Atonic seizures were reduced by 34%, and there was a 19% reduction in overall seizure counts. However, the most striking results of the trial were in global evaluation scores. The felbamate-treated patients displayed marked improvement in alertness, cognition, and overall functional level. This trial marked a major milestone in treating Lennox-Gastaut syndrome, which is usually refractory to any treatment (35,36). Many parents have elected to continue the drug because of its dramatic benefits for these children. In an open trial of 30 children with partial seizures (37), felbamate led to an average 53% decrease in seizure frequency, with a 50% responder rate. The usual felbamate side effects of insomnia and anorexia were reported in about 20% of patients, and weight loss occurred in 57% (37). Felbamate was effective in providing complete control of infantile spasms in three of four patients (38). In a single case of acquired epileptic aphasia, there was complete seizure control and a major restoration of language function (39).

It is difficult to compare felbamate efficacy with that of other new antiepileptic drugs because of the unique trial designs used (40). These were necessitated by the many drug interactions seen with felbamate; a simple add-on trial would lead to excessive side effects and dropouts. The two pivotal studies in adults were unique at the time. In contrast, most other drugs have been studied using add-on, placebo-controlled trial designs. However, most clinicians using felbamate feel it has excellent efficacy compared with other anticonvulsant drugs.

Side Effects

About a third of patients who take felbamate eventually discontinue because of side effects. As previously discussed, felbamate interacts with several drugs, and side effects are much more troublesome when it is used in polypharmacy combinations with these drugs. The most frequently reported adverse effects in trials of felbamate include nausea, anorexia, vomiting, headache, fatigue, insomnia, and weight loss. Increased serum aspartate aminotransferase levels can be seen (9). In a small fraction of patients, irritability or mania develops (41). Agitation develops in many patients. In milder degrees, the insomnia and agitation are perceived in a positive way by patients accustomed to sedation from other drugs.

Unfortunately, within a year of general release, aplastic anemia and hepatic failure were reported with felbamate use. To date, there have been 31 cases of aplastic anemia with 10 deaths (42) and 10 cases of hepatic failure with four deaths (43,44). The mechanisms are not known and risk factors have not been identified. Felbamate is now used only with great caution in highly selected patients. Written informed consent should be obtained, both to impress the patient with the severity of the risk and to protect the physician from lawsuits. A model consent form is now included in the felbamate package insert. Although it is unknown whether blood monitoring can reliably detect changes before irreversible damage is done, blood and liver tests should be performed regularly and often. The risk for aplastic anemia should be taken in perspective. Between 60,000 and 100,000 patients were exposed to felbamate in the first year, implying a risk of about 1/2000 for aplastic anemia and approximately 1/5000 for death. This is comparable with the risk for death resulting from valproate combination therapy in children ages 2 to 15 years, and is much lower than the risk for sudden death if epilepsy is not controlled. For the right patients, felbamate remains a useful drug.

GABAPENTIN

Gabapentin was released in 1994 in the United States and is marketed by Parke-Davis (45–48).

Mechanism

Gabapentin was originally developed as a lipid-soluble, stable analogue of GABA. It does not, however, have any activity at GABA binding sites on the chloride channel. Gabapentin is preferentially accumulated into astrocytes and neurons by an L-amino acid transport system that also transports leucine and other large, neutral α-amino acids (49). In an in vitro study of hipopcampal pyramidal neurons, gabapentin potentiated the action of nipecotic acid by increasing the release of GABA. This effect might be explained by gabapentin-induced increases in cytosolic GABA (50). Recently, magnetic resonance (MR) spectroscopy has shown that gabapentin increases GABA levels in human brain (51,52).

Pharmacology

Gabapentin is a water-soluble compound with chemical properties similar to those of amino acids. It is absorbed and transported by specific systems. Gabapentin levels can be assayed by high-performance liquid chromatography (53). Absorption from the gastrointestinal tract is linear at low doses but is inhibited by gabapentin concentrations at higher doses, leading to a dose-dependent inhibition of absorption that takes effect at doses >1800 mg in adults (54,55). The drug is not protein-bound and is not metabolized. The half-life in healthy adults is 5 to 9 hours.

In modest renal failure, gabapentin clearance is linearly related to creatinine clearance. Renal failure does not affect absorption, and hepatic metabolism of gabapentin does not occur, even in severe renal failure (56). In anuric patients, gabapentin half-life is 135 hours (57). About 30% of the drug is removed with every 4 hours of hemodialysis. Average anuric patients may be loaded with 300 to 400 mg of gabapentin and given an additional 200 to 300 mg for every 4 hours of hemodialysis (57). Typical doses used in pivotal trials were 1200 to 1800 mg/day for adults, but higher doses may be well tolerated and provide improved efficacy. The drug is supplied as 100-, 300-, and 400-mg capsules.

Drug Interactions

There are no significant interactions with other anticonvulsants or with birth control pills (55).

Efficacy

In the International Gabapentin Study, gabapentin was used as add-on therapy at doses of 900 to 1200 mg/d for patients with refractory partial seizures. Gabapentin was associated with a 23% responder rate (at least a 50% decrease in seizure count). No patients became seizure-free. The most common adverse events were central nervous system-related and included somnolence, dizziness, and fatigue in up to 64% of patients (58). One of the most successful trials of gabapentin was by Sivenius et al. (59), who used either 900 or 1200 mg of gabapentin per day as add-on therapy in refractory partial epilepsy. For the 1200-mg arm, median seizure reduction was 57%. The 900-mg daily dose did not produce significant reductions in seizure count. The only important side effect seen was transient drowsiness (59).

Gabapentin benefits may be sustained with long-term follow-up. The U.S. Gabapentin Study Group followed 240 patients in open-label follow-up, and the drug was shown to be well tolerated for up to 2 years. Dropout because of lack of efficacy was seen in 30% of patients (60). Long-term use of gabapentin was studied by Sivenius et al. (61) in patients who completed a short-term, double-blind trial. Of 25 patients who began the trial, 12 showed sufficient benefit to continue in the open-label phase. Of these, seven continued to derive benefit from gabapentin for a total of 4 years, and five (20% of the original cohort) showed a sustained seizure reduction of 50% from baseline.

Gabapentin may be useful as initial monotherapy in partial seizures. In a double-blind study of new-onset epilepsy, gabapentin at up to 1800 mg/d was compared with carbamazepine at 600 mg/d (62). During a 24-week interval, similar numbers of patients completed therapy in both groups. Dropouts were more frequent because of adverse effects from carbamazepine and because of lack of efficacy with gabapentin. A study with doses titrated to maximal tolerated levels (the current accepted definition of a therapeutic range) and longer duration is needed (62). Handforth and Treiman (63) started 23 patients on long-term gabapentin treatment. Sixteen tolerated the drug and continued taking it for up to 4 years. Its benefits did not wear off. When the drug was discontinued, there was no observable rebound effect on seizures. A double-blind, active-control monotherapy study comparing a low dose with a higher dose (2400 mg) of gabapentin showed that some patients were able to achieve and maintain monotherapy successfully with this drug at higher doses (64). Of 35 patients started in an open-label study by Ojemann et al. (65), nine did well enough to try conversion to monotherapy with gabapentin, and five successfully eliminated other anticonvulsants. One of these five became seizure-free.

Fromm (66) found that although most patients improved somewhat on gabapentin, a subgroup with "staring components" to their seizures actually worsened when taking gabapentin. Fromm suggested that these seizures may arise from a unique inhibitory mechanism, and recommends classifying seizures into clinically distinct groups in future trials (66).

Gabapentin has been used in acute intermittent porphyria without precipitation of crises (67,68). Gabapentin has been reported useful in treatment of reflex sympathetic dystrophy and may be useful in other neurogenic pain syndromes as well (69); further studies are under way.

The drug may find best application in niche situations requiring a favorable side effect profile. Ongoing studies are evaluating the utility of gabapentin in benign rolandic epilepsy and in epilepsy in the elderly.

Side Effects

Gabapentin does not cause severe toxicity to any organ system. Side effects are generally mild, especially at doses within the range approved by the Food and Drug Administration of up to 1800 mg/d. Many gabapentin side effects are transient and do not require discontinuation of the drug. Drowsiness and gastrointestinal side effects are sometimes seen.

Twenty-six percent of patients on long-term gabapentin gain >10% of body weight (70). In another survey of add-on use of gabapentin, 36% of patients gained more than 5 lb. Approximately 20% of patients using gabapentin as adjunctive therapy reported irritability and/or dysphoria (71), and hypomania has also been reported rarely with gabapentin (72). Dysphoria can be seen in up to 22% of patients starting gabapentin in open-label use, with 16% requiring discontinuation (73). Mild ataxia develops in occasional patients.

In the combined patient database from five U.S. blinded trials, adverse events occurred only slightly more often in patients taking gabapentin than in the placebo groups (76% vs. 57%), with no serious adverse events caused by gabapentin. The overall safety and tolerability of the drug are noteworthy (74). In a case of massive overdose, gabapentin was not toxic (75). This is probably a result of its self-limited gastrointestinal absorption.

Initial development of gabapentin was delayed because of concern about pancreatic tumors. Fortunately, pancreatic tumors occurred in only one sex and a specific rodent species, and not in other species. Carcinogenic risk to humans is thought to be low (76).

LAMOTRIGINE

Lamotrigine was released in the United States in 1995; it has had a long European track record. It is marketed by Glaxo Wellcome.

Mechanism

Lamotrigine is active in both maximal electroshock and pentylenetetrazol animal models, suggesting a wide spectrum of action (77). Its mechanism of action is inhibition of sustained repetitive action potential firing via inactivation of sodium channels (78–80). Initial reports of action through inhibition of excitatory amino acid release probably refer to an epiphenomenon; any drug that inhibits seizures through any mechanism will reduce excitatory amino acid release. This action may secondarily lead to a reduction in nitric oxide synthesis (81). Lamotrigine is cerebroprotective in several rodent models of ischemia models (78,82,83).

Although lamotrigine was initially developed as a folate antagonist (and tried as a treatment for epilepsy because of a mistaken supposition that phenytoin might exert its anticonvulsant actions through folate antagonism), it does not have significant effects on folate metabolism in humans. This was shown in a study by Sander and Patsalos (84), who followed folate levels during short-term and long-term lamotrigine treatment. No changes in folate levels or red blood cell folate concentrations were noted, and hematologic parameters were not changed.

Pharmacology

Lamotrigine levels can be measured in serum using high-performance liquid chromatography (85). Lamotrigine is 98% absorbed, with time to peak plasma levels of 3 hours following an oral dose. Fifty to sixty percent of the drug is protein-bound (78), and the free fraction easily penetrates the blood-brain barrier. It is metabolized by hepatic glucuronidation (80). The metabolites are excreted in the urine. Elimination is linear, and the half-life of lamotrigine is 20 hours when it is used as monotherapy (86). The half-life is reduced by about half when it is used with enzyme-inducing drugs, and almost doubled when it is combined with valproate. Although the therapeutic range is not clearly established, most studies have shown efficacy between levels of 1 and 4 μg/mL. Higher levels may be tolerated, but an increased response rate with higher levels has not been established. Lamotrigine is supplied in 25-, 100-, 150-, and 200-mg tablets.

Drug Interactions

The most important interaction is with valproate, which blocks the degradation of lamotrigine. The half-life of lamotrigine in this setting is >36 hours (78). The interaction is competition for hepatic glucuronidation. Time of maximal concentration, volume of distribution, and renal clearance are not affected (87). The interaction between lamotrigine and valproate may be used to beneficial effect, as Ferrie and Panayiotopoulos (88) point out in a report of combined treatment that was successful only when the two drugs were used together (88). In a blinded, add-on study of 22 patients taking valproate, addition of 200 mg of lamotrigine per day produced a synergistic effect, with a median decrease of 37% in seizure frequency. Side effects resulting from drug interaction were minimal (89). Beyond the pharmacokinetic change, valproate seems to increase the risk for severe rash induced by lamotrigine. When the drugs are used in combination, initial dosing should be cautious, starting at 25 mg every other day in adults and increasing every other week.

Lamotrigine has no effect on the metabolism of other, standard anticonvulsants. There is a small increase in the fraction of carbamazepine-10,11-epoxide (77,90). Performing single-dose measures in patients on lamotrigine monotherapy and in healthy controls, Pisani et al. (91) found no direct effect of lamotrigine on the metabolism or elimination of carbamazepine-10,11-epoxide. This suggests that alterations in epoxide levels may be caused exclusively by effects of lamotrigine on carbamazepine metabolism. Although the increases in epoxide levels are usually moderate, Warner et al. (92) reported nine patients treated with carbamazepine who experienced clinical toxicity when lamotrigine was begun in association with increases in carbamazepine epoxide levels of up to 45% above baseline. Brodie (93) has suggested a pharmacodynamic as well as a pharmacokinetic interaction. Acetaminophen may lead to 15% reductions in lamotrigine serum levels (94).

Efficacy

Eight double-blind studies of lamotrigine in refractory partial-onset seizures have been performed (95). One of the pivotal lamotrigine studies was by Messenheimer et al. (96). This double-blind, placebo-controlled study compared 400 mg of lamotrigine added to standard anticonvulsant drugs with addition of placebo in 98 patients who had refractory epilepsy. Median seizure reduction was 25%, and seizures were reduced by 50% in approximately 20% of patients. The drug was well tolerated, and only five patients dropped out because of side effects, three of them for rash (96). In a double-blind crossover study, lamotrigine at doses of 150 mg/d or 300 mg/d was compared with placebo in 41 patients who had refractory partial epilepsy (97). Seizures were reduced by at least 50% in 22% of patients; this benefit was mainly seen with complex partial seizures. In fact, secondarily generalized seizures were not significantly reduced. Blood levels in this trial ranged from 1 to 3 μg/mL (97).

Martin and Millac (98) prospectively surveyed 45 patients treated with lamotrigine, and 58% either worsened or did not improve significantly, but 33% achieved a 50% reduction in seizure count. Generalized tonic-clonic seizures seemed to respond better than complex partial seizures, confirming the broad spectrum of action of the drug. Side effects led to discontinuation in 20%.

Lamotrigine was compared with carbamazepine as monotherapy in newly diagnosed epilepsy in a double-blind, randomized, controlled study (99). The study included 151 patients with either primary generalized or partial seizures. Similar fractions of patients became seizure-free with both drugs (39% with lamotrigine, 38% with carbamazepine). Rash was the major side effect leading to withdrawal (9% with lamotrigine, 13% with carbamazepine). Lamotrigine overall was better tolerated, notably with less sedation, and fewer people withdrew because of side effects from lamotrigine than from carbamazepine (99). Initial efficacy was sustained in a long-term open-label study (100).

Lamotrigine has a wide spectrum of action. It is currently indicated only as add-on therapy in partial seizures, but it is potentially effective as monotherapy against partial seizures, primarily generalized tonic-clonic and absence seizures, and drug-resistant seizures in epilepsy syndromes with multiple seizure types (77). Schlumberger et al. (101) summarized three trials of lamotrigine in 120 children with various types of epilepsy. Tolerance was excellent. The drug was most effective against absence seizures, Lennox-Gastaut syndrome, and other symptomatic secondary generalized epilepsies in comparison with epilepsies characterized by localization-related seizures of partial onset. Of the 14 patients who became seizure-free, all but one had generalized epilepsy (101). Low-dose lamotrigine combined with valproate was highly effective against typical absence seizures in a retrospective review of 15 patients. Typical doses were 1.6 to 3.0 mg/kg per day for children and 25 to 50 mg/d for adults (102). In a retrospective review of 12 patients with primary generalized epilepsy inadequately treated with valproate, five became seizure-free and six were improved after switching to lamotrigine (103). Lamotrigine has a broad spectrum of action in children with multiple seizure types; in a survey of 285 children, 50% seizure reductions were found in 30% of those with complex partial seizures and in >50% of those with either typical or atypical absence seizures. Seventy-four percent of children showed global improvement (104). Lamotrigine has been used against infantile spasms with good preliminary results (105). Lamotrigine may be particularly effective in Rett syndrome. In an open trial of four patients, all had at least a 50% reduction in seizures (106).

Side Effects

Side effects of lamotrigine are typically mild and include rash, nausea, vomiting, visual abnormalities (blurred vision, diplopia, and other symptoms), and headache (80,107). Dizziness, fatigue, and similar side effects are more common when lamotrigine is combined with carbamazepine (108). In an overall review of clinical trials, rash appears in 2.3% of patients and is the most common reason for discontinuation. Rash is more common with valproate cotreatment (108). Richens (107) reviewed the dermatologic safety record of lamotrigine in 5800 patient-years of lamotrigine exposure in clinical trials. Rash occurs in about 5% of patients. It occurs more often with a rapid increase in lamotrigine dose and also with coadministration of valproate. Rash can rarely lead to Stevens-Johnson syndrome (107). Initial rash caused by lamotrigine may resolve with gradual reintroduction of the drug and may not be an absolute contraindication to careful use of the drug (109).

In therapeutic doses, diazepam, carbamazepine, and phenytoin all produce adverse effects on oculomotor function (smooth pursuit, saccades, and adaptive tracking). These side effects are not seen with lamotrigine (110).

Cognitive effects have not been a problem, and the drug is mostly nonsedating in the usual dose ranges.

TOPIRAMATE

Topiramate is being developed by the R. W. Johnson Research Institute and McNeil Pharmaceuticals. It has received a letter of approvability from the Food and Drug Administration, and U.S. release is imminent.

Mechanism

Topiramate is effective in a broad range of epilepsy models, suggesting a broad clinical spectrum. Topiramate is effective against both tonic-clonic and absence seizures in DBA/2 mice (111). In contrast, phenytoin and zonisamide were active only against tonic seizures (111). Topiramate prevents amygdaloid kindled seizures in cats (112). The mechanism of action of topiramate is reportedly blockage of excitatory amino acid receptors. Topiramate is active in blocking kainate-evoked currents in patch clamp studies of hippocampal neurons (113). Topiramate may cause desensitization of $GABA_A$ receptors (114). In *Xenopus* oocytes, topiramate caused modulation of expression of various receptor subunits. Whether this is an important in vivo mechanism is unclear (114). The drug is an inhibitor of carbonic anhydrase, and this was originally thought to be part of its action. However, its level of inhibition is a 100-fold less than that of acetazolamide.

Pharmacology

Topiramate is well absorbed. Topiramate is primarily excreted via the kidneys. Some hepatic metabolism takes place. The half-life is long, and twice-daily dosing is feasible. Typical adult doses seem to be 400 mg/d; there may be a plateau effect, with no efficacy gains at higher doses but increased cognitive side effects. Tablets are 100 mg each.

Drug Interactions

Drug interactions do not seem to be a problem with topiramate.

Efficacy

Topiramate was used as add-on therapy in previously intractable epilepsy (115). At doses up to 400 mg/d, the median seizure reduction approached 50%. Side effects were principally related to the central nervous system and included fatigue, altered thinking, and similar complaints (115). In an open study of epilepsy in children at the Minnesota Epilepsy Group, topiramate was effective against multiple seizure types of Lennox-Gastaut syndrome, with 50% to 75% reductions in seizures of generalized tonic-clonic, drop, and atypical absence type (116). Almost 40% of patients became free of drop attack seizures. In study YD (117), doses of 400 mg and 600 mg/d were more effective than doses of 200 mg/d. This was a double-blind, dose-ranging study. The two higher doses achieved similar results, with 46% of patients achieving a 50% seizure reduction (117). Higher doses of topiramate, from 600 to 1000 mg/d, were explored as add-on therapy in study YE. Like study YD, study YE showed an apparent plateau in the dose-response curve. At all doses, about 40% of patients had a 50% seizure reduction. A total of 4% of patients became seizure-free (118). In a blinded, active-control trial, topiramate was shown to be effective in monotherapy at doses of 1000 mg/d. The active control was a low dose (100 mg/d) (119). In the high-dose group, 13% of patients became seizure-free and 46% had a 50% seizure reduction (119).

Side Effects

Major side effects seen with topiramate in double-blind studies are related to central nervous system function. These include somnolence (27%), abnormal thinking (25%), fatigue, and dizziness. Cognitive effects are possibly lessened with gradual escalation of dose (118). Asthenia and weight loss are uncommon problems. In a high-dose monotherapy study, there were four renal stones among 24 patients treated with 1000 mg of topiramate per day (120). Renal stone formation may be related to carbonic anhydrase activity, as it is also seen with zonisamide and acetazolamide.

VIGABATRIN

Vigabatrin has been the focus of a long development effort by Marion Merrell Dow, now Hoechst Marion Rousell, and a new drug application was filed with the Food and Drug Administration more than a year ago. The drug is available in several European countries, Canada, and Mexico. Vigabatrin has been reviewed extensively (121–123).

Mechanism

Vigabatrin irreversibly inhibits GABA transaminase (GABA-T), the key enzyme in the breakdown of GABA. Brain levels of GABA can be measured with MR spectroscopy in vivo. Increased brain levels of GABA were seen using MR spectroscopy in rats treated with vigabatrin (124). In humans, vigabatrin increases brain levels of GABA from an average of 0.9 μMOL/G to 2.6 μmol/g measured by MR spectroscopy. There were minor increases in glutamine and glutamic acid as well (125). Vigabatrin also leads to decreased brain levels of aspartate, glutamate, and alanine (126). In addition to inhibition of GABA-T, vigabatrin also inhibits serum alanine aminotransferase, but Foletti et al. (127) showed that this effect is not metabolically or clinically significant. Patients taking vigabatrin routinely have very low laboratory measures of hepatic function (transaminase enzymes). Vigabatrin is highly effective in pentylenetetrazol models of epilepsy, but only modestly beneficial in maximal electroshock models.

Pharmacology

Vigabatrin kinetics have been reviewed by Rey et al. (128). The drug is absorbed during 1 to 2 hours, with a half-life of 5 to 6 hours in adults. Because its mechanism of action is irreversible inhibition of GABA-T, the duration of action is several days (128). Bioavailability is reduced in children, necessitating a dose increase (typical adult dose, 50 mg/kg per day; typical pediatric dose, 80 mg/kg per day). Cerebrospinal fluid levels are typically only 10% to 20% of blood levels (128). Vigabatrin is not protein-bound and is excreted by the kidneys. Typical daily doses are 3000 to 4000 mg/d, and there may be a plateau effect with no gains in efficacy after further dose increases. Although the effective half-life is long, vigabatrin should be administered twice a day to prevent gastrointestinal side effects associated with massive single doses. Tablets are 500 mg each.

Drug Interactions

Vigabatrin leads to a 20% reduction in phenytoin levels, although the mechanism of the interaction is unclear (128). There may be a potential for beneficial pharmacodynamic interactions with other GABA-active drugs, including tiagabine and gabapentin.

Efficacy

Vigabatrin is highly effective as add-on therapy for partial epilepsy, with 45% to 55% median reductions in seizures and an average 50% responder rate for add-on trials (129). In the U.S. Vigabatrin 024 Study, the responder rate was 43% (130). Ylinen et al. (131) reviewed vigabatrin use in a variety of clinical settings. Vigabatrin led to a 50% reduction in seizures in 55% of 75 patients with refractory complex partial seizures and in 42% of 36 patients with severe epilepsy accompanying mental retardation (131). In an open-label study of 72 patients with refractory partial seizures, vigabatrin seemed to benefit 57%, with 10% becoming seizure-free. Lack of efficacy, including behavioral change and edema, caused 12% to drop out (132). Martin and Millac (133) reported on a 3-year open-label experience with vigabatrin in 57 patients with severe epilepsy. The seizure frequency of 36 of the patients was reduced by 50%. Withdrawal rates were lower than in trials of other new anticonvulsant drugs (133).

Vigabatrin might be useful as monotherapy. Kalviainen et al. (134) studied vigabatrin as monotherapy in patients with newly diagnosed epilepsy using a blinded comparison with carbamazepine. Both drugs have shown similar overall success rates, with dropouts in general caused by side effects with carbamazepine and lack of efficacy with vigabatrin. In another blinded study, 20 patients with stable epilepsy treated with carbamazepine monotherapy were randomized to conversion to vigabatrin monotherapy, and most did well (131). In a double-blind study of 1.5 g of vigabatrin daily in patients with refractory partial seizures, seizures were reduced by 50% in 10 of 20 patients (135).

Long-term use of some anticonvulsants leads to declines in efficacy. Patients who responded to vigabatrin in trials performed by Cocito et al. (136) remained on the drug and were followed for up to 7 years; about a third (39%) continued to improve, about a third (22%) stayed the same, and about a third (39%) deteriorated. In general, the benefits of vigabatrin seem to have been sustained during the 7-year follow-up. No significant adverse effects were seen in this long-term group (136). Long-term treatment in patients completing double-blind studies was reviewed by French et al. (137). Of patients who completed studies 024 and 025, 39% entered open-label extension. Of the original cohort (intent to treat), 8% achieved long-term, seizure-free remission. Tartara et al. (138) studied the long-term use of vigabatrin. Following successful treatment with vigabatrin in a short-term trial, 25 patients were followed on a long-term basis for 4 to 6 years. Fifteen patients showed sustained benefits.

Vigabatrin is spectacularly successful in treating the infantile spasms of West syndrome and spasms associated with tuberous sclerosis; it may emerge as the drug of choice for infantile spasms (139). Vigabatrin was used in 20 children with Lennox-Gastaut syndrome who had not responded to valproate. Eighty-five of the children enjoyed at least a 50% seizure reduction. Only one child suffered a serious side effect (dyskinesia). There were no adverse effects on mood (140). Of 26 infants with infantile spasms, 81% achieved complete remission of spasms on vigabatrin doses averaging 100 mg/kg per day (141). Patients who respond to the drug show seizure reduction in the first 57 days, so prolonged trials may not be necessary. Among 192 children with infantile spasms, 68% achieved complete seizure control with vigabatrin used as first-line monotherapy (141). Gram et al. (142) found that although vigabatrin is effective for infantile spasms, there is no clear dose-response relationship. Effective dose ranges in these studies were 40 to 80 mg/kg per day (142). Children with tuberous sclerosis did particularly well, with 97% achieving complete seizure control (143). Vigabatrin may be especially useful in treating refractory seizures, including infantile spasms, associated with tuberous sclerosis (144). In single case reports, vigabatrin may be effective in Ohtahara syndrome and Aicardi syndrome (145).

The dose-response relationship for vigabatrin is uncertain. In adults, doses >3 g/d do not seem to lead to increased efficacy (146). This was studied by Arteaga et al. (147) in 16 children. Seizure counts decreased as vigabatrin doses were increased up to about 60 mg/kg per day but did not correlate with either serum vigabatrin levels or platelet GABA-T activity (147). Some children improved at doses up to 100 mg/kg per day. Higher doses did not lead to further improvement in children who did not demonstrate at least a partial initial response. Because the half-life of the drug is short but the mechanism of action leads to long-lasting benefits, measurement of serum levels is not necessarily useful with vigabatrin (147). Despite its high cost, vigabatrin is cost-effective because of its marked efficacy (148).

Side Effects

Most patients find vigabatrin to be a pleasant drug, although sedation and nausea are not rare. Attempts to use the drug once daily (suggested by the long duration of transaminase inhibition) are limited by gastrointestinal side effects associated with single massive doses. Twice-daily dosing is usually well tolerated. Fisher and Kerrigan (149) reviewed side effect rates in two combined U.S. double-blind studies. In excess of the rates seen with placebo, drowsiness and dizziness were each seen in 10% more treated patients than placebo patients. Fatigue, vision abnormalities, depression, and paresthesias were seen at excess rates of 7% each. Less common were tremor and confusion (6% and 4%, respectively). The most common side effect in patients continuing the drug long-term was weight gain (138). In the 024 study, mean weight gain was 2.6 kg (130).

Vigabatrin can lead to a variety of motor disturbances, including tremor, athetosis, and dystonia (150). Vigabatrin may induce myoclonus and concomitant paroxysmal electroencephalograhic abnormalities (151). Visual changes range from scintillations to very rare papilledema and visual loss. Lethargy and encephalopathy can occur (149). Visual disorders caused by vigabatrin are uncommon. These include scintillations, scotomata, papilledema, and very rare instances of visual loss (149). Levels of laboratory measures of hepatic function, such as aspartate aminotransferase (SGOT) and alanine aminotransferase (SGPT), are markedly reduced by vigabatrin, but this is usually not associated with symptoms.

Vigabatrin may rarely lead to a worsening of seizure control and emergence of new seizure types (152). In rare cases, status has emerged following the initiation of vigabatrin treatment (153,154). Patients with nonprogressive myoclonic epilepsy may worsen with vigabatrin (155).

Depression is an important side effect of vigabatrin (146). The incidence varies in different studies. Early experiences suggested higher rates than more recent studies, and lower rates are seen in blinded studies than with open-label treatment. In a Dutch study, mood disorders led to discontinuation of vigabatrin in 12% of patients, with an additional 8% experiencing mood disorders not severe enough to lead to discontinuation. In this study, all patients had undergone structured psychiatric evaluation before drug initiation. No single factor or combination of factors was predictive of development of mood problems (156). Depression was reported in 10 patients treated with vigabatrin (157). Previous history of depression seemed to be a predisposing factor. In most patients who became depressed, depression seemed to develop in association with a reduction in seizure frequency (157), suggesting a phenomena similar to "forced normalization."

In early studies, psychosis was reported in 3% to 7% of patients treated with vigabatrin (158,159). With more careful patient selection the rate of psychosis may be reduced. In the global, U.K., U.S., and Canadian databases, psychosis occurred at low rates, ranging from 0.6% to 1.1% (160). Vigabatrin-related psychosis is more common in patients with medically refractory complex partial seizures than in patients with newly diagnosed epilepsy. In double-blind U.S. trials, psychosis developed in the refractory population at an overall rate of 2.9% (160). Sander et al. (161) reported 14 patients in whom psychosis developed following vigabatrin treatment. Nine of these patients had no previous psychiatric history. Mean dose at onset of psychosis was 2580 mg/d. Psychosis in some but not all of these cases seemed to be related to improved seizure control (161). Besides depression and psychosis, severe bipolar disorder has been reported (162). Patients on vigabatrin may also exhibit irritability (146).

Despite occasional psychiatric problems, cognitive side effects are rare. One study showed improved functioning in comparison with patients with newly diagnosed epilepsy taking carbamazepine (134). In a double-blind, add-on study of a range of doses up to 1 g/d, there was essentially no degradation in performance with increasing doses of vigabatrin. Among a battery of tests, declines were seen only on the digit cancellation test (163). In add-on therapy at 2 g/d, vigabatrin led to a reduction in response time on an arithmetic task, with no changes in other cognitive tests (164). Cognitive benefits of vigabatrin were sustained following 1-year long-term follow-up (165). In a double-blind study of 1.5 g of vigabatrin daily in patients with refractory partial seizures, there was a reduction in motor speed and in scores on a design learning task (135). In a trial of vigabatrin in mentally impaired patients, psychologic performance and electroencephalographic pattern were unchanged (166).

In early studies in some species of dogs and rats, vigabatrin led to reversible microvacuole formation in myelin. Whether intramyelinotic edema occurs in humans has been a major safety concern during development of the drug. Changes in T_2 signal on MR imaging are a sensitive indicator of the onset of intramyelinic edema in beagles (167). Early MR imaging signal changes are seen in fornix, thalamus, optic tract, and hypothalamus (168). As demonstrated on quantitative T_2 relaxometry (169), there were no changes in white matter signal characteristics in 45 patients treated with up to 1.5 g of vigabatrin per day (170). Visual and somatosensory evoked potentials can also be used for accurate monitoring of the development of intramyelinic edema in dogs (171). Somatosensory evoked potentials show no major changes in human studies (172). In >60 patients treated with vigabatrin for long periods (up to 5 years) who later came to epilepsy surgery, neuropathologic examination of the resected tissue did not show evidence of myelin vacuolation (173–175).

ZONISAMIDE

Zonisamide is being developed by Dainippon Pharmaceuticals. It is available in Japan, and U.S. development is at an advanced stage (176).

Mechanism

Zonisamide is a weak carbonic anhydrase inhibitor (177), but this is probably not a significant component of its anticonvulsant actions. An analogue, 7-methyl-zonisamide, is equally potent as a carbonic anhydrase inhibitor but has no anticonvulsant activity (178). In a whole-cell patch clamp experiment, zonisamide blocked T-type calcium currents in a dose-dependent fashion, with no effect on L-type currents (179). 7-Methylzonisamide did not demonstrate this effect on calcium currents (179). Zonisamide binding in extracts of rat brain is inhibited by clonazepam and enhanced by GABA; however, this effect is seen at levels of 10^{-3} M, whereas therapeutic levels are in the range of 10^{-4} M (180,181). Zonisamide is neuroprotective in a rat model of ischemia (182).

Pharmacology

Zonisamide is well absorbed. In addition to minimal protein binding, zonisamide is concentrated in erythrocytes in a saturable manner (183). Hepatic clearance produces a half-life of 12 to 20 hours, allowing twice-daily dosing. Zonisamide levels can be determined by high-performance liquid chromatography (184). Effective blood levels of zonisamide are in the range of 10 to 20 μg/mL. Levels >30 mg/L were associated with an increased incidence of side effects in Japanese trials (185). Typical adult daily doses are 400 mg/d. Zonisamide capsules contain 100 mg.

Drug Interactions

Most zonisamide drug interactions are minor. Zonisamide levels are reduced by enzyme-inducing compounds, such as carbamazepine or phenobarbital. Zonisamide leads to a slight increase in phenytoin levels (186), a modest reduction in carbamazepine levels, and increases in the ratio of carbamazepine epoxide to carbamazepine (187).

Efficacy

Zonisamide has been shown to be effective in partial epilepsies in several European and Japanese trials. The results of pivotal U.S. trials are pending. In an older study of 167 patients using a historical-control, open-label design, Leppick et al. (188) found a 52% reduction in seizure frequency. Unfortunately, kidney stones developed in 3.7% of patients (total of four patients) in this trial. Other adverse events were mild (188). Zonisamide monotherapy was used in an open-label trial of 44 children with epilepsy of various types. Doses were titrated upward to either 12 mg/kg per day or until a therapeutic response was seen. The drug produced complete control of seizures in all five children with primary generalized epilepsy and in seven of eight children with secondary generalized epilepsy. Patients with symptomatic partial epilepsy also did well, with more than two thirds becoming seizure-free. The main side effect was transient drowsiness. There were no renal stones in this trial (189). In a European double-blind study of 139 patients with partial-onset seizures, there was an average reduction in seizure count of 28%, with 30% of patients reducing seizures by 50% (190). A seizure-free outcome was seen in 6%. Adverse effects included the usual reports of fatigue, somnolence, dizziness, and ataxia, but these were usually mild and only two patients withdrew because of adverse events. There were no kidney stones (190). In two case reports, zonisamide was effective against absence seizures (191). Besides suggestions of efficacy in absence, atypical absence, and other generalized epilepsies, zonisamide may be useful in progressive myoclonus epilepsy. This was suggested by Henry et al. (192) in a small open study of patients with Lafora's body disease. Zonisamide may be effective in mania, with up to 80% of patients with bipolar disorder showing improvement in one study (193).

Side Effects

Side effects are generally mild and include sedation, tremor, nausea, and other side effects commonly associated with all anticonvulsants. Behavioral disorders have rarely been seen in adults or children (194).

Renal stones were seen in 1.9% of 700 patients in early U.S. trials (185). Predisposing factors seem to include previous history of stones or renal structural abnormality and zonisamide serum levels >30 μg/mL. With appropriate cautions, zonisamide-induced renal stones have not been a clinical problem in Japan, and a repeated set of U.S. trials are nearing completion (185). A reanalysis of the U.S. data showed that stones tended to occur in patients with a predisposition to stones or with exposure to high blood levels.

OXCARBAZEPINE

Oxcarbazepine (195,196) is under U.S. development by Ciba Pharmaceutical Co. following favorable European experience.

Mechanism

The mechanism of action of oxcarbazepine is similar to that of carbamazepine. In rat cortical neuron culture, oxcarbazepine and a metabolite, the monohydroxyl derivative (MHD), suppress sustained high-frequency repetitive firing of sodium-dependent action potentials (197). Oxcarbazepine, but not MHD, may also interact with calcium L-type channels at concentrations of 0.3 mM (198). Besides blocking sodium channels, oxcarbazepine and MHD may act on potassium channels, as the anticonvulsant effect is diminished in vitro when 4-aminopyridine is added (199).

Pharmacology

Oxcarbazepine is a 10-keto analogue of carbamazepine.

Oxcarbazepine is converted to an MHD. The conversion is not altered by enzyme-inducing drugs (200). The MHD is the active compound (200). The MHD is partly renally excreted, accounting for 25% to 30% of its clearance, and the remainder is reduced via glucuronidation (200). Renal impairment has minimal effects on oxcarbamzepine distribution or elimination but causes an accumulation of MHD (201). In severe renal failure, dose adjustment may be required, and toxicity may emerge from unmeasured metabolites. When creatinine clearance is between 10 and 30 mL/min, the oxcarbazepine dose should be reduced 50% (202); with creatinine clearance reduced below 10 mL/min, rational dosing may not be feasible (201). In healthy adults, the MHD has a half-life of about 10 hours, so oxcarbazepine can be administered twice daily (200,203). Food has a minimal effect on oxcarbazepine absorption, causing a 16% increase in AUC (area under curve) for the parent compound (204) and a mild increase in MHD levels (200). Oxcarbazepine doses are about 50% higher than carbamazepine doses (205). Tablets contain 300 or 600 mg.

Drug Interactions

A major advantage of oxcarbazepine is a relative lack of drug interactions in comparison with carbamazepine. Oxcarbazepine does not induce most cytochromes. Doses of other anticonvulsants can be decreased when carbamazepine is converted to oxcarbazepine. The lack of drug interactions with older anticonvulsants was confirmed in a blinded study in which oxcarbazepine was added to the regimen of patients taking phenytoin, carbamazepine, or valproate. No changes in blood levels of the older drugs were seen, and the drug was well tolerated as add-on therapy (206).

Other subtle metabolic abnormalities associated with carbamazepine are not seen with oxcarbazepine. In a prospective study of 12 male patients with epilepsy, replacement of carbamazepine with oxcarbazepine led to a normalization of P_{450} function as measured by antipyrine clearance (207). Cholesterol levels, increased from long-term carbamazepine administration, normalized following the switch to oxcarbazepine, whereas HDL (high-density lipoprotein) cholesterol and triglyceride levels did not change (207). Oxcarbazepine does not share the subtle effect of carbamazepine on thyroid function. In a long-term crossover study, Isojarvi et al. (208) found that carbamazepine was associated with small decreases in circulating thyroid hormone levels and mild impairment of cardiac diastolic function. Conversion to oxcarbazepine reversed these effects. Changing patients from carbamazepine to oxcarbazepine caused normalization of serum sex hormone levels (209). Conversion of carbamazepine to oxcarbazepine can lead to a 50% to 200% increase in the blood levels of neuroleptics (210).

Neither oxcarbazepine nor its MHD interacts with warfarin (211,212) or cimetidine (213). The lack of interaction with erythromycin (214) represents a major improvement over carbamazepine, which shows dramatically increased serum levels and causes clinical toxicity following coadministration of erythromycin.

Although neither oxcarbazepine nor the MHD are major inducers of cytochrome P_{450}, induction of the IIIA subfamily of the P_{450} system occurs (200). This enzyme metabolizes estrogens and dihydropyridine calcium-channel blockers (nifedipine and others) and may lead to an interaction with oral birth control pills (200,211,215). In 13 female patients taking combination oral contraceptive pills, addition of 900 mg of oxcarbazepine per day led to reduced AUC for both ethinyl estradiol and levonorgestrel (215).

Efficacy

In European trials studying replacement of carbamazepine with oxcarbazepine, oxcarbazepine seems to be roughly equivalent to carbamazepine. The largest such study (203) enrolled 165 patients and found the two drugs to be equivalent. Oxcarbazepine was better tolerated than carbamazepine. A study that shows equivalence does not constitute proof of efficacy, and so blinded, controlled studies are under way (216). In a randomized monotherapy study comparing oxcarbazepine with phenytoin, there was no difference in efficacy or neuropsychologic function between the two drugs (217). In another double-blind study, oxcarbazepine and carbamazepine demonstrated similar efficacy against both partial-onset and generalized-onset tonic-clonic seizures (218). Van Parys et al. (219) reviewed their experience with oxcarbazepine in 260 patients who had failed treatment with carbamazepine. One hundred sixty-one patients derived useful benefit from oxcarbazepine. They felt the drug was especially useful in patients who had adverse effects from carbamazepine or who had difficulties with drug interactions on polypharmacy (219). Fisher et al. (220) showed that oxcarbazepine is tolerated and effective in an inpatient-monitoring, unit-based open study of 10 patients. U.S. pivotal trials are under way.

Side Effects

Oxcarbazepine is well tolerated. It does not cause the dose-related nausea, dizziness, visual blurring, and diplopia seen with carbamazepine. Occasional complaints of nausea and anorexia are encountered. Some patients have mood alterations, sometimes euphoric.

Hyponatremia resulting from carbamazepine and oxcarbazepine may be caused by either increased antidiuretic hormone secretion or increased sensitivity of renal tubules to the action of antidiuretic hormone (221). Hyponatremia is more common in patients with mental retardation or psychiatric disturbance (221). It is usually asymptomatic, and drug discontinuation because of hyponatremia is rare (221). Severe hyponatremia can occur (222) and is particularly likely at doses above 30 mg/kg per day (223). Steinhoff et al. reported a patient with serum sodium levels of 115 mEq/L, and coma has been reported (224,225).

Skin eruptions can be seen in patients sensitive to carbamazepine (226). In patients in whom rash does develop, desensitization has been effective in allowing patients eventually to tolerate the medication (227). Modest leukopenia may be seen with either drug (205).

TIAGABINE

Tiagabine is under development by Abbott Laboratories (228).

Mechanism

Tiagabine is an analogue of nipecotic acid, which inhibits GABA uptake. Tiagabine selectively inhibits the GABA transporter GAT-1 (229). Its action is thus analogous to the mechanism of most antidepressants in the serotonin system (230). Tiagabine is active in a pentylenetetrazol model in rodents but not in a maximal electroshock model (231). Activity is seen at levels that do not lead to sedation or behavioral changes (231). Tiagabine is effective against sound-induced seizures in genetically epilepsy-prone rats and against photically induced seizures in *Papio papio* baboons (232). In genetically epilepsy-prone rats, microinjections of tiagabine in the inferior colliculus block sound-induced seizures (233). This block, which is more potent at higher volumes, is felt to be related to increased GABA inhibition at higher volumes (233). Other actions of tiagabine are also possible; nipecotic acid inhibits L-carnitine uptake into rat cortical neurons in culture (234).

Pharmacology

Tiagabine is well absorbed. Half-life is short. The drug is not protein-bound. Kinetics are linear. Metabolism is hepatic. Patients taking enzyme-inducing drugs require higher doses (235). Tiagabine metabolism is not affected by renal dysfunction or hemodialysis (236). Typical doses in U.S. trials range from 32 to 56 mg/d.

Drug Interactions

Tiagabine seems to have no major adverse drug interactions. It does not effect the metabolism of carbamezepine, carbamazepine-10,11-epoxide, or phenytoin. There is a very small (<10%) reduction in valproate AUC (237). There is no appreciable interaction between tiagabine and any of the following compounds: theophylline, warfarin, digoxin, cimetidine (238), oral contraceptives, tirazolam, or ethanol (239).

Tiagabine may exhibit beneficial pharmacodynamic effects with a number of other new anticonvulsants that act on GABA. In vitro, the increased GABA action induced by nipecotic acid seems to "run down" by approximately 50% with prolonged administration (beyond 45 minutes) (50). Interestingly, this run-down effect is reversed by simultaneous administration of gabapentin, suggesting a pharmacodynamic interaction that may hypothetically prove useful clinically (50). Anectodal experience from Europe has suggested that tiagabine and vigabatrin may have synergistic action (240). There is no pharmacokinetic interaction between the two. Leach et al. (240) showed that vigabatrin (at levels of 100 μM) has an additional effect on GABA uptake in rat neurons, supporting a hypothetical pharmacodynamic interaction.

Efficacy

Safety and efficacy were suggested by an open-label trial (241). In the Amery enrichment design, a double-blind study is performed in which only patients who successfully complete an open-label dose titration and achieve a predetermined (typically 25% or 50%) seizure reduction during the open-label phase are enrolled. This process "enriches" the subsequent double-blind study and increases the statistical power to identify subgroups that may benefit from the drug (242). Tiagabine was studied in a double-blind crossover study in a population that was "enriched" by selecting patients who had responded during a prior open-label titration phase. Ninety-four patients were entered into the titration study and 46 were selected as possible responders to the drug, based on a reduction of at least 25% in seizure count during the open-label titration phase. These 46 patients were then entered into a double-blind, placebo crossover study phase. In 26 patients, the total seizure count was reduced by 50% or more (243). Tiagabine does not seem to induce long-term tolerance. Of 1414 patients enrolled in two double-blind, add-on studies, 90 were able to achieve tiagabine monotherapy. Seventy-five patients (5%) became seizure-free (244). About half the patients discontinued, most often because of lack of efficacy. In a group of children ages 2 through 12 years, tiagabine was well tolerated at doses up to 1 mg/kg per day (245). Children with partial seizures responded to the drug, with about 20% achieving a 50% seizure reduction. Children with generalized seizures did not seem to respond to the drug (245). Tiagabine may be effective in children. Wolff et al. (235) conducted an open-label study of 11 children with epilepsy. At 60 mg/d, there was an average seizure reduction of 40%. Adverse events were tolerable but occurred in up to 40% of patients.

Side Effects

Tiagabine is well tolerated by most patients (230). The most common side effects are fatigue, dizziness, and headache (243,244). Tiagabine did not produce cognitive side effects in a double-blind, add-on study (246). In an open trial of 22 patients with refractory partial seizures, tiagabine at doses up to 32 mg produced no measurable effect on neuropsychologic test results. However, in this trial the overall seizure frequency was not reduced (247). In a case report of tiagabine overdose with blood levels 30 times above the usual range, there was acute depression of consciousness with full recovery (248).

Tiagabine increased the number and duration of generalized spike-and-wave discharges in rats with absence epilepsy and so might not be useful in generalized disorders (249). Although tiagabine was modestly effective in stopping experimental status epilepticus in a rodent model, it produced an undesirable syndrome of hyporeactivity and high-amplitude electroencephalographic paroxysmal discharges, suggesting that tiagabine may not be useful in human status (250).

A use for tiagabine other than epilepsy treatment was suggested by Gao et al. (251), who found that it inhibits haloperidol-induced oral dyskinesias in rodents.

UCB LO59

UCB LO59 is now known as levetiracetam and is under preliminary U.S. development.

Mechanism

Levetiracetam is a member of the racetam family, which includes piracetam. These drugs may act to potentiate ion flux through non-L-type voltage-dependent calcium channels or to decrease potassium efflux. A broad variety of clinical actions are ascribed to these "nootropic" drugs, including reversal of anticholinergic-induced amnesia and reduction in sedation caused by barbiturates (252). In rats, levetiracetam inhibits pentylenetretrazol-induced, audiogenic seizures as well as kindled and NMDA-induced seizures (253). It does not confer protection against maximal electroshock-induced seizures (253), although some studies support a modest effect (254).

Pharmacology

Levetiracetam exhibits linear kinetics and is well tolerated at doses of 1000 to 3000 mg/d (255).

Drug Interactions

No drug interactions have been observed.

Efficacy

Following 1 week of therapy in a single-blind, dose-escalation, add-on study of levetiracetam, there were no measurable cognitive side effects (256).

Side Effects

Levetiracetam is reportedly very well tolerated, although results of large, blinded trials are not available. In animals, toxicity is minimal, with only mild sedation at doses 50 to 100 times higher than anticonvulsant doses (254).

STIRIPENTOL

Mechanism

Stiripentol is an alcohol that is active against animal models of absence epilepsy (257).

Pharmacology

Rat gastrointestinal tract can convert the (*R*)-enantiomer of stiripentol to the (*S*)-form. The (*R*)- and (*S*)-forms are eliminated via different pathways (258,259). Chiral inversion of stiripentol is unidirectional: the (*S*)-enantiomer is converted to the (*R*)-enantiomer, but not vice versa (259). Pregnancy (in rats) does not affect the distribution or metabolism of stiripentol (260).

Drug Interactions

Stiripentol blocks cytochrome P_{450}. Stiripentol shows the intriguing potential of blocking the conversion of carbamazepine to carbamazepine epoxide. The effect takes about 7 to 10 days to develop. Carbamazepine epoxide clearance is not altered (261). This suggests that "rational polypharmacy" using the two drugs together might lead to decreased side effects. This was investigated in a monkey model by Lockard et al. (262). Stiripentol may prevent phenytoin-induced teratogenesis, as suggested by studies in a mouse model (263,264).

Efficacy

An open-label study suggested efficacy against partial seizures (265). The principal utility of the drug seems to be against absence, both typical and atypical. In an open trial, stiripentol was effective against previously resistant atypical absence in 10 children (266). Doses ranging from 1000 to 3000 mg/d led to effective serum levels ranging from 4 to 22 μg/mL. All patients improved, with an average decrease of 70% in seizure count.

Side Effects

Sedation and gastrointestinal problems seem to be the major issues. In a pediatric study of 10 patients, one discontinued because of vomiting; other patients experienced anorexia, nausea, and lethargy but did not discontinue the medication (266).

LORECLEZOLE

Loreclezole is in an early development stage (267) at Janssen Pharmaceutica.

Mechanism

Loreclezole is a triazole derivative that modulates the β-subunit of the GABA receptor, and the specific binding site has been mapped to an individual amino acid (268). Loreclezole acts to increase chloride flux. In an amygdala kindled cat model, flumazenil (a benzodiazepine antagonist) reversed the efficacy of benzodiazepines but had no effect on either loreclezole or barbiturates. Based on these findings, Ashton et al. (269) suggested that loreclezole acts more like a barbiturate than a benzodiazepine. Loreclezole increases extracellular brain serotonin in genetically epilepsy-prone rats (270). In a hippocampal slice, a low-magnesium loreclezole preparation inhibited development of epileptic bursts (271). In genetically epilepsy-prone rats, loreclezole reduced absence seizures and reduced electroencephalographic spike-and-wave discharges. There were no other behavioral changes and no changes in electroencephalographic background activity (272).

Efficacy

Preliminary studies suggest modest efficacy. In a double-blind, add-on study, 19% of patients experienced a 50% seizure reduction (273). Efficacy was preserved in long-term follow-up (274). Loreclezole may be useful in monotherapy. In nine patients who had previously responded to loreclezole as add-on therapy, Rentmeester and Hulsman (275) tapered the older anticonvulsants. Six patients tolerated the transition to monotherapy without deterioration in seizure control, with one of the six improving as other drugs were removed.

LOSIGAMONE

Losigamone is in an early stage of development, and few published human data are available (276,277).

Mechanism

The mechanism of action of losigamone is unknown.

Pharmacology

No pharmacologic data have been published for losigamone.

Interactions

Losigamone does not induce hepatic enzymes and shows no evidence of interaction with standard anticonvulsants (276).

Efficacy

In an open-label trial, patients were treated with 600 to 1800 mg of losigamone per day, producing levels of 10 to 20 μg/mL. The responder rate was 55%.

Side Effects

The principal side effects relate to the central nervous system.

REMACEMIDE

Remacemide is a novel anticonvulsant at an early stage of development (278,279).

Mechanism

Remacemide acts to inhibit rapid firing of sodium channels. Its desglycinated metabolite has similar activity and also binds at the NMDA receptor complex (280).

Pharmacology

Remacemide is hepaticaly converted to a desglycinated metabolite; both are cleared by the liver. The half-life of the parent compound is 3 to 4 hours, and the half-life of the metabolite is 12 to 19 hours (279,281).

Drug Interactions

Remacemide is a potential inducer of hepatic metabolism.

Efficacy

In a double-blind, placebo-controlled crossover study, remacemide led to a median seizure reduction of one third, and seizures were reduced by 50% in one third of patients.

Side Effects

The principal side effects in a double-blind trial were dizziness and gastrointestinal complaints; these were mild (282). In that study, there were no measurable cognitive side effects.

CLOBAZAM

Clobazam is a benzo-1,5-diazepine. It is supposedly less sedating and less habituating than the more traditional benzo-1,4-diazepines. Development in the United States has been halted because of a perceived small market and intimations by the Food and Drug Administration that benzodiazepine development is not a high priority. Clobazam is available in Canada and some other countries where it is widely used in severe childhood epilepsies. In the Canadian experience of 1300 patients, responder rates were in the 40% to 50% range (283), and in a review of all placebo-controlled trials, the responder rates were >50%, with 16% to 21% of patients becoming seizure-free (284). In a double-blind crossover study of refractory childhood epilepsy with mental retardation, clobazam produced a 52% responder rate (285). As add-on therapy in refractory partial epilepsy, it was modestly effective, and sedation was a mild problem (286). Clobazam may potentiate phenytoin toxicity (287). A major concern is development of habituation and loss of responsiveness, which occur in one third to one half of patients maintained on the drug for 1 to 6 months (288).

ETEROBARB

Eterobarb (289) has been in development for many years, as a barbiturate with purportedly less sedation than phenobarbital. Development in the United States is moving forward slowly.

A large number of drugs have fallen by the wayside and are dormant at the present time (Table 4).

SUMMARY

Between 30% and 60% of patients with epilepsy have not achieved adequate control with current medications, and side effects are a significant problem. In the past 2 years, three drugs for epilepsy have been approved. At least six more drugs are in the final stages of development, and there is an active "pipeline." None of the new drugs are panaceas, but many have special advantages and meet important specific needs. Felbamate, despite a high incidence of aplastic anemia and hepatic failure, remains useful because of its lack of sedative effects and high efficacy. Gabapentin is remarkable for its favorable side effect profile, lack of interac-

TABLE 4. *Dormant drugs*

Drug	Drug type	Reason dormant
Clobazam	1,5-benzodiazepine	Market insufficient
Dezinamide	Sodium-channel drug	Development costs
Flunarizine (291)	Calcium-channel blocker	Mild efficacy
Milacemide	Glycine agonist	Marginal efficacy (292)
MK801	NMDA antagonist	Psychosis
Nafimidone	Phenytoin-like drug	Narrow therapeutic range
Nitrazepam	Benzodiazepine	Market insufficient
ORG 6370		Anticholinergic side effects, may increase some seizures
Progabide (293)	GABA prodrug	Poor efficacy, hepatotoxic
Ralitoline (294)	Phenytoin-like drug (295)	Short half-life

tions, and straightforward kinetics. Lamotrigine is also nonsedating and may be especially useful in generalized epilepsies. Topiramate and vigabatrin are both highly effective, although each is associated with a variety of cognitive or psychiatric side effects that may limit utility. Oxcarbazepine shares the efficacy of carbamazepine, with fewer side effects or drug interactions. Zonisamide seems to be effective and cause mild side effects, although the risk for renal stones indicates a need for cautious use. Tiagabine, like gabapentin, is a mild drug with a favorable side effect profile. New forms of old drugs will make for easier administration; fosphenytoin will increase the safety of parenchymal phenytoin use. The best of the new drugs help, at most, 10% of previously uncontrolled patients to become seizure-free. The development of new drugs remains an important need.

REFERENCES

1. Mattson RH, Cramer JA, Collins JF, et al. Comparison of carbamazepine, phenobarbital, phenytoin, and primidone in partial and secondary generalized tonic-clonic seizures. *N Engl J Med* 1985;313:145–151.
2. Vickrey B. A procedure for developing a quality-of-life measure for epilepsy surgery patients. *Epilepsia* 1993;S34:13–S27.
3. Engel JJ. The progressive nature of epilepsy. In: Engel JJ, ed. *Seizures and Epilepsy*. Philadelphia: FA Davis; 1989:229–232.
4. Rausch R, Mattson RH, Cramer JA, et al. Neuropsychological and psychosocial follow-up of patients with temporal lobectomy surgery for intractable epilepsy: results at 1 year and 10 years. Comparison of carbamazepine, phenobarbital, phenytoin, and primidone in partial and secondary generalized tonic-clonic seizures. *Epilepsia* 1995;36:145–151.
5. Thakker KM, Mangat S, Garndtt WR, Levy R, Kochak GM. Comparative bioavalibility and steady-state fluctuations of Tegretol commercial and carbamazepine oros tablets in adult and pediatric epilepsy patients. *Biopharm Drug Dispos* 1992;13:559–569.
6. Leppik I, Boucher B, Wilder B, et al. Pharmacokinetics and safety of a phenytoin prodrug given i.v. or i.m. in patients. *Neurology* 1990;40:456–460.
7. Smith R, Brown B, Maher R, Matier W. Pharmacology of ACC-9653 (phenytoin prodrug). *Epilepsia* 1989; 30(Suppl 2):S15–S21.
8. Sofia RD, Kramer L, Perhach JL, Rosenberg A. Felbamate (review). *Epilepsy Res Suppl* 1991;3:103–108.
9. Wagner ML. Felbamate: a new antiepileptic drug (review). *Am J Hosp Pharm* 1994;51:1657–1666.
10. Taylor LA, McQuade RD, Tice MA. Felbamate, a novel antiepileptic drug, reverses *N*-methyl-D-aspartate/glycine-stimulated increases in intracellular Ca^{2+} concentration. *Eur J Pharmacol* 1995;289:229–233.
11. Coffin V, Cohen-Williams M, Barnett A. Selective antagonism of the anticonvulsant effects of felbamate by glycine. *Eur J Pharmacol* 1994;256:R9–R10.
12. Domenici MR, Sagratella S, Ongini E, Longo R, Scotti de Carolis A. Felbamate displays in vitro antiepileptic effects as a broad-spectrum excitatory amino acid receptor antagonist. *Eur J Pharmacol* 1994;271:259–263.
13. White HS, Harmsworth WL, Sofia RD, Wolf HH. Felbamate modulates the strychnine-insensitive glycine receptor. *Epilepsy Res* 1995;20:41–48.
14. Subramaniam S, Rho JM, Penix L, Donevan SD, Fielding RP, Rogawski MA. Felbamate block of the *N*-methyl-D-aspartate receptor. *J Pharmacol Exp Ther* 1995;273:878–886.
15. Wallis RA, Panizzon KL, Nolan JP. Glycine-induced CA1 excitotoxicity in the rat hippocampal slice. *Brain Res* 1994;664:115–125.
16. Chronopoulos A, Stafstrom C, Thurber S, Hyde P, Mikati M, Holmes GL. Neuroprotective effect of felbamate after kainic acid-induced status epilepticus. *Epilepsia* 1993;34:359–366.
17. Wallis RA, Panizzon KL, Fairchild MD, Wasterlain CG. Protective effects of felbamate against hypoxia in the rat hippocampal slice. *Stroke* 1992;23:547–551.
18. Wasterlain CG, Adams LM, Hattori H, Schwartz PH. Felbamate reduces hypoxic-ischemic brain damage in vivo. *Eur J Pharmacol* 1992;212:275–278.
19. Wallis RA, Panizzon KL. Glycine reversal of felbamate hypoxic protection. *Neuroreport* 1993;4: 951–954.
20. Wallis RA, Panizzon KL, Nolan JP. Glycine-induced CA1 excitotoxicity in the rat hippocampal slice (corrected and republished in *Brain Res* 1995 Jul 10;685: 115–125). *Brain Res* 1994;664:115–125.
21. Rho JM, Donevan SD, Rogawski MA. Mechanism of action of the anticonvulsant felbamate: opposing effects on *N*-methyl-D-aspartate and gamma-aminobutyric acid A receptors (see comments). *Ann Neurol* 1994;35:229–234.
22. Greenfield LJ, Kume A, Albin RL, Macdonald RL. Felbamate inhibits [^{3}H]butylbicyclo-orthobenzoate (TBOB) binding and enhances chloride current at $GABA_A$ receptors. *Epilepsia* 1995;36(Suppl 4):S48.
23. Serra M, Ghiani CA, Spano S, Biggio G. Felbamate antagonizes isoniazid- and FG 7142-induced reduction of $GABA_A$ receptor function in mouse brain. *Eur J Pharmacol* 1994;265:185–188.
24. Annesley TM, Clayton LT. Determination of felbamate in human serum by high-performance liquid chromatography. *Ther Drug Monit* 1994;16:419–424.
25. Poquette MA. Isothermal gas chromatographic method for the rapid determination of felbamate concentration in human serum. *Ther Drug Monit* 1995;17: 168–173.
26. Graves N, Holmes G, Fuerst R, Leppik I. Effect of felbamate on phenytoin and carbamazepine serum concentrations. *Epilepsia* 1989;30:225–229.
27. Gidal BE, Zupanc ML. Potential pharmacokinetic interaction between felbamate and phenobarbital. *Ann Pharmacother* 1994;28:455–458.

28. Wagner ML, Graves NM, Leppik IE, et al. The effect of felbamate on valproic acid disposition. *Clin Pharmacol Ther* 1994;56:494–502.
29. Wagner ML, Remmel RP, Graves NM, Leppik IE. Effect of felbamate on carbamazepine and its major metabolites. *Clin Pharmacol Ther* 1993;53:536–543.
30. Tisdel KA, Israel DS, Kolb KW. Warfarin-felbamate interaction: first report (letter). *Ann Pharmacother* 1994;28:805.
31. Glue P, Banfield CR, Colucci RD, Perhach JL. Comment: warfarin-felbamate interaction (letter). *Ann Pharmacother* 1994;28:1412–1413.
32. Sachdeo R, Kramer LD, Rosenberg A, Sachdeo S. Felbamate monotherapy: controlled trial in patients with partial-onset seizures (see comments). *Ann Neurol* 1992;32:386–392.
33. Bourgeois B, Leppik IE, Sackellares JC, et al. Felbamate: a double-blind controlled trial in patients undergoing presurgical evaluation of partial seizures. *Neurology* 1993;43:693–696.
34. Leppik IE, Dreifuss FE, Pledger GW, et al. Felbamate for partial seizures: results of a controlled clinical trial. *Neurology* 1991;41:1785–1789.
35. Anonymous. Efficacy of felbamate in childhood epileptic encephalopathy (Lennox-Gastaut syndrome). The Felbamate Study Group in Lennox-Gastaut Syndrome (see comments). *N Engl J Med* 1993;328:29–33.
36. Jensen PK. Felbamate in the treatment of Lennox-Gastaut syndrome. *Epilepsia* 1994;35(Suppl 5):S54–S57.
37. Carmant L, Holmes GL, Sawyer S, Rifai N, Anderson J, Mikati MA. Efficacy of felbamate in therapy for partial epilepsy in children. *J Pediatr* 1994;125:481–486.
38. Hurst DL, Rolan TD. The use of felbamate to treat infantile spasms. *J Child Neurol* 1995;10:134–136.
39. Glauser TA, Olberding LS, Titanic MK, Piccirillo DM. Felbamate in the treatment of acquired epileptic aphasia. *Epilepsy Res* 1995;20:85–89.
40. Bourgeois BF. Felbamate in the treatment of partial-onset seizures (review). *Epilepsia* 1994;35(Suppl 5):S58–S61.
41. Hill RR, Stagno SJ, Tesar GE. Secondary mania associated with the use of felbamate. *Psychosomatics* 1995;36:404–406.
42. Pennell PB, Ogaily MS, Macdonald RL. Aplastic anemia in a patient receiving felbamate for complex partial seizures. *Neurology* 1995;45(3 Pt 1):456–460.
43. Wallace Laboratories. *Felbamate-Induced Hepatic Failure*. 1995.
44. Anonymous. Acute liver failure linked to felbamate use (news). *Am J Hosp Pharm* 1994;51:2882.
45. Chadwick D. Gabapentin. *Epilepsy Res Suppl* 1991;3:183–186.
46. Chadwick D. Gabapentin (review; see comments). *Lancet* 1994;343:89–91.
47. Foot M, Wallace J. Gabapentin (review). *Epilepsy Res Suppl* 1991;3:109–114.
48. Ramsay RE. Clinical efficacy and safety of gabapentin (review). *Neurology* 1994;44(6 Suppl 5):S23–S30.
49. Su TZ, Lunney E, Campbell G, Oxender DL. Transport of gabapentin, a gamma-amino acid drug, by system L-alpha-amino acid transporters: a comparative study in astrocytes, synaptosomes, and CHO cells. *J Neurochem* 1995;64:2125–2131.
50. Honmou O, Kocsis JD, Richerson GB. Gabapentin potentiates the conductance increase induced by nipecotic acid in CA1 pyramidal neurons in vitro. *Epilepsy Res* 1995;20:193–202.
51. Petroff OAC, Rothman KL, Behar KL, Lamoureux D, Mattson RH. Gabapentin increases GABA in human brain. *Epilepsia* 1995;36(Suppl 4):S89.
52. Petroff OAC, Rothman DL, Behar KL, Lamoureux D, Mattson RH. The effect of gabapentin on brain gamma-aminobutyric acid in patients with epilepsy. *Ann Neurol* 1996;39:95–99.
53. Lensmeyer GL, Kempf T, Gidal BE, Wiebe DA. Optimized method for determination of gabapentin in serum by high-performance liquid chromatography. *Ther Drug Monit* 1995;17:251–258.
54. Andrews CO, Fischer JH. Gabapentin: a new agent for the management of epilepsy (review). *Ann Pharmacother* 1994;28:1188–1196.
55. McLean MJ. Clinical pharmacokinetics of gabapentin (review). *Neurology* 1994;44(6 Suppl 5):S17–S22.
56. Blum RA, Comstock TJ, Sica DA, et al. Pharmacokinetics of gabapentin in subjects with various degrees of renal function. *Clin Pharmacol Ther* 1994;56:154–159.
57. Wong MO, Eldon MA, Keane WF, et al. Disposition of gabapentin in anuric subjects on hemodialysis. *J Clin Pharmacol* 1995;35:622–626.
58. Anhut H, Ashman P, Feuerstein TJ, Sauermann W, Saunders M, Schmidt B. Gabapentin (Neurontin) as add-on therapy in patients with partial seizures: a double-blind, placebo-controlled study. The International Gabapentin Study Group. *Epilepsia* 1994;35:795–801.
59. Sivenius J, Kalviainen R, Ylinen A, Riekkinen P. Double-blind study of gabapentin in the treatment of partial seizures. *Epilepsia* 1991;32:539–542.
60. Anonymous. The long-term safety and efficacy of gabapentin (Neurontin) as add-on therapy in drug-resistant partial epilepsy. The U.S. Gabapentin Study Group. *Epilepsy Res* 1994;18:67–73.
61. Sivenius J, Ylinen A, Kalviainen R, Riekkinen PJ, Sr. Long-term study with gabapentin in patients with drug-resistant epileptic seizures. *Arch Neurol* 1994;51:1047–1050.
62. Anhut H, Greiner MJ, Murray GH, the International GBP Monotherapy Study Group 94577/78. Double-blind, fixed-dose comparison study of gabapentin and carbamazepine monotherapy in newly diagnosed partial epilepsy. *Epilepsia* 1995;36(Suppl 4):S67.
63. Handforth A, Treiman DM. Efficacy and tolerance of long-term, high-dose gabapentin: additional observations. *Epilepsia* 1994;35:1032–1037.
64. Hayes AF, Garofalo EA, Greeley CA, et al. A double-blind, multicenter study of gabapentin monotherapy in patients with medically refractory partial seizures. *Epilepsia* 1995;36(Suppl 4):S89.
65. Ojemann LM, Wilensky AJ, Temkin NR, Chmelir T, Ricker BA, Wallace J. Long-term treatment with gabapentin for partial epilepsy. *Epilepsy Res* 1992;13:159–165.
66. Fromm GH. Gabapentin: discussion (review). *Epilepsia* 1994;35(Suppl 5):S77–S80.
67. Tatum WO 4th, Zachariah SB. Gabapentin treatment of seizures in acute intermittent porphyria. *Neurology* 1995;45:1216–1217.
68. Krauss GL, Simmons-O'Brien E, Campbell M. Suc-

cessful treatment of seizures and porphyria with gabapentin. *Neurology* 1995;45(3 Pt 1):594–595.
69. Mellick LB, Mellick GA. Successful treatment of reflex sympathetic dystrophy with gabapentin (letter). *Am J Emerg Med* 1995;13:96.
70. Asconape J, Collins T. Weight gain associated with the use of gabapentin. *Epilepsia* 1995;36(Suppl 4):S72.
71. Shantz D, Towbin JA, Spitz MC. Changes in mood and affect in patients on gabapentin. *Epilepsia* 1995; 36(Suppl 4):S73.
72. Short C, Cooke L. Hypomania induced by gabapentin (letter). *Br J Psychiatry* 1995;166:679–680.
73. King J, Bayles R. Weight gain during add-on therapy using gabapentin. *Epilepsia* 1995;36(Suppl 4):S72.
74. Leiderman DB. Gabapentin as add-on therapy for refractory partial epilepsy: results of five placebo-controlled trials. *Epilepsia* 1994;35(Suppl 5):S74–S76.
75. Fischer JH, Barr AN, Rogers SL, Fischer PA, Trudeau VL. Lack of serious toxicity following gabapentin overdose. *Neurology* 1994;44:982–983.
76. Sigler RE, Gough AW, de la Iglesia FA. Pancreatic acinar cell neoplasia in male Wistar rats following 2 years of gabapentin exposure. *Toxicology* 1995;98:73–82.
77. Pellock JM. The clinical efficacy of lamotrigine as an antiepileptic drug (review). *Neurology* 1994;44(11 Suppl 8):S29–S35.
78. Meldrum BS. Lamotrigine—a novel approach (review). *Seizure* 1994;3(Suppl A):41–45.
79. Cheung H, Kamp D, Harris E. An in vitro investigation of the action of lamotrigine on neuronal voltage-activated sodium channels. *Epilepsy Res* 1992;13: 107–112.
80. Burstein AH. Lamotrigine (review). *Pharmacotherapy* 1995;15:129–143.
81. Lizasoain I, Knowles RG, Moncada S. Inhibition by lamotrigine of the generation of nitric oxide in rat forebrain slices. *J Neurochem* 1995;64:636–642.
82. Smith SE, Meldrum BS. Cerebroprotective effect of lamotrigine after focal ischemia in rats. *Stroke* 1995; 26:117–121.
83. Wiard RP, Dickerson MC, Beek O, Norton R, Cooper BR. Neuroprotective properties of the novel antiepileptic lamotrigine in a gerbil model of global cerebral ischemia. *Stroke* 1995;26:466–472.
84. Sander JW, Patsalos PN. An assessment of serum and red blood cell folate concentrations in patients with epilepsy on lamotrigine therapy. *Epilepsy Res* 1992; 13:89–92.
85. Fraser AD, MacNeil W, Isner AF, Camfield PR. Lamotrigine analysis in serum by high-performance liquid chromatography. *Ther Drug Monit* 1995;17:174–178.
86. Ramsay R, Pellock J, Garnett W, et al. Pharmacokinetics and safety of lamotrigine (Lamictal) in patients with epilepsy. *Epilepsy Res* 1991;10:191–200.
87. Yuen AW, Land G, Weatherley BC, Peck AW. Sodium valproate acutely inhibits lamotrigine metabolism. *Br J Clin Pharmacol* 1992;33:511–513.
88. Ferrie CD, Panayiotopoulos CP. Therapeutic interaction of lamotrigine and sodium valproate in intractable myoclonic epilepsy. *Seizure* 1994;3:157–159.
89. Stolarek I, Blacklaw J, Forrest G, Brodie MJ. Vigabatrin and lamotrigine in refractory epilepsy. *J Neurol Neurosurg Psychiatry* 1994;57:921–924.
90. Rambeck B, Wolf P. Lamotrigine clinical pharmacokinetics (review). *Clin Pharmacokinet* 1993;25:433–443.
91. Pisani F, Xiao B, Fazio A, Spina E, Perucca E, Tomson T. Single-dose pharmacokinetics of carbamazepine-10,11-epoxide in patients on lamotrigine monotherapy. *Epilepsy Res* 1994;19:245–248.
92. Warner T, Patsalos PN, Prevett M, Elyas AA, Duncan JS. Lamotrigine-induced carbamazepine toxicity: an interaction with carbamazepine-10,11-epoxide. *Epilepsy Res* 1992;11:147–150.
93. Brodie MJ. Lamotrigine—an update. *Can J Neurol Sci* 1996;23:56–9.
94. Depot M, Powell JR, Messenheimer JA, Cloutier G, Dalton MJ. Kinetic effects of multiple oral doses of acetominophen on a single oral dose of lamotrigine. *Clin Pharmacol Ther* 1990;48:346–355.
95. Yuen AW. Lamotrigine: a review of antiepileptic efficacy (review). *Epilepsia* 1994;35(Suppl 5):S33–S36.
96. Messenheimer J, Ramsay RE, Willmore LJ, et al. Lamotrigine therapy for partial seizures: a multicenter, placebo-controlled, double-blind, crossover trial. *Epilepsia* 1994;35:113–121.
97. Schapel GJ, Beran RG, Vajda FJ, et al. Double-blind, placebo controlled, crossover study of lamotrigine in treatment-resistant partial seizures. *J Neurol Neurosurg Psychiatry* 1993;56:448–453.
98. Martin PJ, Millac PA. Impact of lamotrigine on patients with refractory epilepsy: the Leicester experience. *Seizure* 1994;3:209–213.
99. Brodie MJ, Richens A, Yuen AW. Double-blind comparison of lamotrigine and carbamazepine in newly diagnosed epilepsy. UK Lamotrigine/Carbamazepine Monotherapy Trial Group (published erratum appears in *Lancet* 1995 Mar 11;345:662; see comments). *Lancet* 1995;345:476–479.
100. Pisani F, Russo M, Trio R, et al. Lamotrigine in refractory epilepsy: a long-term open study. *Epilepsy Res Suppl* 1991;3:187–191.
101. Schlumberger E, Chavez F, Palacios L, Rey E, Pajot N, Dulac O. Lamotrigine in treatment of 120 children with epilepsy. *Epilepsia* 1994;35:359–367.
102. Ferrie CD, Robinson RO, Knott C, Panayiotopoulos CP. Lamotrigine as an add-on drug in typical absence seizures. *Acta Neurol Scand* 1995;91:200–202.
103. Philbrook B, Martinez OA, Callerame KJ, Toledo C, Gonzalez JG, Ramsey RE. Efficacy of lamotrigine in patients with primary generalized epilepsy: a retrospective study. *Epilepsia* 1995;36(Suppl 4):S66.
104. Wallace SJ. Lamotrigine—a clinical overview (review). *Seizure* 1994;3(Suppl A):47–51.
105. Veggiotti P, Cieuta C, Rex E, Dulac O. Lamotrigine in infantile spasms (letter). *Lancet* 1994;344:1375–1376.
106. Uldall P, Hansen FJ, Tonnby B. Lamotrigine in Rett syndrome. *Neuropediatrics* 1993;24:339–340.
107. Richens A. Safety of lamotrigine (review). *Epilepsia* 1994;35(Suppl 5):S37–S40.
108. Gilman JT. Lamotrigine: an antiepileptic agent for the treatment of partial seizures (review; see comments). *Ann Pharmacother* 1995;29:144–151.
109. Tavernor SJ, Wong IC, Newton R, Brown SW. Rechallenge with lamotrigine after initial rash. *Seizure* 1995; 4:67–71.
110. Peck AW. Clinical pharmacology of lamotrigine (review). *Epilepsia* 1991;32(Suppl 2):S9–S12.
111. Nakamura J, Tamura S, Kanda T, et al. Inhibition by topiramate of seizures in spontaneously epileptic rats and DBA/2 mice. *Eur J Pharmacol* 1994;254:83–89.

112. Nakamura F, Hiyoshi T, Kudo T, Yagi K, Seino M. Anticonvulsant effect of topiramate [2,3:4,5-bis-*O*-(1-methylethylidene)-beta-D-fructopyranose sulfamate] on amygdaloid kindled seizures in the cat. *Jpn J Psychiatry Neurol* 1993;47:394–395.
113. Severt L, Coulter DA, Somati S, DeLoernzo RJ. Topiramate selectively blocks kainate currents in cultured hippocampal neurons. *Epilepsia* 1995;36(Suppl 4): S38.
114. Gordey M, Delorey TM, Olsen RW. Topiramate modulates GABA receptor responses in *Xenopus* oocytes expressing several recombinant receptor subunit combinations. *Epilepsia* 1995;36(Suppl 4):S48.
115. Ben-Menachem E, Dam M, Mikkelsen M, et al. Topiramate add-on treatment in patients with intractable partial epilepsy: a multicenter study. *Epilepsia* 1993; 34:109.
116. EspeLillo J, Ritter F, Frost MD, Spiegel RH, Reiffe R. Topiramate in childhood epilepsy: titration, adverse events, and efficacy in multiple seizure types. *Epilepsia* 1995;36(Suppl 4):S56.
117. Faught E, Wilder BJ, Ramsey RE, et al. Topiramate dose-ranging trial in refractory parital epilepsy. *Epilepsia* 1995;36(Suppl 4):S33.
118. Privatera M, Fincham R, Penry JK, et al. Dose-ranging trial with higher doses of topiramate in patients with resistant partial seizures. *Epilepsia* 1995;36(Suppl 4):S33.
119. Sachdeo SK, Sachdeo RC, Reiffe RA, Lim P, Pledger G. Topiramate: double-blind trial as monotherapy. *Epilepsia* 1995;36(Suppl 4):S33.
120. Reiff RA, Lim P, Pledger G. Topiramate: side effect profile in double-blind studies. *Epilepsia* 1995; 36(Suppl 4):S34.
121. Michelucci R, Tassinari CA. Vigabatrin. *Epilepsy Res Suppl* 1991;3:193–196.
122. Mumford JP, Lewis PJ. Vigabatrin (review). *Epilepsy Res Suppl* 1991;3:161–168.
123. Mattson RH, Petroff O, Rothman D, Behar K. Vigabatrin: effects on human brain GABA levels by nuclear magnetic resonance spectroscopy (review). *Epilepsia* 1994;35(Suppl 5):S29–S32.
124. Preece NE, Jackson GD, Houseman JA, Duncan JS, Williams SR. Nuclear magnetic resonance detection of increased cortical GABA in vigabatrin-treated rats in vivo. *Epilepsia* 1994;35:431–436.
125. Petroff OA, Rothman DL, Behar KL, Mattson RH. Initial observations on effect of vigabatrin on in vivo ^{1}H spectroscopic measurements of gamma-aminobutyric acid, glutamate, and glutamine in human brain. *Epilepsia* 1995;36:457–464.
126. Löscher W, Horstermann D. Differential effects of vigabatrin, gamma-acetylenic GABA, amino-oxyacetic acid, and valproate on levels of various amino acids in rat brain regions and plasma. *Naunyn Schmiedebergs Arch Pharmacol* 1994;349:270–278.
127. Foletti GB, Delisle MC, Bachmann C. Reduction of plasma alanine aminotransferase during vigabatrin treatment. *Epilepsia* 1995;36:804–809.
128. Rey E, Pons G, Olive G. Vigabatrin. Clinical pharmacokinetics (review). *Clin Pharmacokinet* 1992;23: 267–278.
129. Connelly JF. Vigabatrin (review). *Ann Pharmacother* 1993;27:197–204.
130. French JA, Mosier M., Walker S, Sommerville K, Sussman N, Vigabatrin protocol 024 investigators cohort. A double-blind, placebo-controlled study of gabapentin 3 g/day in patients with uncontrolled complex partial seizures. *Neurology* 1996;46:54–61.
131. Ylinen A, Sivenius J, Pitkanen A, et al. Gamma-vinyl GABA (vigabatrin) in epilepsy: clinical, neurochemical, and neurophysiologic monitoring in epileptic patients. *Epilepsia* 1992;33:917–922.
132. Buchanan N. Vigabatrin use in 72 patients with drug-resistant epilepsy. *Seizure* 1994;3:191–196.
133. Martin PJ, Millac PA. Vigabatrin: a 3-year clinical analysis. *Seizure* 1993;2:137–140.
134. Kalviainen R, Aikia M, Partanen J, et al. Randomized controlled pilot study of vigabatrin versus carbamazepine monotherapy in newly diagnosed patients with epilepsy: an interim report. *J Child Neurol* 1991; 2(Suppl 2):S60–S69.
135. Grunewald RA, Thompson PJ, Corcoran R, Corden Z, Jackson GD, Duncan JS. Effects of vigabatrin on partial seizures and cognitive function. *J Neurol Neurosurg Psychiatry* 1994;57:1057–1063.
136. Cocito L, Maffini M, Loeb C. Vigabatrin in chronic epilepsy: a 7-year follow-up study of responder patients. *Seizure* 1993;2:301–307.
137. French JA, Brodie MA, Dollar L, The Vigabatrin 024 and 025 Study Group. Long-term follow-up of partial seizure patients treated with vigabattrin. *Epilepsia* 1995;36(Suppl 4):S32.
138. Tartara A, Manni R, Galimberti CA, et al. Six-year follow-up study on the efficacy and safety of vigabatrin in patients with epilepsy. *Acta Neurol Scand* 1992;86: 247–251.
139. Schmitt B, Wohlrab G, Boltshauser E. Vigabatrin in newly diagnosed infantile spasms (letter; review). *Neuropediatrics* 1994;25:54.
140. Feucht M, Brantner-Inthaler S. Gamma-vinyl-GABA (vigabatrin) in the therapy of Lennox-Gastaut syndrome: an open study. *Epilepsia* 1994;35:993–998.
141. Appleton RE, Nicolaides P, Montiel Viesca F. Vigabatrin monotherapy for infantile spasms. *Epilepsia* 1995; 36(Suppl 4):S32.
142. Gram L, Sabers A, Dulac O. Treatment of pediatric epilepsies with gamma-vinyl GABA (vigabatrin). *Epilepsia* 1992;33(Suppl 5):S26–S29.
143. Aicardi J. Vigabatrin as first-line monotherapy in infantile spasms. *Epilepsia* 1995;36(Suppl 4):S32.
144. Curatolo P. Vigabatrin for refractory partial seizures in children with tuberous sclerosis (letter). *Neuropediatrics* 1994;25:55.
145. Baxter PS, Gardner-Medwin D, Barwick DD, Ince P, Livingston J, Murdoch-Eaton D. Vigabatrin monotherapy in resistant neonatal seizures. *Seizure* 1995;4: 57–59.
146. Reynolds EH. Gamma-vinyl GABA (vigabatrin): clinical experience in adult and adolescent patients with intractable epilepsy (review). *Epilepsia* 1992;33(Suppl 5):S30–S34.
147. Arteaga R, Herranz JL, Valdizan EM, Armijo JA. Gamma-vinyl GABA (vigabatrin): relationship between dosage, plasma concentrations, platelet GABA-transaminase inhibition, and seizure reduction in epileptic children. *Epilepsia* 1992;33:923–931.
148. O'Neill BA, Trimble MR, Bloom DS. Adjunctive therapy in epilepsy: a cost-effectiveness comparison of alternative treatment options (review). *Seizure* 1995;4: 37–44.

149. Fisher RS, Kerrigan JF. Vigabatrin toxicity. In: Levy RH, Mattson RH, Meldrum BS, eds. *Antiepileptic Drugs*. 4th ed. New York: Raven Press; 1995:931–940.
150. Jongsma MJ, Laan LA, van Emde Boas W, Meinardi H. Reversible motor disturbances induced by vigabatrin (letter). *Lancet* 1991;338:893.
151. Marciani MG, Maschio M, Spanedda F, Iani C, Gigli GL, Bernardi G. Development of myoclonus in patients with partial epilepsy during treatment with vigabatrin: an electroencephalographic study. *Acta Neurol Scand* 1995;91:1–5.
152. Lortie A, Chiron C, Mumford J, Dulac O. The potential for increasing seizure frequency, relapse, and appearance of new seizure types with vigabatrin (review). *Neurology* 1993;43(11 Suppl 5):S24–S27.
153. Rogers D, Bird J, Eames P. Complex partial status after starting vigabatrin (see comments). *Seizure* 1993;2: 155–156.
154. de Krom MC, Verduin N, Visser E, Kleijer M, Scholtes F, De Groen JH. Status epilepticus during vigabatrin treatment: a report of three cases. *Seizure* 1995;4: 159–162.
155. Appleton RE. Vigabatrin in the management of generalized seizures in children (review). *Seizure* 1995;4: 45–48.
156. Aldenkamp AP, Vermeulen J, Mulder OG, et al. Gamma-vinyl GABA (vigabatrin) and mood disturbances. *Epilepsia* 1994;35:999–1004.
157. Ring HA, Crellin R, Kirker S, Reynolds EH. Vigabatrin and depression. *J Neurol Neurosurg Psychiatry* 1993;56:925–928.
158. Trimble MR. *The Psychosis of Epilepsy*. New York: Raven Press; 1991:109–135.
159. Ferrie CD, Robinson RO, Panayiotopolos CP. Psychotic and severe behavioral reactions with vigabatrin. *Acta Neurologica Scand*, 1996;93:1–8.
160. Levinson DF, Mumford JP, Devinsky O. Vigabatrin and psychosis. *Epilepsia* 1995;36(Suppl 4):S32.
161. Sander JW, Hart YM, Trimble MR, Shorvon SD. Vigabatrin and psychosis. *J Neurol Neurosurg Psychiatry* 1991;54:435–439.
162. Naumann M, Supprian T, Kornhuber J, Lange KW, Reiners K. Bipolar affective psychosis after vigabatrin (letter). *Lancet* 1994;343:606–607.
163. Dodrill CB, Arnett JL, Sommerville KW, Sussman NM. Effects of differing dosages of vigabatrin (Sabril) on cognitive abilities and quality of life in epilepsy. *Epilepsia* 1995;36:164–173.
164. McGuire AM, Duncan JS, Trimble MR. Effects of vigabatrin on cognitive function and mood when used as add-on therapy in patients with intractable epilepsy. *Epilepsia* 1992;33:128–134.
165. Aikia M, Kalviainen R, Sivenius J, Halonen T, Riekkinen P. Cognitive effects of oxcarbazepine and phenytoin monotherapy in newly diagnosed epilepsy: 1-year follow-up. *Epilepsy Res* 1992;11:199–203.
166. Pitkanen A, Ylinen A, Matilainen R, et al. Long-term antiepileptic efficacy of vigabatrin in drug-refractory epilepsy in mentally retarded patients. A 5-year follow-up study. *Arch Neurol* 1993;50:24–29.
167. Peyster RG, Sussman NM, Hershey BL, et al. Use of ex vivo magnetic resonance imaging to detect onset of vigabatrin-induced intramyelinic edema in canine brain. *Epilepsia* 1995;36:93–100.
168. Weiss KL, Schroeder CE, Kastin SJ, et al. MRI monitoring of vigabatrin-induced intramyelinic edema in dogs. *Neurology* 1994;44:1944–1949.
169. Jackson GD, Williams SR, Weller RO, et al. Vigabatrin-induced lesions in the rat brain demonstrated by quantitative magnetic resonance imaging. *Epilepsy Res* 1994;18:57–66.
170. Jackson GD, Grunewald RA, Connelly A, Duncan JS. Quantitative MR relaxometry study of effects of vigabatrin on the brains of patients with epilepsy. *Epilepsy Res* 1994;18:127–137.
171. Schroeder CE, Gibson JP, Yarrington J, Heydorn WE, Sussman NM, Arezzo JC. Effects of high-dose gamma-vinyl GABA (vigabatrin) administration on visual and somatosensory evoked potentials in dogs. *Epilepsia* 1992;33(Suppl 5):S13–S25.
172. Hammond EJ, Rangel RJ, Wilder BJ. Evoked potential monitoring of vigabatrin patients. *Br J Clin Pract Symp Suppl* 1988;61:16–23.
173. Hammond EJ, Ballinger WE Jr, Lu L, Wilder BJ, Uthman BM, Reid SA. Absence of cortical white matter changes in three patients undergoing long-term vigabatrin therapy. *Epilepsy Res* 1992;12:261–265.
174. Sivenius J, Paljarvi L, Vapalahti M, Nousiainen U, Riekkinen P. Vigabatrin (gamma-vinyl-GABA): neuropathologic evaluation in five patients. *Epilepsia* 1993;34:193–196.
175. Agosti R, Yasargil G, Egli M, Wieser H, Wiestler O. Neuropathology of a human hippocampus following long-term treatment with vigabatrin: lack of microvacuoles. *Epilepsy Res* 1990;6:166–170.
176. Seino M, Miyazaki H, Ito T. Zonisamide (review). *Epilepsy Res Suppl* 1991;3:169–174.
177. Masuda Y, Karasawa T. Inhibitory effect of zonisamide on human carbonic anhydrase in vitro. *Arzneimittelforschung* 1993;43:416–418.
178. Masuda Y, Noguchi H, Karasawa T. Evidence against a significant implication of carbonic anhydrase inhibitory activity of zonisamide in its anticonvulsive effects. *Arzneimittelforschung* 1994;44:267–269.
179. Suzuki S, Kawakami K, Nishimura S, et al. Zonisamide blocks T-type calcium channel in cultured neurons of rat cerebral cortex. *Epilepsy Res* 1992;12: 21–27.
180. Mimaki T, Suzuki Y, Tagawa T, Karasawa T, Yabuuchi H. Interaction of zonisamide with benzodiazepine and GABA receptors in rat brain. *Med J Osaka Univ* 1990; 39:13–17.
181. Mimaki T, Suzuki Y, Tagawa T, Karasawa T, Yabuuchi H. [^{3}H]Zonisamide binding in rat brain. *Med J Osaka Univ* 1990;39:19–22.
182. Hayakawa T, Higuchi Y, Nigami H, Hattori H. Zonisamide reduces hypoxic-ischemic brain damage in neonatal rats irrespective of its anticonvulsive effect. *Eur J Pharmacol* 1994;257:131–136.
183. Nishiguchi K, Ohnishi N, Iwakawa S, et al. Pharmacokinetics of zonisamide: saturable distribution into human and rat erythrocytes and into rat brain. *J Pharmacobiodynamics* 1992;15:409–415.
184. Furuno K, Oishi R, Gomita Y, Eto K. Simple and sensitive assay of zonisamide in human serum by high-performance liquid chromatography using a solid-phase extraction technique. *J Chromatogr B Biomed Appl* 1994;656:456–459.
185. Peters DH, Sorkin EM. Zonisamide. A review of its pharmacodynamic and pharmacokinetic properties,

and therapeutic potential in epilepsy (review). *Drugs* 1993;45:760–787.
186. Kimura M, Tanaka N, Kimura Y, Miyake K, Kitaura T, Fukuchi H. Pharmacokinetic interaction of zonisamide in rats. Effect of other antiepileptics on zonisamide. *J Pharmacobiodynamics* 1992;15:631–639.
187. Minami T, Ieiri I, Ohtsubo K, et al. Influence of additional therapy with zonisamide (Excegran) on protein binding and metabolism of carbamazepine. *Epilepsia* 1994;35:1023–1025.
188. Leppik IE, Willmore LJ, Homan RW, et al. Efficacy and safety of zonisamide: results of a multicenter study. *Epilepsy Res* 1993;14:165–173.
189. Kumagai N, Seki T, Yamawaki H, et al. Monotherapy for childhood epilepsies with zonisamide. *Jpn J Psychiatry Neurol* 1991;45:357–359.
190. Schmidt D, Jacob R, Loiseau P, et al. Zonisamide for add-on treatment of refractory partial epilepsy: a European double-blind trial. *Epilepsy Res* 1993;15: 67–73.
191. Kotani H, Hirai K, Nishiki T, et al. Zonisamide monotherapy against absence attacks: report of two cases (in Japanese). *No to Hattatsu (Brain and Development)* 1994;26:349–354.
192. Henry T, Leppik I, Gumnit R, Jacobs M. Progressive myoclonus epilepsy treated with zonisamide. *Neurology* 1988;38:928–931.
193. Kanba S, Yagi G, Kamijima K, et al. The first open study of zonisamide, a novel anticonvulsant, shows efficacy in mania. *Prog Neuropsychopharmacol Biol Psychiatry* 1994;18:707–715.
194. Kimura S. Zonisamide-induced behavior disorder in two children. *Epilepsia* 1994;35:403–405.
195. Jensen PK, Gram L, Schmutz M. Oxcarbazepine (review). *Epilepsy Res Suppl* 1991;3:135–140.
196. Grant SM, Faulds D. Oxcarbazepine. A review of its pharmacology and therapeutic potential in epilepsy, trigeminal neuralgia and affective disorders (review). *Drugs* 1992;43:873–888.
197. Wamil AW, Schmutz M, Portet C, Feldmann KF, McLean MJ. Effects of oxcarbazepine and 10-hydroxycarbamazepine on action potential firing and generalized seizures. *Eur J Pharmacol* 1994;271:301–308.
198. Schmutz M, Brugger F, Gentsch C, McLean MJ, Olpe HR. Oxcarbazepine: preclinical anticonvulsant profile and putative mechanisms of action. *Epilepsia* 1994; 35(Suppl 5):S47–S50.
199. McLean MJ, Schmutz M, Wamil AW, Olpe HR, Portet C, Feldmann KF. Oxcarbazepine: mechanisms of action (review). *Epilepsia* 1994;35(Suppl 3):S5–S9.
200. Lloyd P, Flesch G, Dieterle W. Clinical pharmacology and pharmacokinetics of oxcarbazepine (review). *Epilepsia* 1994;35(Suppl 3):S10–S13.
201. Rouan MC, Lecaillon JB, Godbillon J, et al. The effect of renal impairment on the pharmacokinetics of oxcarbazepine and its metabolites. *Eur J Clin Pharmacol* 1994;47:161–167.
202. Schwabe S. Oxcarbazepine: clinical development program. *Epilepsia* 1994;35(Suppl 5):S51–S53.
203. Dam M, Ekberg R, Loyning Y, Waltimo O, Jakobson K. A double-blind study comparing oxcarbazepine and carbamazepine in patients with newly diagnosed previously untreated epilepsy. *Epilepsy Res* 1989;3: 70–76.
204. Degen PH, Flesch G, Cardot JM, Czendlik C, Dieterle W. The influence of food on the disposition of the antiepileptic oxcarbazepine and its major metabolites in healthy volunteers. *Biopharm Drug Dispos* 1994; 15:519–526.
205. Dam M. Practical aspects of oxcarbazepine treatment. *Epilepsia* 1994;35(Suppl 3):S23–S25.
206. McKee PJ, Blacklaw J, Forrest G, et al. A double-blind, placebo-controlled interaction study between oxcarbazepine and carbamazepine, sodium valproate, and phenytoin in epileptic patients. *Br J Clin Pharmacol* 1994;37:27–32.
207. Isojarvi JI, Pakarinen AJ, Rautio A, Pelkonen O, Myllyla VV. Liver enzyme induction and serum lipid levels after replacement of carbamazepine with oxcarbazepine. *Epilepsia* 1994;35:1217–1220.
208. Isojarvi JI, Airaksinen KE, Mustonen JN, et al. Thyroid and myocardial function after replacement of carbamazepine by oxcarbazepine. *Epilepsia* 1995;36: 810–816.
209. Isojarvi JI, Pakarinen AJ, Rautio A, Pelkonen O, Myllyla VV. Serum sex hormone levels after replacing carbamazepine with oxcarbazepine. *Eur J Clin Pharmacol* 1995;47:461–464.
210. Raitasuo V, Lehtovaara R, Huttunen MO. Effect of switching carbamazepine to oxcarbazepine on the plasma levels of neuroleptics. A case report. *Psychopharmacology* 1994;116:115–116.
211. Baruzzi A, Albani F, Riva R. Oxcarbazepine: pharmacokinetic interactions and their clinical relevance (review). *Epilepsia* 1994;35(Suppl 3):S14–S19.
212. Kramer G, Tettenborn B, Klosterskov-Jensen P, Menge GP, Stoll KD. Oxcarbazepine does not affect the anticoagulant activity of warfarin. *Epilepsia* 1992;33: 1145–1148.
213. Keranen T, Jolkkonen J, Klosterskov-Jensen P, Menge GP. Oxcarbazepine does not interact with cimetidine in healthy volunteers. *Acta Neurol Scand* 1992;85: 239–242.
214. Keranen T, Jolkkonen J, Jensen PK, Menge GP, Andersson P. Absence of interaction between oxcarbazepine and erythromycin. *Acta Neurol Scand* 1992;86: 120–123.
215. Klosterskov-Jensen P, Saano V, Haring P, Svenstrup B, Menge GP. Possible interaction between oxcarbazepine and an oral contraceptive. *Epilepsia* 1992;33: 1149–1152.
216. Schwabe S. Clinical development outlook of oxcarbazepine. *Epilepsia* 1994;35(Suppl 3):S2–S4.
217. Aikia M, Kalviainen R, Sivenius J, Halonen T, Riekkinen PJ. Cognitive effects of oxcarbazepine and phenytoin monotherapy in newly diagnosed epilepsy: 1-year follow-up. *Epilepsy Res* 1992;11:199–203.
218. Reinikainen K, Keranen T, Halonen T, Komulainen H, Riekkinen P. Comparison of oxcarbazepine and carbamazepine: a double-blind study. *Epilepsy Res* 1987;1: 284–289.
219. Van Parys JA, Meinardi H. Survey of 260 epileptic patients treated with oxcarbazepine (Trileptal) on a named-patient basis. *Epilepsy Res* 1994;19:79–85.
220. Fisher RS, Eskola J, Blum DE, Kerrigan JF, Drazkowski J, Duncan B. An open-label pilot study of oxcarbazepine for inpatients under evaluation for epilepsy surgery. *Drug Dev Res* 1996;38:43–49.
221. Van Amelsvoort T, Bakshi R, Devaux CB, Schwabe S. Hyponatremia associated with carbamazepine and ox-

carbazepine therapy: a review (review). *Epilepsia* 1994;35:181–188.
222. Johannessen A, Nielsen O. Hyponatremia induced by oxcarbazepine. *Epilepsy Res* 1987;1:155–156.
223. Pendlebury S, Moses D, Eadie M. Hyponatraemia during oxcarbazepine therapy. *Hum Toxicol* 1989;8: 337–344.
224. Nielsen O, Johannessen A, Bardrum B. A cross-sectional study. Oxcarbazepine-induced hyponatremia. *Epilepsy Res* 1988;2:269–271.
225. Steinhoff BJ, Stoll KD, Stodieck SR, Paulus W. Hyponatremic coma under oxcarbazepine therapy. *Epilepsy Res* 1992;11:67–70.
226. Beran RG. Cross-reactive skin eruption with both carbamazepine and oxcarbazepine. *Epilepsia* 1993;34: 163–165.
227. Watts D, Bird J. Oxcarbazepine sensitivity treated by desensitisation (letter). *J Neurol Neurosurg Psychiatry* 1991;54:376.
228. Pierce MW, Suzdak PD, Gustavson LE, Mengel HB, McKelvy JF, Mant T. Tiagabine (review). *Epilepsy Res Suppl* 1991;3:157–160.
229. Borden LA, Murali Dhar TG, Smith KE, Weinshank RL, Branchek TA, Gluchowski C. Tiagabine, SK&F 89976-A, CI-966, and NNC-711 are selective for the cloned GABA transporter GAT-1. *Eur J Pharmacol* 1994;269:219–224.
230. Mengel H. Tiagabine (review). *Epilepsia* 1994; 35(Suppl 5):S81–S84.
231. Nielsen EB, Suzdak PD, Andersen KE, Knutsen LJ, Sonnewald U, Braestrup C. Characterization of tiagabine (NO-328), a new potent and selective GABA uptake inhibitor. *Eur J Pharmacol* 1991;196:257–266.
232. Smith SE, Parvez NS, Chapman AG, Meldrum BS. The gamma-aminobutyric acid uptake inhibitor, tiagabine, is anticonvulsant in two animal models of reflex epilepsy. *Eur J Pharmacol* 1995;273:259–265.
233. Faingold CL, Randall ME, Anderson CA. Blockade of GABAuptake with tiagabine inhibits audiogenic seizures and reduces neuronal firing in the inferior colliculus of the genetically epilepsy-prone rat. *Exp Neurol* 1994;126:225–232.
234. Anonymous. Gabapentin—a new antiepileptic drug. *Drug Ther Bull* 1994;32:29–30.
235. Wolff D, Leppik I, So E, et al. A pharmacokinetic study of tiagabine HCL in patients at various steady-state doses. Efficacy of tiagabine in older pediatric patients with refractory partial seizures. *Neurology* 1995; 45(Suppl 4):A249.
236. Cato A, Qian JX, Gustavson LE, et al. Pharmacokinetics and safety of tiagabine in subjects with various degrees of renal function. *Epilepsia* 1995;36(Suppl 3):S159.
237. Gustavson LE, Cato A, Guenther HJ, et al. Lack of clinically important drug interactions between tiagabine and carbamazepine, phenytoin, or valproate. *Epilepsia* 1995;36(Suppl 3):S159.
238. Snel S, Jonkman JHG, Van Heiningen PNM, Jansen JA, Mengel HB. Tiagabine: evaluation of the risk of interaction with cimetidine in healthy male volunteers. *Epilepsia* 1994;35:74.
239. Jansen JA, Sommerville KW, Jonkman JHG, et al. Tiagabine: evaluation of the risk of interaction with theophylline, warfarin, digoxin, cimetidine, oral contraceptives, tirazolam, or ethanol. *Epilepsia* 1995;36 (Suppl 3):S160.
240. Leach JP, Sills G, Thompson G, Forrest G, Butler E, Brodie MJ. Concentration-related effects of vigabatrin on GABA uptake in cultured rodent astrocytes. *Epilepsia* 1995;36(Suppl 4):S33.
241. Richens A, Chadwick D, Duncan J, et al. Safety and efficacy of tiagabine HCl as adjunctive treatment for complex partial seizures. *Epilepsia* 1992;33:119.
242. Gram L. Tiagabine: a novel drug with a GABAergic mechanism of action. *Epilepsia* 1994;35(Suppl 5): S85–S87.
243. Richens A, Chadwick DW, Duncan JS, et al. Adjunctive treatment of partial seizures with tiagabine: a placebo-controlled trial. *Epilepsy Res* 1995;21:37–42.
244. Sachdeo RC, Biton V, Boellner SW, et al. Long-term safety of tiagabine HCl. *Epilepsia* 1995;36(Suppl 4): S55.
245. Uldall P, Bulteau C, Pedersen SA, Dullac O, Meinild H, Lassen LC. Single-blind study of safety, tolerability, and preliminary efficacy of tiagabine as adjunctive treatment of children with epilepsy. *Epilepsia* 1995; 36(Suppl 3):S147.
246. Glauser TA, Olberding LS. Lamotrigine use in refractory infantile spasms and the Lennox-Gastaut syndrome. *Epilepsia* 1995;36(Suppl 4):S89.
247. Sveinbjornsdottir S, Sander JW, Patsalos PN, Upton D, Thompson PJ, Duncan JS. Neuropsychological effects of tiagabine, a potential new antiepileptic drug. *Seizure* 1994;3:29–35.
248. Leach JP, Stolarek I, Brodie MJ. Deliberate overdose with the novel anticonvulsant tiagabine. *Seizure* 1995; 4:155–157.
249. Coenen AML, Van Luijtelaar ELJM, Blezer E. Effects of tiagabine on spike-wave discharges, behavior, and spectral content of the EEG in rats with absence epilepsy. *Epilepsia* 1995;36(Suppl 3):S45.
250. Walton NY, Gunawan S, Treiman DM. Treatment of experimental status epilepticus with the GABA uptake inhibitor, tiagabine. *Epilepsy Res* 1994;19:237–244.
251. Gao XM, Kakigi T, Friedman MB, Tamminga CA. Tiagabine inhibits haloperidol-induced oral dyskinesias in rats. *J Neural Transm Gen Sect* 1994;95:63–69.
252. Gouliaev AH, Senning A. Piracetam and other structurally related nootropics (review). *Brain Res Brain Res Rev* 1994;19:180–222.
253. Löscher W, Hönack D. Profile of UCB L059, a novel anticonvulsant drug, in models of partial and generalized epilepsy in mice and rats. *Eur J Pharmacol* 1993; 232:147–158.
254. Gower AJ, Noyer M, Verloes R, Gobert J, Wulfert E. UCB L059, a novel anti-convulsant drug: pharmacological profile in animals (published erratum appears in *Eur J Pharmacol* 1993 Jan 19;230:389). *Eur J Pharmacol* 1992;222:193–203.
255. Patsallos P, Walker, Ratnaraj N, Sander JWAS, Shorvon SD. The pharmacokinetics of levetiracetam (UCB LO59) in patients with intractable epilepsy. *Epilepsia* 1995;36(Suppl 4):S52.
256. Neyens LG, Alpherts WC, Aldenkamp AP. Cognitive effects of a new pyrrolidine derivative (levetiracetam) in patients with epilepsy. *Prog Neuropsychopharmacol Biol Psychiatry* 1995;19:411–419.
257. Vincent JC. Stiripentol (review). *Epilepsy Res Suppl* 1991;3:153–156.
258. Tang C, Zhang K, Lepage F, Levy RH, Baillie TA. Metabolic chiral inversion of stiripentol in the rat. II.

Influence of route of administration. *Drug Metab Dispos* 1994;22:554–560.
259. Zhang K, Tang C, Rashed M, et al. Metabolic chiral inversion of stiripentol in the rat. I. Mechanistic studies. *Drug Metab Dispos* 1994;22:544–553.
260. Maurizis JC, Rapp M, Madelmont JC, et al. Disposition of stiripentol in the pregnant and non-pregnant female rat. *Xenobiotica* 1993;23:1335–1343.
261. Kerr BM, Martinez-Lage JM, Viteri C, Tor J, Eddy AC, Levy RH. Carbamazepine dose requirements during stiripentol therapy: influence of cytochrome P_{450} inhibition by stiripentol. *Epilepsia* 1991;32:267–274.
262. Lockard J, Levy R, Loiseau P, Strube E, Tor J, Dodrill C. Carbamazepine plus stiripentol: is polytherapy by design possible? Neurophysiological and therapeutic evaluation of stiripentol in epilepsy: preliminary results. *Epilepsia* 1988;144:165–172.
263. Finnell RH, Van Waes M, Musselman A, Kerr BM, Levy RH. Differences in the patterns of phenytoin-induced malformations following stiripentol coadministration in three inbred mouse strains. *Reprod Toxicol* 1993;7:439–448.
264. Finnell RH, Kerr BM, Van Waes M, Steward RL, Levy RH. Protection from phenytoin-induced congenital malformations by coadministration of the antiepileptic drug stiripentol in a mouse model. *Epilepsia* 1994;35:141–148.
265. Rascol O, Squalli A, Montastruc J, et al. A pilot study of stiripentol. *Clin Neuropharmacol* 1989;12:119–123.
266. Farwell JR, Anderson GD, Kerr BM, Tor JA, Levy RH. Stiripentol in atypical absence seizures in children: an open trial. *Epilepsia* 1993;34:305–311.
267. De Beukelaar F, Tritsmans L. Loreclezole (review). *Epilepsy Res Suppl* 1991;3:125–128.
268. Wingrove PB, Wafford KA, Bain C, Whiting PJ. The modulatory action of loreclezole at the gamma-aminobutyric acid type A receptor is determined by a single amino acid in the beta 2 and beta 3 subunit. *Proc Natl Acad Sci U S A* 1994;91:4569–4573.
269. Ashton D, Fransen J, Heeres J, Clincke GH, Janssen PA. In vivo studies on the mechanism of action of the broad-spectrum anticonvulsant loreclezole. *Epilepsy Res* 1992;11:27–36.
270. Dailey JW, Seo DO, Yan QS, Ko KH, Jo M, Jobe PC. The anticonvulsant effect of the broad-spectrum anticonvulsant loreclezole may be mediated in part by serotonin in rats: a microdialysis study (published erratum appears in *Neurosci Lett* 1994 Oct 24;180:294). *Neurosci Lett* 1994;178:179–183.
271. Zhang CL, Heinemann U. Effects of the triazole derivative loreclezole (R72063) on stimulus-induced ionic and field potential responses and on different patterns of epileptiform activity induced by low magnesium in rat entorhinal cortex-hippocampal slices. *Naunyn Schmiedebergs Arch Pharmacol* 1992;346:581–587.
272. Ates N, van Luijtelaar EL, Drinkenburg WH, Vossen JM, Coenen AM. Effects of loreclezole on epileptic activity and on EEG and behaviour in rats with absence seizures. *Epilepsy Res* 1992;13:43–48.
273. Rentmeester T, Janssen A, Hulsman J, et al. A double-blind, placebo-controlled evaluation of the efficacy and safety of loreclezole as add-on therapy in patients with uncontrolled partial seizures. *Epilepsy Res* 1991;9:59–64.
274. Rentmeester T, Janssen A, Hulsman J, et al. Long-term evaluation of the efficacy and safety of loreclezole as add-on therapy in patients with uncontrolled partial seizures: a 1-year open follow-up. *Epilepsy Res* 1991;9:65–70.
275. Rentmeester TW, Hulsman JA. Loreclezole monotherapy in patients with partial seizures. *Epilepsy Res* 1992;11:141–145.
276. Stein U, Klessing K, Chatterjee SS. Losigamone (review). *Epilepsy Res Suppl* 1991;3:129–133.
277. Kramer G, Wad N, Bredel-GieBler A, Biber A, Dienel A. Losigamone valproate interaction: a placebo-controlled, double-blind study in healthy volunteers. *Epilepsia* 1995;36(Suppl 4):S53.
278. Muir KT, Palmer GC. Remacemide (review). *Epilepsy Res Suppl* 1991;3:147–152.
279. Clark B, Hutchison JB, Jamieson V, Jones T, Palmer GC, Scheger RD. Remacemide hydrochloride. In: Levy RH, Mattson RH, Meldrum BS, eds. *Antiepileptic Drugs*. 4th ed. New York: Raven Press; 1995: 1035–1042.
280. Palmer GC, Murray RT, Wilson TCM, Fisons Pharmaceuticals. Biologic profile of the metabolites and potential metabolites of the anticonvulsant remacemide. *Epilepsy Res* 1992;12:19–20.
281. Stagnitto ML, Palmer GC, Ordy JM. Preclinical profile of remacemide: a novel anticonvulsant effective against maximal electroshock seizures in mice. *Epilepsy Res* 1990;7:11–28.
282. Fisons Pharmaceuticals. CR2065: a double-blind, placebo-controlled study of the safety, tolerability, and pharmacokinetics of remacemide tablets in epileptic patients, comparing twice and four times daily dosing with placebo for a period of 1 month. Internal report 1996.
283. Canadian CCG. Clobazam in treatment of refractory epilepsy: the Canadian experience—a retrospective study. *Epilepsia* 1991;32:407–16.
284. Schmidt D, Kramer G. The new anticonvulsant drugs. Implications for avoidance of adverse effects (review). *Drug Saf* 1994;11:422–431.
285. Keene D, Whiting S, Humphreys P. Clobazam as an add-on drug in the treatment of refractory epilepsy of childhood. *Can J Neurol Sci* 1990;17:317–319.
286. Allen J, Oxley J, Robertson M, Trimble M, Richens A, Jawad S. Clobazam as adjunctive treatment in refractory epilepsy. *Br Med J (Clin Res Ed)* 1983;286: 1246–1247.
287. Zifkin B, Sherwin A, Andermann F. Phenytoin toxicity due to interaction with clobazam. *Neurology* 1991;41: 313–314.
288. Remy C. Clobazam in the treatment of epilepsy: a review of the literature. *Epilepsia* 1994;35:S88–S91.
289. Wolter KD. Eterobarb (review). *Epilepsy Res Suppl* 1991;3:99–102.
290. Mattson RH, Cramer JA, Collins JF, VA Cooperative Study Group 264. A comparison of valproate with carbamazepine for the treatment of complex partial and secondarily generalized tonic-clonic seizures in adults. *N Engl J Med* 1992;327:765–771.
291. Battaglia A, Ferrari A, Guerrini R. Double-blind placebo-controlled trial of flunarizine as add-on therapy in refractory childhood epilepsy. *Brain Dev* 1991; 13:217–222.

292. Houtkooper M, van OC, Rentmeester T, Hoppener P, Onkelinx C. Double-blind study of milacemide in hospitalized therapy-resistant patients with epilepsy. *Epilepsia* 1986;27:255–262.
293. Morselli PL, Lloyd KG, Palminteri R. Progabide. In: Levy RH, Mattson RH, Meldrum BS, eds. *Antiepileptic Drugs*. 4th ed. New York: Raven Press; 1995: 997–1009.
294. Anhut H, Satzinger G, von HA. Ralitoline. *Epilepsy Res Suppl* 1991;3:141–145.
295. Rock D, McLean M, Macdonald R, Catterall W, Taylor C. Ralitoline (CI-946) and ci-953 block sustained repetitive sodium action potentials in cultured mouse spinal cord neurons and displace batrachotoxinin a 20-alpha-benzoate binding in vitro. *Epilepsy Res* 1991;8: 197–203.

Antiepileptic Drug Development.
Advances in Neurology, Vol. 76,
edited by J. French, I. Leppik, and M. A. Dichter.
Lippincott–Raven Publishers, Philadelphia © 1998.

7

AED Doses: From Animals to Humans

Ilo E. Leppik

MINCEP Epilepsy Care, Minneapolis, Minnesota 55416.

INTRODUCTION

Determining the appropriate dose to be used in clinical trials is not a simple task, and the consequences of choosing incorrectly can be substantial. Picking a dose that is too low may make an otherwise effective agent appear to be inactive, and using a dose that is too high may lead to unacceptable toxicity. In the former case, years of research efforts may be erroneously discarded, and in the latter, adverse events during the drug trial may result in an effective drug being judged too toxic for clinical use.

The details encountered in interspecies scaling of dose are more complicated than it might appear initially. A number of factors must be taken into account. They can be considered under two broad areas: pharmacodynamic activity, or concentrations needed at the receptor sites, and pharmacokinetic factors, or doses needed to maintain appropriate concentrations over time.

In the last few decades, the process of scaling up animal doses for human use has been greatly refined. Phenytoin was the first antiepileptic drug discovered through testing in animals. During the winter of 1937, Merritt and Putnam (1) experimented with cats given phenytoin and subjected to electrical shocks. "Diphenylhydantoin in doses of 25 to 40 mg daily raised the animal's threshold until it was impossible to obtain a convulsion. The animal was not poisoned by these doses" (1). As reported in a later article, Merritt and Putnam started patients on "a dose of 0.1 g three times a day, increased up to a maximum of 0.2 g three times a day" (2). It is not clear from their articles how they progressed from the cat to human doses. A less fortunate outcome of scaling up the doses effective in cats to larger mammals was the use of LSD (lysergic acid diethylamide) in an elephant. Based on the fact that doses of 0.5 mg/kg were needed to produce effects in the rhesus macaque and intravenous doses of at least 0.15 mg/kg in cats, a dose of 0.1 mg of LSD per kilogram, or 297 mg of LSD, was given to Tusko, an elephant weighing 6500 to 7000 lb. The investigators expected this dose to be of borderline effectiveness, but Tusko trumpeted, fell heavily onto his right side, defecated, and went into status epilepticus 5 minutes after the intramuscular injection had been administered (3). This unfortunate experience highlighted the problems associated with scaling up doses. Fortunately, considerable progress has been made in the rational selection of doses to be used in humans for the first time (4).

ISSUES OF INTERSPECIES DRUG DEVELOPMENT

Use of animals in developing drugs for human epilepsy is based on the premise that observations in other species will be predictive of outcomes in humans. This would be true if both the effects and the concentrations needed to produce such effects were similar across species, so that the compound could be tested for effectiveness in animals, followed by determination of the appropriate concentrations at the receptor site. Scaling the dose then would become a matter of determining the pharmacokinetics of the agent in humans and calculating the doses required to produce the desired concentrations in persons with epilepsy. Fortunately, all forms of life on earth share an impressive array of biochemical similarities. These include left-handed amino acids (L-amino acids), DNA/RNA-based genetic programs, ATP (adenosine triphosphate) as the energy-storing molecule, and cellular mechanisms for membrane conduction (5).

For animal studies to be useful, the activity in animal models should be predictive of action in the human disorder. For epilepsy, a number of animal models have been developed to test drugs, and in general a good correlation has been shown between activity in animal models and human epilepsy (6).

This still leaves the issue of drug metabolism. Organ systems among species have many commonalities. For example, a human liver cell resembles a rat or frog liver cell more than it resembles a human skin or gastrointestinal cell, allowing for interspecies predictions of metabolism (5). The applicability of using animals to predict drug metabolism has been extensively studied. The rat provides a good or fair qualitative model of human drug metabolism 41% of the time, other nonprimates (dog, rabbit, guinea pig) 59% of the time, and rhesus monkey 92% of the time (7,8).

DOSES AND CONCENTRATIONS IN ANIMAL MODELS AND HUMANS

It is useful to evaluate animal studies in epilepsy and how their results relate to human doses and concentrations (Table 1). A number of reported measures of drug effect in animals report doses required for effect. Fewer studies have evaluated concentrations. These include the use of maximal electroshock (MES) seizures, sustained repetitive firing (SRF), and measurement of the protective index (PI), which is derived from the median effective dose (ED_{50}) and the median toxic dose (TD_{50}).

One of the first studies of phenytoin concentrations in brain and plasma used MES in the rat. Doses used were identical to those described in earlier studies (9). Measurement of concentrations indicated that the plasma concentrations effective for these drugs in this model approximated those seen in humans and that no synergistic effect occurred between phenytoin and phenobarbital (10).

The potency of antiepileptic agents can be estimated using the SRF model. The effective unbound (free) concentrations in this model are approximately 2 mg/L for phenytoin, 2 mg/L for carbamazepine, and 3 mg/L for valproate (11,12,13). These are similar to the unbound concentrations seen to be effective in humans, again supporting the notion that biologic models derived from nonhuman tissue can correlate with concentrations useful in humans.

TABLE 1. *Some comparisons between animal and human doses or concentrations in standard models*

Drug	Animal model	Dose or level for similar effect: Animal	Dose or level for similar effect: Human
Phenytoin	ED_{50} MES	9 mg/kg (rat)	20 mg/kg loading dose
Carbamazepine	ED_{50} MES	8.5 mg/kg (rat)	8 mg/kg loading dose
Phenytoin	SRF	2 mg/L unbound	2 mg/L unbound
Carbamazepine	SRF	2 mg/L unbound	2 mg/L unbound
Phenytoin	TD_{50} rotorod	65 mg/kg	30 mg/kg loading dose
Carbamazepine	TD_{50} rotorod	71 mg/kg	20 mg/kg loading dose

ED_{50}, median effective dose; MES, maximal electroshock; SRF, sustained repetitive firing; TD_{50}, median toxic dose.

The PI is calculated by dividing the dose at which 50% of the animals show toxic signs (TD_{50}) by the dose at which 50% of the animals show the desired therapeutic effect (ED_{50}). A standard measure of toxicity is the rotorod, on which the rats or mice must balance as the rod is rotated. The balance of rats or mice is assumed to correlate with human balance, and poor balance can be considered to correspond to ataxia. These animal studies are performed as single-dose studies, and results may correspond with the loading dose rather than long-term doses in humans. Also, they would correspond to initial concentrations seen in humans. For phenytoin, when the rotorod test is used to determine toxicity and MES seizures the therapeutic effect, the PI is approximately 7, suggesting a sevenfold range between effective and toxic levels. In humans, the range between effective levels and levels at which ataxia is seen may be threefold or fourfold, which, although not the same as the PI, is at least in the same general range. For carbamazepine, the PI is approximately 8, again approximating the general range in humans. Thus, it appears that use of the PI in animals may give some estimation of the "therapeutic window" in humans.

Toxicity as measured by the rotorod test indicates that the acute dose of phenytoin is 65 mg/kg. For carbamazepine the TD_{50} is 71 mg/kg. For valproate, the TD_{50} is 426 mg/kg. This appears to correlate with experience in humans, in whom ataxia is a prominent sign of neurotoxicity associated with phenytoin or carbamazepine; ataxia is not prominent with valproate.

To measure the ED_{50}, rodents are administered the medicine intraperitoneally, leading to rapid absorption. For carbamazepine, the ED_{50} is 8.5 mg/kg in the rat and 15 mg/kg in the mouse. Interestingly, the human loading dose is about 8 mg/kg (14). For phenytoin, the ED_{50} in rat is 9 mg/kg, and it is 30 mg/kg in mouse. The loading dose for humans in status epilepticus is 20 mg/kg (15). In the rat, the dose for felbamate is 48 mg/kg, in comparison with a human daily dose of 40 mg/kg per day. It thus appears that persons with epilepsy tolerate doses twice those tolerated by human volunteers. When the drugs are finally used in human, the doses may eventually be twice those tolerated in clinical trials.

Allometry is the study of size and its consequences; it can be used to predict doses or clearances of drugs for various body sizes (7). One consideration that modifies a simple allometric scaling of a dose is the fact that all organ masses do not increase proportionately with body mass. Blood volume in terrestrial mammals is approximately 8.5% of body mass, regardless of size (16). In regard to the skeletal system, larger mammals have more of their body mass dedicated to bone. Only 5% of the body mass of the shrew consists of bone, whereas 27% of the body mass of the elephant comprises bone (17). One major discrepancy that arises in scaling using body mass relates to brain mass. Whereas an equation relating brain mass to body mass is quite predictive of brain weight among primates, the human brain mass is actually 3.9-fold greater than predicted (18). In addition to body mass, major discrepancies are found among metabolic rates. Vertical allometry gives good correlation for diazepam clearance among rat, dog, rabbit, and guinea pig. However, this equation indicates that human clearance of diazepam should be 900 mL/min, which is about 35-fold greater than the observed clearance of 26 mL/min (7). Nevertheless, the allometric equation provides overall a quite reasonable first approximation. According to the allometric equation with cat and human data inserted, the dose for Tusko should have been 5.4 to 19 mg of LSD, rather than the 297 mg actually administered (7).

FIRST-TIME-IN-HUMAN DOSES

During the last quarter of a century, an effective system of preclinical testing has been developed for antiepileptic drugs; it is described in detail in Chapters 2 and 3 of this book. Once an effective and safe compound has been developed and detected by animal studies, the issue of designing the appropriate clinical trials begins. Present methodology is to take a compound through staged clinical trials: phases I, II, and III. These phases are described in detail in many publications (19). In phase I, the human dose must be approximated from animal studies. Phases II and III rely on human data from phase I.

Three variables from animal studies have been used to determine the first-time-in-human doses: the LD_{50}, which is the median dose lethal to 50% of the animals; the no-observed-effect level (NOEL), which is the maximal dose causing no discernible biologic activity in 15- to 30-day studies; and the no-toxic-effect level (NTEL), which is the maximal dose causing no discernible toxicity in 15- to 30-day studies (7). These doses can be allometrically scaled to human doses, which are usually given in single rising-dose tolerance (SRDT) studies (20). The dose selected may be a fraction (1/10 to 1/1000) of the maximal NOEL dose. Subsequently, the dose is cautiously escalated to encompass the anticipated human therapeutic dose (20).

Ideally, one should be able to use animal unbound blood levels of the NOEL and NTEL studies to determine the human dose. This would assume that effective concentrations in animals correspond to those effective in humans. One could then use the predicted pharmacokinetic parameters to design doses that would approximate in humans the concentrations in animals. However, this approach rests on a number of assumptions about the predictability of pharmacodynamic and pharmacokinetic parameters that cannot be adequately tested until the first doses are given to humans.

In most cases, toxic drug manifestations observed in animals are predictive for humans. However, it is not possible to predict undetermined, rare events, be they stock market crashes, or unexpected toxicities such as aplastic anemia from felbamate.

In scaling to the final daily doses useful in clinical practice, the doses used in clinical trials may be too low. This has been the experience with the latest drugs introduced for the treatment of epilepsy (Table 2). Usually, patients with epilepsy tolerate doses twice those

TABLE 2. *Doses of newer antiepileptic drugs used in clinical trials and in clinical practice*

Drug	Dose in clinical trials	Doses in use
Felbamate	2400 mg/d	4800 mg/d
Gabapentin	900–1500 mg/d	4800 mg/d
Lamotrigine	200–400 mg/d	800 mg/d

that human volunteers tolerate. The doses used may also depend on the kinetics of the drug and its interactions. These may not be detected in initial trials. For example, in the study of MK801, a drug that was barred from additional trials because of its potential to cause toxic effects, the maximal dose tolerated in human volunteers was 1 to 2 mg/d (21). In a dose-ascension study in persons with epilepsy, it was found that some patients tolerated doses of 2 to 4 mg/d. Others tolerated 8 to 14 mg/d. Initially, blood levels were not available, so dosing was empiric. When the data were analyzed, it was found that persons on valproate monotherapy were the ones who tolerated only 2 to 4 mg/d. On the other hand, those tolerating 8 to 16 mg were receiving phenytoin or carbamazepine. Blood levels were similar in both groups, indicating that the major factor in differences in dose was the state of induction of the liver.

CONCLUSIONS

Animal models are essential in developing new drugs for the treatment of epilepsy. A critical stage is deciding on the first dose in humans. With improved methods of scaling from small animals to humans, this has become a more rational process. Single rising-dose tolerance studies appear to be the best way of scaling up, as they provide an estimate of tolerated doses in human volunteers. In epilepsy, however, the general experience has been that persons with epilepsy in phase II and phase III studies often tolerate doses double those tolerated by volunteers. Furthermore, once a drug is introduced into practice, doses that are needed to control seizures and that are tolerated may also double. New antiepileptic drugs should be tested in doses that are accompanied by some degree of toxicity. Although this may lead to an unfavorable adverse events profile, it will ensure that adequate doses have been used to elicit any antiseizure activity that may be present. It will prevent rejection of a compound as not efficacious. Also, it will provide information regarding the potential side effects of a compound, which will be useful in guiding both physicians and patients.

REFERENCES

1. Merritt H, Putnam T. A new series of anticonvulsant drugs tested by experiments on animals. *Arch Neurol Psychiatry* 1938;39:1003–1015.
2. Merritt H, Putnam T. Sodium diphenyl hydantoinate in the treatment of convulsive disorders. *JAMA* 1938; 111:1068–1073.
3. West LJ, Pierce CM, Thomas WD. Lysergic acid diethylamide: its effects on a male Asiatic elephant. *Science* 1962;138:1100–1103.
4. Colburn WA. Controversy V: phase I, first-time-in-man studies. *J Clin Pharmacol* 1990;30:210–222.
5. Luria SE, Gould SJ, Singer S. *A View of Life*. Menlo Park, CA: Benjamin/Cummings Publishing; 1981.
6. Löscher W, Schmidt D. Strategies in antiepileptic drug development: is rational drug design superior to random screening and structural variation? *Epilepsy Res* 1994;17:95–134.
7. Boxenbaum H, DiLea C. First-time-in-human dose selection: allometric thoughts and perspectives. *J Clin Pharmacol* 1995;35:57–66.
8. Caldwell J. The current status of attempts to predict species differences in drug metabolism. *Drug Metab Rev* 1981;12:221–237.
9. Weaver LC, Swinyard EA, Woodbury LA, Goodman LS. Studies on anticonvulsant drug combinations: phenobarbital and diphenylhydantoin. *J Pharmacol Exp Ther* 1955;113:359–370.
10. Leppik IE, Sherwin AL. Anticonvulsant activity of phenobarbital and phenytoin in combination. *J Pharmacol Exp Ther* 1977;200:570–575.
11. McLean MJ, Macdonald RL. Multiple actions of phenytoin on mouse spinal cord neurons in cell culture. *J Pharmacol Exp Ther* 1983;227:779–789.
12. McLean MJ, Macdonald RL. Sodium valproate, but not ethosuximide, produces use- and voltage-dependent limitation of high-frequency repetitive firing of action potential of mouse central neurons in cell culture. *J Pharmacol Exp Ther* 1986;237:1001–1011.
13. McLean MJ, Macdonald RL. Carbamazepine and 10,11-epoxycarbamazepine produce use- and voltage-dependent limitation of high-frequency repetitive firing of action potential of mouse central neurons in cell culture. *J Pharmacol Exp Ther* 1986;238:727–738.
14. Leppik IE, Pascual-Leone A, Dhuna A. Oral loading with carbamazepine: a pilot study. *Epilepsia* 1988;29: 699–700.
15. Leppik IE. Status epilepticus: the next decade. *Neurology* 1990;40(Suppl 2):4–9.
16. Prothero J. Scaling of body proportions in adult terrestrial mammals. *Am J Physiol* 1992;29:961–966.
17. Prange HD, Anderson JF, Rahn H. Scaling of skeletal muscle mass to body mass in birds and animals. *Am Naturalist* 1979;113:103–122.
18. Harvey PH, Clutton-Brock TH. Life history variations in primates. *Evolution* 1985;39:210–212.
19. Cereghino JJ, Kupferberg HJ. Preclinical testing. *Epilepsy Res Suppl* 1993;10:19–30 (*New Antiepileptic Drug Development: Preclinical and Clinical Aspects*).
20. Posvar EL, Sedman AJ. New drugs: first time. *J Clin Pharmacol* 1989;29:961–966
21. Leppik IE, Marienau KJ, Graves NM, Rask CA. MK 801 for epilepsy: a pilot study. *Neurology* 1988;38: 405.

Antiepileptic Drug Development.
Advances in Neurology, Vol. 76,
edited by J. French, I. Leppik, and M. A. Dichter.
Lippincott–Raven Publishers, Philadelphia © 1998.

8

Assessing Pharmacokinetic and Pharmacodynamic Interactions in Clinical Trials of Antiepileptic Drugs

Ross A. Reife

Global Clinical Research and Development, R. W. Johnson Pharmaceutical Research Institute, Raritan, New Jersey 08861, and Thomas Jefferson University, Philadelphia, Pennsylvania 19107.

CLINICAL PHARMACOKINETCS/ PHARMACODYNAMICS

In the practice of clinical medicine, an understanding of the pharmacokinetic profile and pharmacodynamic effects of a drug is essential for a physician to use a drug appropriately. Information about pharmacokinetics and pharmacodynamics, therefore, generally is required before regulatory agencies will approve a drug for use. In the clinical development of a new chemical entity (NCE), these data are obtained in a semi-orderly fashion as drug development progresses from phase I to phase III.

In phase I, basic clinical pharmacokinetic assessments are performed. Clinical pharmacokinetics has been defined as the study of the time course of a drug and its metabolites in humans. The goal is a quantitative description of what happens to the drug once it enters the human body. The parameters studied primarily are absorption, distribution, metabolism, and excretion. Once a pharmacokinetic profile of an NCE has been obtained in several animal species, a human pharmacokinetic profile is obtained as soon as the drug is introduced in humans. It is essential to obtain this information during phase I, often in healthy subjects, so that clinical development can continue in the populations expected to benefit from the drug based on an estimate of appropriate dosing in respect to safety, tolerability, and efficacy.

Phase II generally consists of studies in which the pharmacodynamic effects of the drug are assessed. Typically, these are dose-ranging trials. Pharmacodynamics has been described as "the study of the biochemical and physiologic *effects* of drugs and their *mechanisms of action*" (1). The latter generally are assessed in the preclinical arena, the goal being the identification of the primary mode of action of the drug through an understanding of its effects on receptors. In humans, physiologic effects, as opposed to mechanism of action, have been the more accessible area of study. Within clinical pharmacodynamic studies, attempts are made to describe the relationship of both concentration and time to effect.

For some classes of drugs, pharmacodynamic assessments can be made rapidly, depending on the effect being studied. For example, the effect of warfarin on coagulation can be studied within a short period of time, whereas a much longer time is needed to substantiate the claim that warfarin decreases the rate of re-thrombosis. In epilepsy, antiepileptic drugs are assessed by their ability to reduce seizures during a given period of time. No immediate or short-term assessment of their pharmacodynamic effects in terms of efficacy can be made. In some cases, surrogate markers are used for a quick assessment of a pharmacodynamic relationship. In general, however, these surrogates are not substitutes for clinical endpoints, and surrogates are not available for antiepileptic drugs. The assessments of the pharmacodynamic effects of a drug continue into phase III, during which the drug is used in a larger population of patients in longer studies.

Thus, in common parlance, clinical pharmacokinetics is the study of the effects of humans on a drug, whereas clinical pharmacodynamics is the study of a drug's effects on humans. Throughout the classic phases of development, studies relating to pharmacokinetics and pharmacodynamics are performed. At some time point, depending on the class of a drug, studies are begun to investigate the interaction potential of the drug. In the practice of clinical medicine, the knowledge of drug interactions is of unquestioned importance. Each time a drug is prescribed for a patient, the physician must assess the effect that other drugs the patient is taking may have on the new drug (and vice versa) and the effect that the new drug, in combination with the other drugs, may have on the patient.

INTERACTIONS

In performing clinical trials with an NCE, just as there is a need to learn about the safety and efficacy of the new potential drug, there is also a need to learn about its likelihood for interactions. Indeed, without knowing about the interaction potential of a drug, one can be misled in terms of its safety and efficacy. On the other hand, the amount of this information necessary to determine that an NCE is effective and relatively safe for use is subject to question.

A drug interaction occurs when one drug alters the clinical pharmacokinetics or clinical pharmacodynamics of another drug. One drug can change the time course of another and/or its metabolites within the body (a pharmacokinetic interaction). One drug also can modify the effects of another, either enhancing or inhibiting it (predominantly through a pharmacodynamic interaction, possibly occurring via altered pharmacokinetics). Two drugs used together can also produce effects not entirely attributable to either drug alone—that is, a new effect (again, predominantly through a pharmacodynamic interaction, perhaps secondary to a pharmacokinetic interaction).

Two drugs given together may or may not have pharmacokinetic interactions. If there is an interaction, it can be caused either by the effect of one drug on the binding of another to plasma proteins (displacement) or by an induction or inhibition of enzymatic metabolism. The result of such pharmacokinetic interactions is either an increase or a decrease in free drug concentration, a change in the concentration of metabolites of the drug, or no change at all.

Similarly, two drugs given together may or may not have pharmacodynamic interactions. At the receptor level, a drug may be a partial or full agonist, inverse agonist, or modulator; drug interactions depend on these intrinsic properties of each drug. The results of interactions at the receptor level may be seen clinically as synergistic, additive, subadditive, decreased, or new effects, or there may be no clinical manifestations.

Because of ethical considerations, antiepileptic drugs generally are developed first as adjunctive therapy. Thus, the question of interaction potential attains great importance. The standard design of a phase II/III antiepileptic drug trial is a randomized, double-blind, placebo-controlled trial of the new drug as add-on therapy for patients with re-

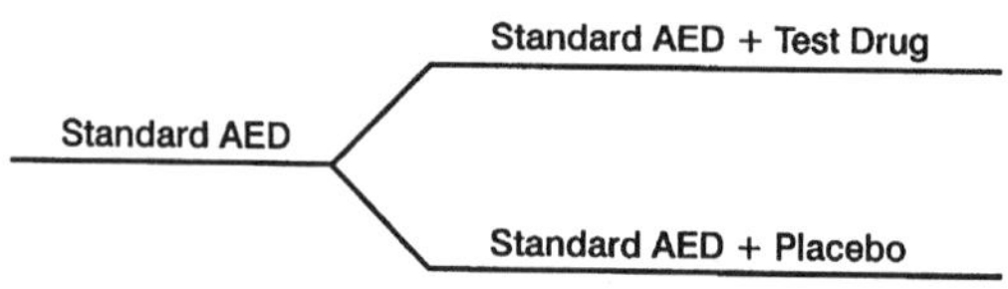

FIG. 1. Standard efficacy trial design for antiepileptic drugs.

fractory epilepsy. The basic trial design is shown in Fig. 1. This design, or a variation of it, has been used in the development of drugs such as felbamate (2), gabapentin (3–5), lamotrigine (6), tiagabine (7), valproate (8), topiramate (9,10), and vigabatrin (11).

In retrospect, it is obvious that any trial that employs this design must take into account the potential for interaction between the NCE and the standard antiepileptic drug. Even with an awareness of the potential for interaction, this trial design can lead to difficulties in the interpretation of results. Examples of such problems and attempts to overcome them can be found in trials with, for example, chlorazepate (12), progabide (13), oxcarbazepine (14), and felbamate (15).

Pharmacokinetic Interactions

The study of felbamate performed by the National Institutes of Health in conjunction with Carter-Wallace, Inc. (15) is particularly illustrative of the need to understand pharmacokinetic interactions. This was a double-blind, three-period, crossover study in which patients with refractory epilepsy who were taking carbamazepine remained on carbamazepine but were randomized to one of four sequences of add-on treatment with felbamate or placebo. The study design is shown in Fig. 2.

The investigators found that "the study failed to detect a significant effect of (felbamate) on seizure frequency at the 0.05 level." At the time the study was designed, however, only preliminary information existed about the pharmacokinetic interaction between felbamate and carbamazepine. This study helped to define that interaction: "There was a definite interaction between felbamate and carbamazepine; carbamazepine levels decreased 24% . . . when patients were receiving felbamate" (15). Based on this information, the authors performed a repeated analysis with the carbamazepine level added to the statistical model as an explanatory variable. The result based on the repeated analysis was a statistically significant estimated felbamate effect.

This study illustrates the pitfalls inherent in the lack of a robust understanding of the pharmacokinetic interaction potential of a drug. The implication is that if such interactions are known, they can be controlled. For example, if specific medications are known to interact

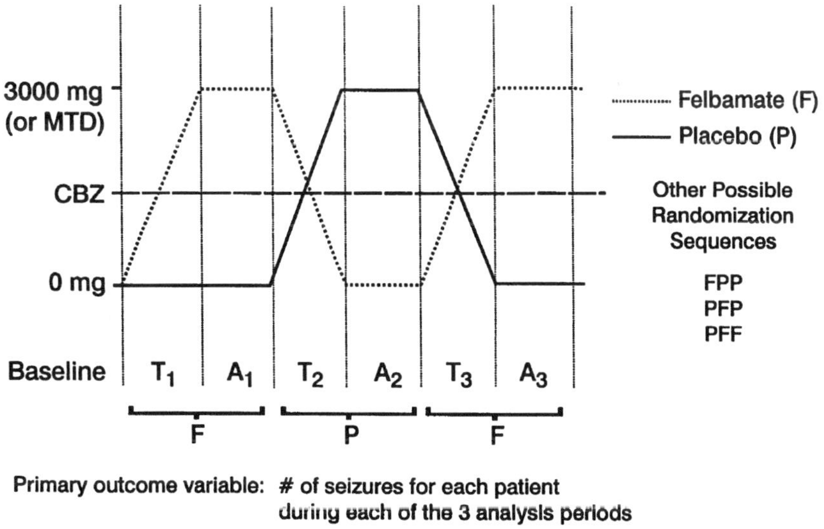

FIG. 2. Pharmacokinetic interactions in double-blind trials: representative randomization sequence in a placebo (*P*)-controlled efficacy study of felbamate (*F*) with concomitant carbamazepine (*CBZ*). *A*, analysis; *MTD*, maximal tolerated dose; *T*, titration. (Reprinted with permission from Theodore et al., ref 15.)

with the drug being tested, patients taking those medications can be excluded from clinical trials. Alternatively, novel techniques have been employed to control for the interactions. If an interaction is thought to exist but is not quite so well described, it can be controlled using a blinded and an unblinded observer. A placebo-controlled trial of valproate as add-on therapy successfully employed this technique two decades ago (16). For known interactions, predetermined dosage adjustments can be made. In a study of felbamate (17), the recognized interaction between felbamate and phenytoin was controlled by a 20% reduction in the phenytoin dose when felbamate was added.

Awareness of the need to understand pharmacokinetic interactions and the availability of the proper tools to do the required assessments has led to several clinical pharmacokinetic interaction study designs. The standard pharmacokinetic interaction design involves titrating a study drug in a patient stabilized on another standard drug (i.e., a patient in whom another drug is at steady state and generally is considered to be within the therapeutic range). This design is shown in Fig. 3.

The plasma concentrations of both the add-on drug and the concomitant standard drug are measured at several time points after each titration, including a time point at which the add-on drug should be at steady state. This gives information about the interaction at several doses of the new drug as it is added to a standard.

Another design, which has been called the "up-the-down-staircase" design, has been used in several trials with some new drugs (18). This design has the advantage of allowing for the assessment of the interaction at several doses of the new drug and at several doses of the concomitant antiepileptic drug. It replicates the clinical situation in which one drug is added to another and the first drug is then down-titrated when efficacy is attained. An example of this study design is shown in Fig. 4.

Pharmacodynamic Interactions

Although analytic methodology has advanced to a level that makes clinical studies of pharmacokinetic interactions relatively straightforward, such is not the case for the investigation of clinical pharmacodynamic interactions. The conclusion that clinical pharmacodynamic interactions exist is based essentially on common-sense assumptions. The arguments for rational polypharmacy rest on the assumption that these interactions exist. The labeling for antiepileptic drugs suggests that regulatory agencies make the same assumption. Antiepileptic drugs shown to be effective only in add-on trials, for example, generally are not labeled for use as monotherapy. In addition, adverse events seen in add-on clinical trials are often attributed to pharmacodynamic interactions. In a study in which either felbamate or valproate was used for adjunctive therapy and then for monotherapy, the adverse event rates of these drugs were compared under both conditions, as shown in Table 1 (19). The increase in adverse event rates when these

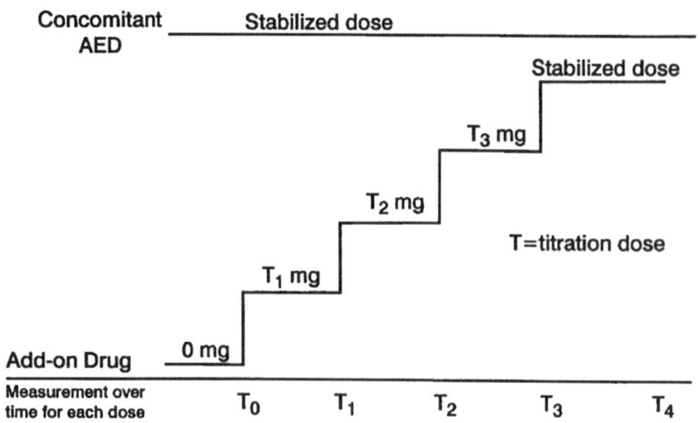

FIG. 3. Standard pharmacokinetic trial design for add-on therapy.

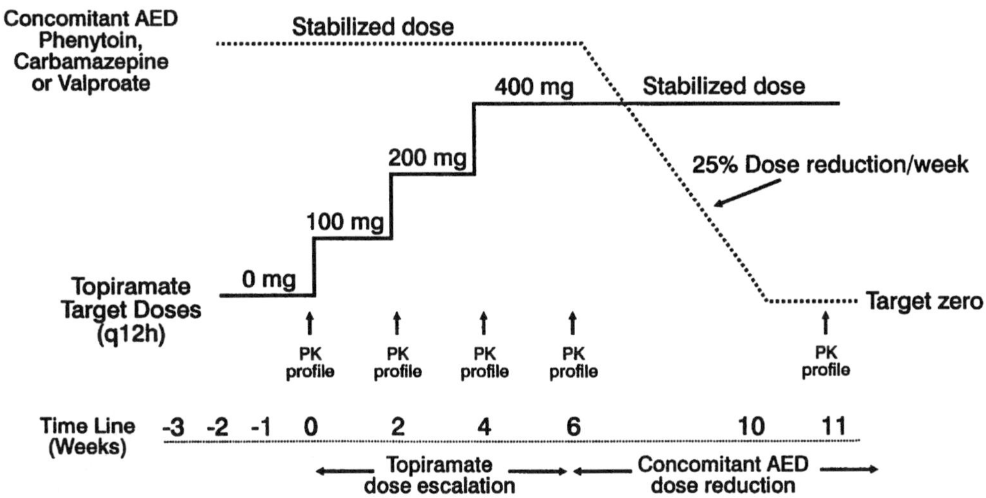

FIG. 4. Pharmacokinetic (*PK*) interaction of topiramate with traditional concomitant drugs (*AEDs*): study design. (Reprinted with permission from Sachdeo et al., ref. 18.)

drugs are given as polytherapy versus monotherapy is often explained by presumed pharmacodynamic interactions under such conditions.

Preclinical evidence also supports the notion of pharmacodynamic interactions. Using animal models of efficacy, such as the maximal electroshock (MES) test, the effects of each of two antiepileptic drugs, given alone and together in various ratios, can be plotted on isobolograms (20). These graphs then indicate the degree of additive, synergistic, or other effects. An example using topiramate in combination with several standard antiepileptic drugs at fixed ratios is shown in Fig. 5 (21).

A clinical trial with a factorial design would most directly assess the presence of a pharmacodynamic relationship between two drugs (22). In this type of study, each drug is considered a factor and is examined in the presence and absence of the other drug. As seen in Fig. 6, there are four possible cells in a two-factor approach. An interaction could be said to exist if the effect of drug X given alone (X – placebo) is not the same as the effect of drug X when given with drug Y (XY – Y).

TABLE 1. *Incidence of treatment emergent adverse events in monotherapy trials: first occurrence in adjunctive phase versus monotherapy phase*

	Adjunctive therapy		Monotherapy	
	Felbamate, % (n = 78)	Valproate, % (n = 77)	Felbamate, % (n = 58)	Valproate, % (n = 50)
Headache	28	19	4	9
Nausea	27	28	1	1
Vomiting	12	14	5	2
Somnolence	18	7	1	2
Dizziness	13	9	1	2
Dyspepsia	8	11	5	1
Diarrhea	5	12	3	0
Anorexia	15	2	1	1
Insomnia	8	3	5	2
Abdominal pain	4	7	1	1

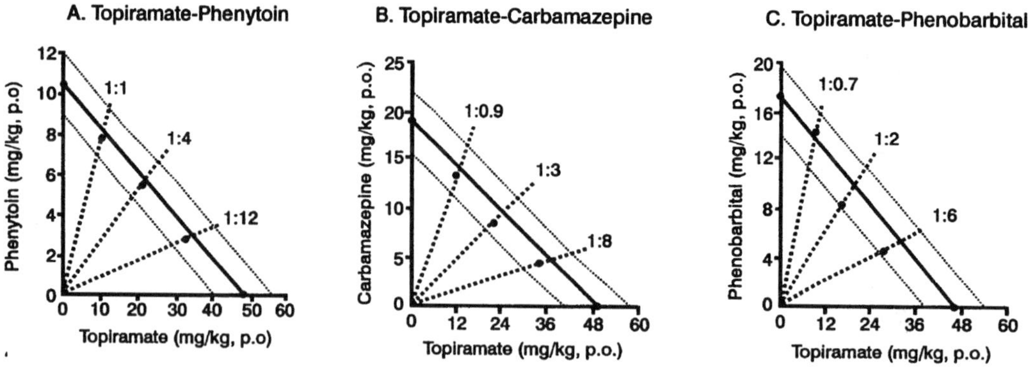

FIG. 5. Fixed-ratio drug interactions in the mouse MES test. The anticonvulsant activity of topiramate and phenytoin in combination was additive. The anticonvulsant activity of topiramate combined with carbamazepine or phenobarbital was synergistic ($p < 0.01$). *Dotted lines* connect the 95% fiducial limits for each anticonvulsant; *dashed lines* relate to ratio of drug doses. (Reprinted with permission from Swinyard et al., ref 20.)

This type of design could be employed in a clinical trial to test for the existence of a pharmacodynamic interaction between two antiepileptic drugs. To look for a pharmacodynamic interaction between valproate and phenytoin, for example, these drugs could be substituted for drug X and drug Y in Fig. 7. In the context of an add-on trial in patients with refractory epilepsy, typically performed early in antiepileptic drug development, a background drug would normally be present. If this were presumed to be carbamazepine, the basic add-on trial design to evaluate the interaction between valproate and phenytoin would look like that shown in Fig. 7A. Figure 7B shows the four cells that exist in this factorial design.

As designated in the diagram, carbamazepine (CBZ), as the background drug, exists in all the cells. According to the same reasoning that was used previously for drug X and drug Y, an interaction between phenytoin (PHT) and valproate (VPA) exists if the effect of either drug alone is not the same as the effect when the drugs are given concomitantly. Summarizing this in terms of Fig. 7, an interaction would exist if the following were true:

[PHT + CBZ] – [Placebo + CBZ]
[(VPA + PHT) + CBZ] – [VPA + CBZ]

There are several reasons why this straightforward trial has never been conducted with antiepileptic drugs. Many of the reasons are logistic: the trial would probably have to be a large one; recruitment of patients who fulfill just the right criteria might be difficult; and the study would probably be costly. All these logistic issues, however, could probably be

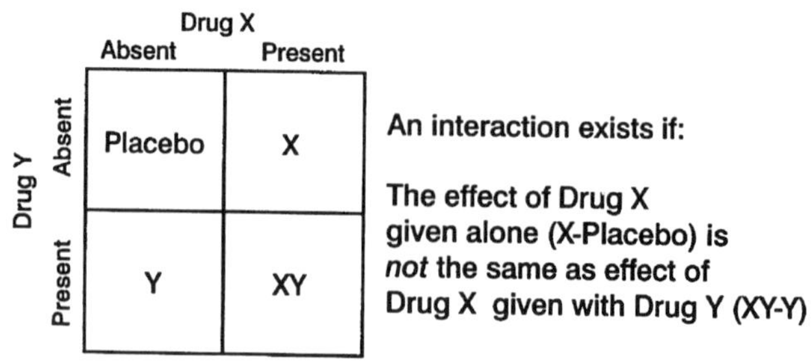

FIG. 6. Pharmacodynamic interaction trial to determine whether drug X and drug Y interact.

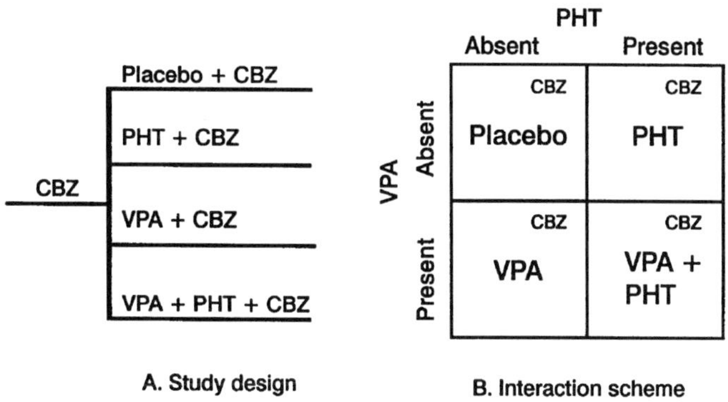

FIG. 7. A: Pharmacodynamic interaction trial to determine whether phenytoin (*PHT*) and valproate (*VPA*) interact in the presence of carbamazepine (*CBZ*). **B:** Cells of the factorial design.

overcome if there were an overwhelming need or desire for this type of information. It seems as if this is not the case, despite all the actions that are rooted in the assumptions of pharmacodynamic interactions.

This lack of motivation to perform clinical pharmacodynamic interaction trials may be reasonable. According to the pharmacology of antiepileptic drugs, it seems unlikely that any two would modulate in opposing directions. Simplistically speaking, antiepileptic drugs tend to enhance inhibitory systems or inhibit excitatory systems; the basic mechanisms by which they work are enhancement of the effects of GABA (τ-aminobutyric acid), reduction of the effects of glutamate, down-regulation of sodium or calcium channels, or some combination of these. It is unlikely that the effect of any antiepileptic drug would be the opposite of another antiepileptic drug in any one of these systems. Thus, any interaction in these systems is likely to result in positive pharmacodynamic effects in regards to efficacy. The question to be answered then is the following: If an interaction exists, what is its magnitude? This question leads to a greater degree of predictability and is easier for the clinician to address than the question of opposing directions.

In addition, the initial claims and uses of most antiepileptic drugs are as add-on therapy for patients with refractory epilepsy. By the time an antiepileptic drug is marketed, the results of multiple add-on trials usually are available, as are at times the results of monotherapy trials. Although these results do not allow for a direct assessment of pharmacodynamic interactions, they do allow for an indirect assessment. If results are consistent when the drug is used concomitantly across all antiepileptic drugs and when the drug is used as monotherapy, it is unlikely that its effects are the result of pharmacodynamic interactions.

SUMMARY AND CONCLUSIONS

An understanding of the pharmacokinetic and pharmacodynamic properties of a drug is a basic requirement for its clinical use. The investigations of these properties and their timing are fairly clearly defined in the drug development process. Without fundamental knowledge of the pharmacokinetics and pharmacodynamics of a drug, a physician could not use it appropriately, nor would a regulatory agency be likely to approve its use.

Information about the interactions of a new antiepileptic drug with other antiepileptic drugs also aids a physician and is required, in varying degrees, by regulatory agencies. The amount of this information that is needed depends, in part, on the class of drug and the population for which the agent is intended. Because antiepileptic drugs are often used as polytherapy and generally are developed first for this use, their interaction potential must be part of the thought process in their development. The correct time to obtain this information, however, is not clearly defined.

The analytic methodology to investigate the pharmacokinetic profile of an NCE exists and is fairly sophisticated. This methodology has enabled the development of study designs to investigate pharmacokinetic interactions. Because the plasma concentration of an antiepileptic drug may be increased or decreased as a result of pharmacokinetic interactions with concomitant antiepileptic drugs, it is of great importance to know about the specific interaction potential of an antiepileptic drug early in its development. Recent studies have confirmed the importance of investigating pharmacokinetic interactions in phase I before proceeding into phases II and III. Without this information, study results are often difficult to interpret; with this knowledge, study designs can be modified to minimize the confounding effect.

A methodology exists to investigate the pharmacodynamic effects of an antiepileptic drug at receptors in cell cultures and in animal models of seizures; however, no procedure has been established to evaluate the short-term or immediate clinical pharmacodynamic effect of an antiepileptic drug, as has been done for other classes of drugs and other diseases. The clinical effect that is sought in trials with antiepileptic drugs is a reduction in seizures with little toxicity. The methodology to investigate the effect of seizure reduction over time has been used repeatedly with minor variations in the development of all the new antiepileptic drugs.

However, no study has evaluated the effect of pharmacodynamic interactions among antiepileptic drugs on seizure reduction. Some studies have purported to show an interaction effect on adverse events, and assumptions are made about pharmacodynamic interactions. Although the information regarding pharmacodynamic interactions is important and existing trial designs could evaluate this, there has been no perceived need to carry out such trials. This information is less accessible than pharmacokinetic interaction information. Moreover, pharmacodynamic interactions, as opposed to pharmacokinetic interactions, are probably unidirectional and lead only to increased effects. Although it would be preferable to have this knowledge, an antiepileptic drug can be used effectively without it; over time, the information about pharmacodynamics will be inferred.

Thus, conducting pharmacokinetic interaction studies with antiepileptic drugs early in their development as part of phase I is essential, whereas obtaining pharmacodynamic interaction information can be deferred.

REFERENCES

1. Benet LZ. Introduction. In: Hardman JG, Limbird LE, eds. *Goodman and Gilman's Pharmacological Basis of Therapeutics*. 9th ed. New York: McGraw-Hill; 1996.
2. Jensen PK. Felbamate in the treatment of refractory partial-onset seizures. *Epilepsia* 1993;34(Suppl 7): S25–S29.
3. U.S. Gabapentin Study Group No. 5. Gabapentin as add-on therapy in refractory partial epilepsy: a double-blind, placebo controlled, parallel-group study. *Neurology* 1993;43:2292–2298.
4. U.K. Gabapentin Study Group. Gabapentin in partial epilepsy. *Lancet* 1990;335:1114–1117.
5. Anhut H, Ashman P, Feuerstein TJ, Sauermann W, Saunders M, Schmidt B. Gabapentin (Neurontin) as add-on therapy in patients with partial seizures: a double-blind, placebo-controlled study. The International Gabapentin Study Group. *Epilepsia* 1994;35:795–801.
6. Matsuo F, Bergen D, Faught E, et al. Placebo-controlled study of the efficacy and safety of lamotrigine in patients with partial seizures. U.S. Lamotrigine Protocol 0.5 Clinical Trial Group. *Neurology* 1993;43: 2284–2291.
7. Ben-Menachem E. International experience with tiagabine add-on therapy. *Epilepsia* 1995;36(Suppl 6): S14–S21.
8. Willmore LJ, Shu V, Wallin B. Efficacy and safety of add-on divalproex sodium in the treatment of complex partial seizures. The M88-194 Study Group. *Neurology* 1996;46:49–53.
9. Faught E, Wilder BJ, Ramsay RE, et al. Topiramate placebo-controlled dose-ranging trial in refractory partial epilepsy using 200-, 400-, and 600-mg daily dosages. *Neurology* 1996;46:1684–1690.
10. Privitera M, Fincham R, Penry J, et al. Topiramate placebo-controlled dose-ranging trial in refractory partial epilepsy using 600-, 800-, and 1,000-mg daily dosages. *Neurology* 1996;46:1678–1683.
11. French JA, Mosier M, Walker S, Sommerville K, Sussman N. A double-blind, placebo-controlled study of vi-

gabatrin 3 g/day in patients with uncontrolled complex partial seizures. Vigabatrin Protocol 024 Investigative Cohort. *Neurology* 1996;46:54–61.
12. Wilensky AJ, Ojemann LM, Temkin NR, Troupin AS, Dodrill CB. Clorazepate and phenobarbital as antiepileptic drugs: a double-blind study. *Neurology* 1981;31:1271–1276.
13. Martínez-Lage JM, Bossi L, Morales G, Martinez Vila E, Orofiamma B, Viteri C. Progabide treatment in severe epilepsy: a double-blind cross-over trial versus placebo. *Epilepsia* 1984;25:586–593.
14. Reinikainen KJ, Keränen T, Halonen T, Komulainen H, Riekkinen PJ. Comparison of oxcarbazepine and carbamazepine: a double-blind study. *Epilepsy Res* 1987;1: 284–289.
15. Theodore WH, Raubertas RF, Porter RJ, et al. Felbamate: a clinical trial for complex partial seizures. *Epilepsia* 1991;32:392–397.
16. Gram L, Wulff K, Rasmussen KE, et al. Valproate sodium: a controlled clinical trial including monitoring of drug levels. *Epilepsia* 1977;18:141–148.
17. Graves NM, Holmes GB, Fuerst RH, Leppik IE. Effect of felbamate on phenytoin and carbamazepine serum concentrations. *Epilepsia* 1989;30:225–229.
18. Sachdeo RC, Sachdeo SK, Walker SA, Kramer LD, Nayak RK, Doose DR. Steady-state pharmacokinetics of topiramate and carbamazepine in patients with epilepsy during monotherapy and concomitant therapy. *Epilepsia* 1996;37:774–780.
19. Kramer LD, Pledger GW, Kamin M. Prototype antiepileptic drug clinical development plan. *Epilepsia* 1993;34:1075–1084.
20. Swinyard EA, Woodhead JH, Wolf HH. Use of isobolograms in predicting drug interactions. In: Pitlick W, ed. *Antiepileptic Drug Interactions*. Bethesda, MD: National Institutes of Health; 1989.
21. Shank RP, Gardocki JF, Vaught JL, et al. Topiramate: preclinical evaluation of a structurally novel anticonvulsant. *Epilepsia* 1994;35:450–460.
22. Pledger GW. Drug interactions in clinical trials: statistical considerations. In: Pitlick WH, ed. *Antiepileptic Drug Interactions*. New York: Demos; 1989.

Antiepileptic Drug Development.
Advances in Neurology, Vol. 76,
edited by J. French, I. Leppik, and M. A. Dichter.
Lippincott–Raven Publishers, Philadelphia © 1998.

9

Novel Methods for Studying New Antiepileptic Drug Pharmacology

Richard H. Mattson, Richard D. Scheyer, Ognen A. C. Petroff,
Matthew J. During, Theresa L. Collins, and Dennis Spencer

Department of Neurology, Yale University School of Medicine, New Haven, Connecticut 06510, Department of Molecular Medicine, University of Auckland School of Medicine, Auckland, New Zealand.

INTRODUCTION

In early studies of the pharmacology of investigational antiepileptic drugs, screening for efficacy and toxicity in animal models is followed by studies of tolerability and pharmacokinetics in human volunteers (1). The absorption, distribution, metabolism, and elimination are defined using both direct measurements of blood and tissue quantities after oral or parenteral administration together with labeled or stable isotope forms of the compounds (2,3). These standard and traditional techniques provide important information for an understanding of the frequency and quantity of doses needed to achieve a desired clinical effect. Carbamazepine and phenytoin are believed to exert a direct use-dependent action on sodium channels, and phenobarbital a neuromodulatory effect, at least in part, at the $GABA_A$ (τ-aminobutyric acid) receptor (4). The clinical effects of carbamazepine closely parallel the concentration of free drug at the site of action in the central nervous system (5). However, considerable evidence suggests that several new antiepileptic drugs exert their pharmacodynamic effect indirectly.

GABAergic compounds have been developed in an effort to inhibit epileptic excitability (6,7) (Fig. 1). However, many of these appear to act indirectly rather than at a receptor or ion channel. Consequently, a close correlation may not exist between the timing of doses and blood or brain concentrations. For example, in experimental animal studies, gabapentin and vigabatrin have little immediate effect (8,9). Warnil and McLean (10) have demonstrated that the effect of gabapentin on sustained repetitive firing in a cellular preparation of the fetal rat spinal cord neuron slowly increases with incubation up to 12 to 24 hours. Similarly, Welty et al. (8) found that seizure threshold in the rodent model continued to rise at a time when blood and brain concentrations of gabapentin were decreasing (Fig. 2). Although in part this can be explained by the time delay required for active uptake by the L-amino acid transporter, it is likely that this may also represent the result of effects on intracellular amino acid metabolism (11). Löscher found clear evidence of increased turnover of GABA in gabapentin-treated animals (12).

Vigabatrin, another new antiepileptic drug, was also developed to have a GABA-mediated action (9). It is a compound closely related to GABA but possesses a terminal vinyl group (Fig. 1) that binds irreversibly to GABA transaminase (GABA-T), resulting in a blockage of metabolic degradation and an accumulation of GABA in the cell (9,13,14). The pharmacodynamic effects of vigabatrin depend on the length of time required for the cells to resynthesize GABA-T rather than the length of time required for the systemic clearance of vigabatrin.

Tiagabine, another new antiepileptic drug, is related to nipecotic acid and was developed specifically to inhibit GABA reuptake into glia and/or nerve terminals (15,16). Such an effect should result in increased extracellular GABA concentrations and associated inhibition. The effect may be delayed because of this secondary action.

Thus, it can be seen that for perhaps three of the new antiepileptic drugs, traditional pharmacokinetic measures of blood or even brain concentrations may be less useful in predicting pharmacodynamic effects than for the older, standard antiepileptic drugs. With these new drugs, it may be more important to measure the neurotransmitters rather than the antiepileptic drugs themselves. New methods of microdialysis and nuclear mag-

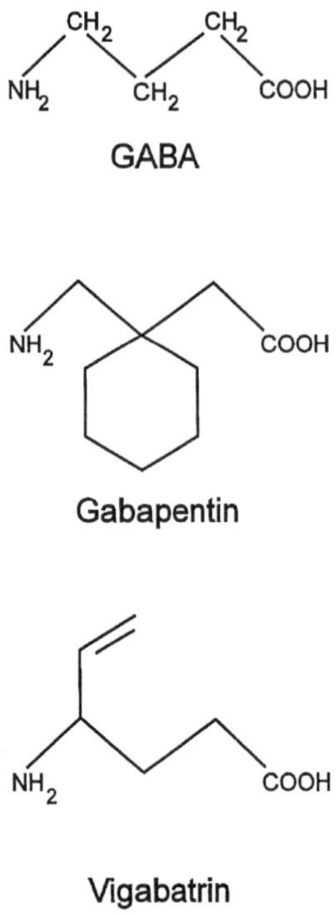

FIG. 1. The structural similarity of GABA and the putative GABAergic drugs gabapentin and vigabatrin.

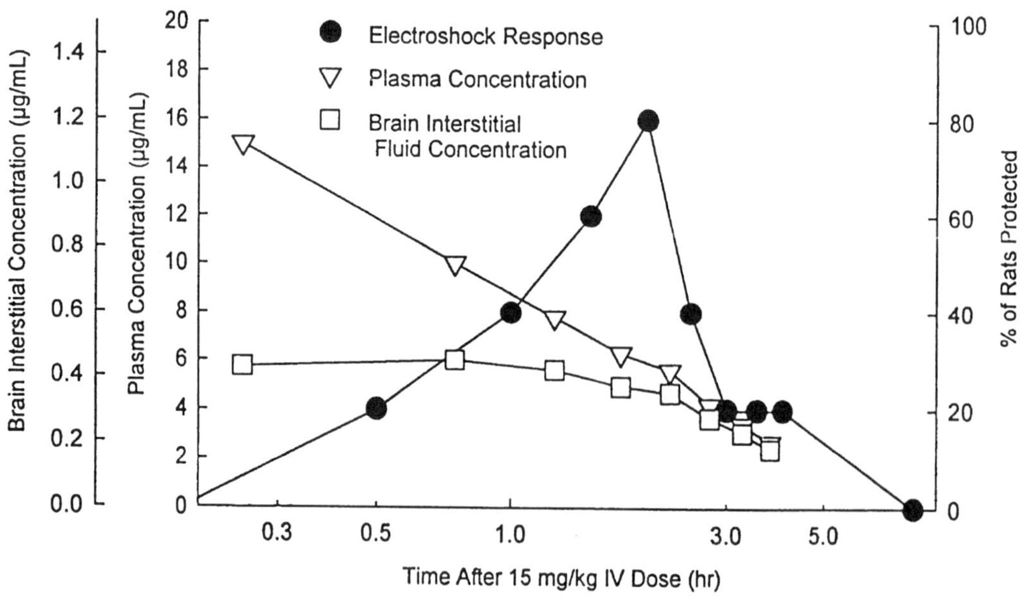

FIG. 2. Seizure threshold in the rodent model continues to rise at a time when blood and brain concentrations of gabapentin are decreasing (Welty et al.) (8).

netic resonance (MR) spectroscopy have provided opportunities to measure the neurochemical effects of some of these compounds.

MICRODIALYSIS

The technique of microdialysis has been utilized in animal experimental models for more than a decade (5,17,18). Insertion of a collection tube into the brain of animals allows continual perfusion of artificial extracellular fluid into the intracerebral extracellular space. A semipermeable membrane is located along this tubing; electrolytes and other chemicals can pass across the membrane, depending on the physical characteristics of the membrane itself. Most commonly used membranes readily allow molecules of <8000 d to cross freely. Amino acid neurotransmitters, including GABA and glutamate, readily cross the semipermeable membrane, so that samples of the constituents of the extracellular fluid can be collected as continuous perfusion occurs. The semipermeable membrane also allows substances such as antiepileptic drugs to be introduced into the extracellular space by way of the continuous perfusion. The perfusion fluid is sterile, but even a contaminating infectious agent cannot cross the membrane owing to its size.

Although extensively used for animal studies, microdialysis was developed to study patients with epilepsy by Dr. Matthew During, working in collaboration with Dr. Dennis Spencer. This team developed an electrode, the "Spencer dialatrode," consisting of a typical depth electrode used for intracranial recording during presurgical electrographic evaluation (Fig. 3). Workers in Sweden also studied human epilepsy by similar methods (19). Joined to the dialatrode is a very small tubing containing an input and output, with an area of semipermeable membrane near the tip. The microdialysis apparatus adds only approximately a 50th of the mass of the depth electrode and consequently is relatively small compared with the depth electrode itself. The depth electrode provides the usual clinically indicated recordings of intracranial electrical events (electroencephalographic spikes and seizures) needed for presurgical localization of a seizure focus and at the same time allows continuous, 24-h/d perfusion of artificial extracellular fluid and collection of constituents of the intracerebral compartment. Perfusion rates are adjustable; the more slowly perfusion is carried out, the more complete is equilibrium of substances across the membrane. Very slow perfusion necessitates longer periods of time to collect sufficient samples for chemical analysis.

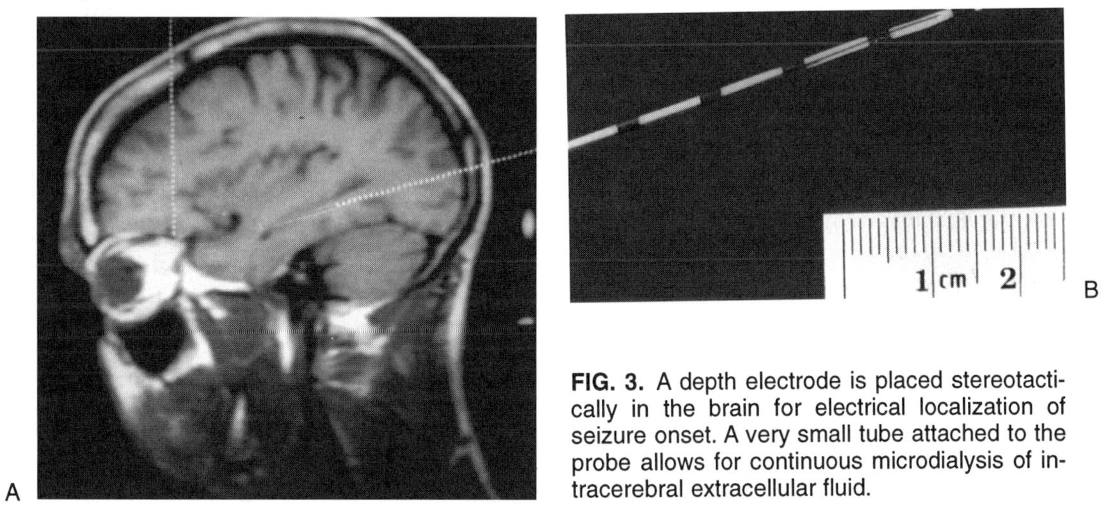

FIG. 3. A depth electrode is placed stereotactically in the brain for electrical localization of seizure onset. A very small tube attached to the probe allows for continuous microdialysis of intracerebral extracellular fluid.

A perfusion rate of 2.5 μL/min allows 25 μL of fluid to be collected each 10 minutes. This rate allows moderate equilibrium to occur and provides a sample during a time course that is appropriate for many pharmacologic studies. On the other hand, for measurement of changes during a seizure or for detection of rapid penetration of drugs into the brain following systemic administration, a more rapid perfusion rate is required. The flow rate at which 50% recovery is obtained is different for each antiepileptic drug. This correlates with the lipid solubility of the antiepileptic drug and probably relates to how rapidly it crosses the blood-brain barrier (Fig. 4).

Sampling of amino acid concentrations has confirmed the putative action of tiagabine as an inhibitor of GABA uptake (15). Both Fink-Jensen et al. (20), studying rats, and During et al. (21), studying humans, found that administration of tiagabine leads to an increase in concentration of extracellular GABA as measured in microdialysis fluid. The half-life of tiagabine in blood when coadministered with enzyme-inducing drugs is shorter than the duration of GABA elevation in the brain. This raises the possibility that the clinical effect may outlast the effects predicted from tiagabine half-life and blood levels.

Limitations

Although microdialysis and sampling of fluid perfused through the brain provide a remarkable opportunity to observe the dynamic chemical changes occurring in the intracerebral extracellular space, multiple technical issues require that interpretation of results be conservative. The placement of the dialysis tubing intracellularly represents a traumatic event that at least temporarily can be expected to distort normal functions (22). The procedure can be expected to disturb the blood-brain barrier and produce changes in the microdialysis fluid that might actually represent effects caused by abnormal penetration of substances from the blood, confounding interpretation. Animal as well as human studies provide evidence that the blood-brain barrier is restored within 24 hours or, in some animal studies, considerably earlier (17). In addition, in human studies of epilepsy, Scheyer et al. (Fig. 4) found a different rate of recovery of various antiepileptic drugs during in vivo microdialysis than during vitro microdialysis, adding strong supportive evidence of a restored barrier (5). The difficulty in obtaining absolute concentrations has been referred to above. Full equilibrium is obtained only under circumstances of no flow, but this, of course, provides no sample for analysis, so that some compromise is required regarding the rate of flow needed to obtain adequate samples for analysis in an investigationally relevant period of time, and equilibrium across the semipermeable membrane is then less than complete. It has been possible to perform analyses at various flow rates and establish a curve with a calculated concentration at a no-flow condition.

A final caveat is that the microdialysis samples chemical concentrations in the extracellular fluid, and only by inference does such sampling indicate what is occurring at the level of the synapse. The dialyzed fluid is, of course, only a gross measure of the microenvironment of the synapse. The limitations in

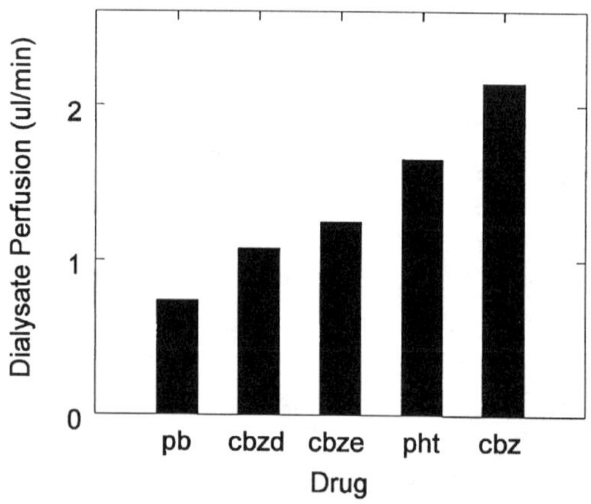

FIG. 4. The microdialysis perfusion rate at which 50% antiepileptic drug recovery is obtained correlates with lipid solubility. *PB*, phenobarbital; *CBZ-D*, carbamazepine diol; *CBZ-E*, carbamazepine epoxide; *PHT*, phenytoin (5).

interpretation of findings must be kept in mind.

Applications

Microdialysis provides opportunities to assess mechanisms and pharmacodynamic effects of antiepileptic drugs, and in particular several of the new compounds having GABA-related actions. Tiagabine, a GABA reuptake inhibitor, should cause an increase in extracellular GABA concentrations. As noted above, Fink-Jensen and colleagues (20) administered tiagabine to rats. Using microdialysis, they analyzed GABA concentration in extracellular fluid and found an increase in GABA following drug administration that correlated with dose and effectiveness in preventing experimental seizures. During et al. (21) observed similar changes in GABA concentration in people undergoing microdialysis and simultaneous cranial electrographic recording before possible resective epilepsy surgery. The experiments confirmed the changes in neurotransmitter concentration, but the study results were insufficient to provide data of clinical/electrographic antiepileptic effect. Similar, related studies using drugs such as gabapentin and vigabatrin, which might alter extracellular fluid concentrations, warrant further consideration. Changes in GABA concentrations that follow administration of these compounds are primarily intracellular and may not be apparent in microdialysis samples (14,23,24) unless paroxysmal stimulation or spontaneous seizures occur. Microdialysis of animal preparations indicates promoted release of nonvesicular GABA with paroxysmal discharge (25). Such findings can be further studied in epilepsy patients during presurgical intensive monitoring with closed-circuit television and electroencephalography. Changes in GABA concentration found in microdialysis fluid in response to seizures or electrical stimulation may be greater when patients are given vigabatrin or gabapentin. Such findings might provide insights into the pharmacodynamic effects of these antiepileptic drugs.

Although such systemic administration may provide important information, these drug effects, of course, affect the entire brain and not necessarily just regions near the epilepsy focus. If the drugs are perfused through the microdialysis system, very localized effects might be studied and compared with those observed in the absence of drug or when the drug is administered systemically.

NUCLEAR MAGNETIC RESONANCE SPECTROSCOPY

Nuclear MR spectroscopy, sometimes referred to as a noninvasive metabolic biopsy, is a revolutionary technique that provides insights into many aspects of science and medicine. Although imaging of the brain has been the best-appreciated advance, nuclear MR spectroscopy can also be used to measure chemical constituents of the brain noninvasively. Nuclear MR spectroscopists have developed methods for measuring levels of brain neurotransmitters, including GABA and glutamate (26) (Fig. 5). Changes in inhibition associated with GABA and excitation caused by glutamate have long been thought to play a role in epilepsy pathogenesis, and these

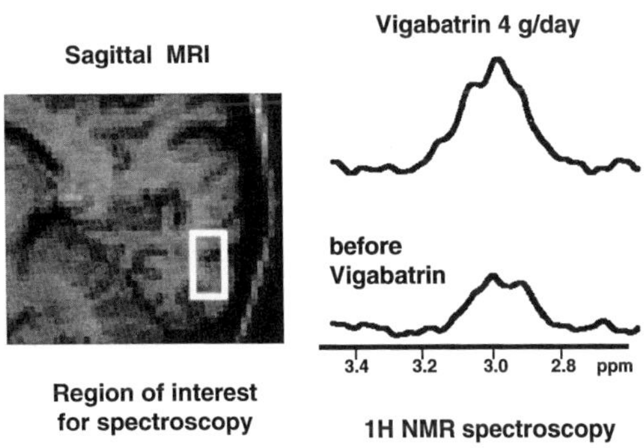

FIG. 5. Left: MR image of the area of occipital brain analyzed for GABA (or other chemicals) using nuclear MR spectroscopy. **Right:** Elevated GABA peak after long-term administration of 4g vigabatrim per day.

changes are considered to representing a site for action of antiepileptic drugs. Few antiepileptic drugs have been developed that directly alter excitatory amino acid function, but several GABA-active drugs have been developed and marketed. Tiagabine, mentioned earlier, is a GABA uptake inhibitor, and administration leads to increased extracellular concentrations based on microdialysis studies. Nuclear MR spectroscopic measurements of whole-brain GABA concentrations in a few patients have failed to reveal any difference compared with concentrations in patients not given tiagabine. This may be explained by shifts in concentration in the extracellular space, which is small compared with intracellular volume. In contrast, vigabatrin is an effective new antiepileptic drug (27,28) that acts as a GABA-T inhibitor. After vigabatrin is administered, total levels of GABA in the brain should be elevated. Vigabatrin has been shown to elevate brain GABA levels based on determination of concentrations in the brains of rodents treated with this drug (9). Indirect evidence of vigabatrin-induced elevation of brain GABA in humans has also been obtained by Ben-Menachem and others (29–33). Analysis of cerebral spinal fluid concentrations demonstrated a rise proportional to dosage. Petroff et al. (13,14,34), in a series of studies at Yale, have performed nuclear MR spectroscopy on a cubic centimeter of occipital lobe and found elevations in brain GABA proportional to increasing doses of vigabatrin. GABA concentrations were found to be more than double those measured in controls or patients treated with other drugs (carbamazepine, phenytoin, or valproate). These same studies disclosed an associated modest decrease of glutamate concentrations. Nuclear MR spectroscopy not only allows noninvasive measurement of neurotransmitters altered by administration of antiepileptic drugs, but also permits measurements to be repeated over time to provide a dynamic assessment of pharmacologic effect. Recent studies (35) have suggested that after a single 50-mg dose of vigabatrin per kilogram, GABA levels rise within 2 hours and remain elevated for up to a

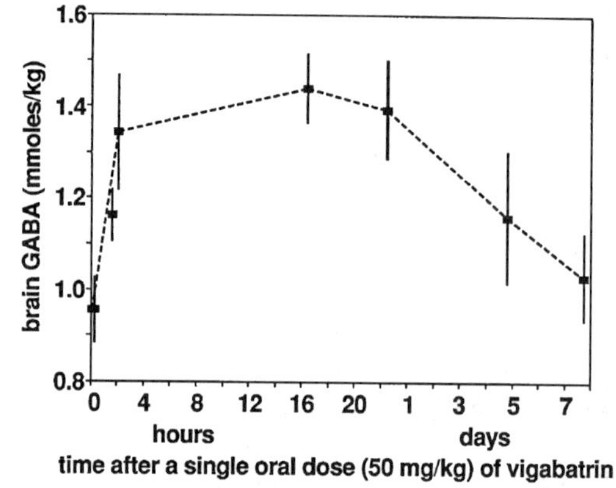

FIG. 6. A single 3-g dose of vigabatrin results in approximately a 150% increase in brain levels of GABA, which only slowly return to predose levels during the next week (35).

week before returning to baseline values (Fig. 6), confirming earlier studies of cerebrospinal fluid by Ben-Menachem et al. (30). Such findings suggest that the pharmacodynamic effect of vigabatrin may be quite prolonged, in contrast to its relatively short half-life in pharmacokinetic studies (30) (Fig. 7), and may provide valuable information for the optimal clinical use of this drug.

The pharmacology of gabapentin has also been investigated using nuclear MR spectroscopy, and modest but significant elevations of brain GABA levels have been revealed that have correlated with gabapentin

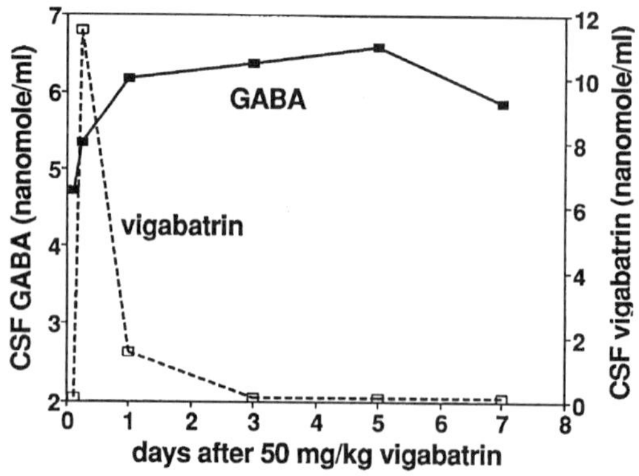

FIG. 7. GABA levels in the cerebrospinal fluid remain elevated for at least a week, even though vigabatrin levels drop rapidly in 24 hours (30).

dose (23). The potential exists for comparison of serum drug levels and central nervous system neurotransmitter levels as measured by nuclear MR spectroscopy and microdialysis following oral or locally perfused gabapentin, tiagabine, and vigabatrin.

Limitations

The absolute nuclear MR spectroscopic measures of neurotransmitter concentration are based on indirect methods but have been standardized using brain extract methods (12,14). The pharmacologic studies also sample only a limited portion of the brain, and the assumption that similar changes occur in other parts of the brain and in the epileptic focus must be made cautiously.

SUMMARY

A number of new antiepileptic drugs act by indirect mechanisms and thus produce effects that may not best be measured by traditional blood studies of the drugs and their metabolites. Study of the indirect action of these drugs on GABA-mediated inhibition by microdialysis and nuclear MR spectroscopy has proved more relevant. These new investigative techniques may also prove valuable as compounds affecting glutamate or other excitatory neurotransmitters are developed.

REFERENCES

1. White HS, Woodhead JH, Franklin MR, Swinyard EA, Wolf HH. Experimental selection, quantification, and evaluation of antiepileptic drugs. In: Levy RH, Mattson RH, Meldrum BS, eds. *Antiepileptic Drugs*. 4th ed. New York: Raven Press; 1995:99–110.
2. Johannessen S. Laboratory monitoring of antiepileptic drugs. In: Levy RH, Mattson RH, Meldrum BS, eds. *Antiepileptic Drugs*. 4th ed. New York: Raven Press; 1995:179–187.
3. Browne TR, Szubo GK, Evans JF, Evans BA, Greenblatt DJ, Schumacher GE. Studies of nonlinear pharmacokinetics with stable isotope-labeled phenytoin. In: Baillie TA, Jones JP, eds. *Synthesis and Applications of Iso topically Labeled Compounds*. Amsterdam: Elsevier; 1994:157–162.
4. Macdonald RL. Benzodiazepines: mechanisms of action. In: Levy RH, Mattson RH, Meldrum BS, eds. *Antiepileptic Drugs*. 4th ed. New York: Raven Press; 1995:491–498.
5. Scheyer RD, During MJ, Cramer JA, Toftness BR, Hochholzer JM, Mattson RH. Simultaneous HPLC analysis of carbamazepine and carbamazepine epoxide in human brian microdialysate. *J Liquid Chromatogr* 1994;17(Suppl 7):1567–1576.
6. Dichter MA, Ayala GF. Cellular mechanisms of epilepsy: a status report. *Science* 1987;237:157–164.
7. Roberts E, Frankel S. Gamma-aminobutyric acid in brain: its formation from glutamic acid. *J Biol Chem* 1950:187:55–63.
8. Welty DF, Schielke GP, Vartanian MG, Taylor CP. Gabapentin anticonvulsant action in rats: disequilibrium with peak drug concentration in plasma and brain microdialysate. *Epilepsy Res* 1993;16:175–181.
9. Schecter PJ. Clinical pharmacology of vigabatrin. *Br J Clin Pharmacol* 1989;27(Suppl 1):195–225.
10. Wamill AW, McLean MJ. Limitation by gabapentin of high-frequency action potential firing by mouse central neurons in cell culture. *Epilepsy Res* 1994;17:1–11.
11. Taylor CP. Gabapentin: mechanisms of action. In: Levy RH, Mattson RH, Meldrum BS, eds. *Antiepileptic Drugs*. 4th ed. New York: Raven Press;1995:829–841.
12. Löscher W. Valproate enhances GABA turnover in the substantia nigra. *Brain Res* 1989;501:198–203.
13. Rothman D, Petroff O, Behar K, Mattson R. Localized ^{1}H NMR measurements of τ-aminobutyric acid in human brain in vivo. *Proc Natl Acad Sci U S A* 1993:90: 5662–5666.
14. Petroff OAC, Rothman DL, Behar KL, Mattson RH. Initial observations on the effect of vigabatrin on the in vivo ^{1}H spectroscopic measurements of GABA, glutamate, and glutamine in human brain. *Epilepsia* 1995; 36:457–464.
15. Ostergaard LH, Gram L, Dam M. Potential antiepileptic drugs: tiagabine. In: Levy RH, Mattson RH, Meldrum BS, eds. *Antiepileptic Drugs*. 4th ed. New York: Raven Press; 1995:1057–1061.
16. Kroogsgard-Larsen P, Falch E, Larsson OM, Schousboe A. GABA uptake inhibitors: relevance to antiepileptic drug research. *Epilepsy Res* 1987;1:77–93.
17. Beneniste H, Huttemeier PC. Microdialysis: theory and application. *Prog Neurobiol* 1990;351:195–215.
18. During MJ, Spencer DD. Extracellular hippocampal glutamate and spontaneous seizure in the conscious human brain. *Lancet* 1993;341:1607–1613.
19. Carlson H, Ronne-Engstrom E, Ungerstedt U, Hillered L. Seizure-related elevations of extracellular amino acids in human focal epilepsy. *Neurosci Lett* 1992;140:30–32.
20. Fink-Jensen A, Suzdak PD, Swedberg MDB, Judge ME, Hansen L, Nielsen PG. The τ-aminobutyric acid (GABA) uptake inhibitor tiagabine increases extracellular brain levels of GABA in awake rats. *Eur J Pharmacol* 1992;20:197–201.
21. During MJ, Mattson RH, Scheyer R. The effect of tiagabine HCl on extracellular GABA levels in the human hippocampus. *Epilepsia* 1992;33:83.
22. Westergren I, Nystrom B, Hamberger A, Johansson BB. Intracerebral dialysis and the blood-brain barrier. *J Neurochem* 1995;64:229–234.
23. Petroff OAC, Rothman DL, Behar KL, Lamoureux D, Mattson R. The effect of gabapentin on brain gamma-aminobutyric acid in patients with epilepsy. *Ann Neurol* 1996;39:95–99.
24. Honmou O, Kocsis JD, Richerson GB. Gabapentin potentiates the conductance increase induced by nipecotic

acid in CA1 pyramidal neurons in vitro. *Epilepsy Res* 1995;20:193–202.
25. Kocsis JD, Mattson RH. GABA levels in the brain: a target for new antiepileptic drugs. *Neuroscientist* 1996; 2:S326–3340.
26. Rothman DL, Behar KL, Hetherington HP, Shulman RG. Homonuclear ^{1}H double-resonance difference spectroscopy of the rat brain in vivo. *Proc Natl Acad Sci U S A* 1984;81:6330–6334.
27. Browne TR, Mattson RH, Penry JK, et al. Multicenter long-term safety and efficacy study of vigabatrin for refractory complex partial seizures in the United States. *Br J Clin Pharmacol* 1989;27(Suppl 1):955–1005.
28. French JA, Mosier M, Walker S, Sommerville K, Sussman N. Vigabatrin Protocol 024 Investigational Cohort. Double-blind placebo-controlled study of vigabatrin 3 grams per day in patients with uncontrolled complex partial seizures. *Neurology* 1996;46:54–61.
29. Ben-Menachum, Persson LI, Schecter PJ, et al. The effect of different vigabatrin treatment regimens on CSF biochemistry and seizure control in epileptic patients. *Br J Clin Pharmacol* 1989;27(Suppl 1):79S–85S.
30. Ben-Menachem E, Perrson LI, Schecter PJ, et al. Effects of single doses of vigabatrin on CSF concentrations of GABA, homocarnosine, homovanillic acid, and 5-hydroxyindoleacetic acid in patients with complex partial epilepsy. *Epilepsy Res* 1988;2:96–101.
31. Kalviainen R, Halonen T, Pitkanen A, Reikkinen PJ. Amino acid levels in the cerebrospinal fluid of newly diagnosed epileptic patients: effect of vigabatrin and carbamazepine monotherapies. *J Neurochem* 1993;60: 1244–1250.
32. Reikkinen PJ, Ylinen A, Halonen T, Sivenius J, Pitkanan A. Cerebrospinal fluid GABA and seizure control with vigabatrin. *Br J Clin Pharmacol* 1989;27(Suppl 1): 87S–94S.
33. Jung MJ, Palfreyman MG. Vigabatrin: mechanisms of action. In: Levy RH, Mattson RH, Meldrum BS, eds. *Antiepileptic Drugs*. 4th ed. New York: Raven Press; 1995:903–913.
34. Mattson RH, Petroff O, Rothman D, Behar K. Vigabatrin: effects on human brain GABA levels by nuclear magnetic resonance spectroscopy. *Epilepsia* 1994:35 (Suppl 5):S29–S32.
35. Petroff OAC, Rothman DL, Behar KL, Collins TL, Mattson RH. Human brain GABA levels rise rapidly after initiation of vigabatrin therapy. *Neurology* 1996;47: 1567–1571.

Antiepileptic Drug Development.
Advances in Neurology, Vol. 76,
edited by J. French, I. Leppik, and M. A. Dichter.
Lippincott–Raven Publishers, Philadelphia © 1998.

10

The Art of Antiepileptic Trial Design

Jacqueline A. French

Department of Neurology, University of Pennsylvania, Philadelphia, Pennsylvania 19104.

INTRODUCTION

Antiepileptic drug trials stand as among the most difficult to perform. The reasons for this are numerous. They include the extreme variability and unpredictability of the condition for which drug treatment is being attempted, the requirement that all patients with diagnosed epilepsy receive therapy (thereby eliminating the possibility of any comparison group receiving placebo), and the complex pharmacokinetic interactions so commonly seen with this class of drugs. Standard designs have been developed to circumvent many of these difficulties, but no single trial design will be appropriate for all drugs or all populations of patients with epilepsy.

When a pharmaceutical company is creating a drug development plan for a new antiepileptic drug, certain standard trials, with well-characterized designs, almost always will be used. However, every antiepileptic drug has unique characteristics. Plans for specific drugs may require alteration or even, in some cases, complete redesign of standard protocols. In addition, the spectrum of activity or appropriateness for monotherapy may lead to decisions about testing in alternative populations or situations, in which case novel protocol designs are necessary. Therefore, it is very unusual for the development plan for two different compounds to be exactly alike.

This chapter addresses the alternatives available for antiepileptic drug protocol design, and the pros and cons of each. It also discusses how drug characteristics may lead to selection of one alternative over another.

SELECTION OF POPULATION

The first decision that must be made when a protocol is designed concerns the choice of population for study; this choice greatly influences protocol design and implementation. When a population is selected, three major characteristics must be addressed: seizure/epilepsy type, degree of intractability, and age.

The first studies in patients of a new drug are usually performed in adults with intractable partial seizures. Adults are chosen because of the risks involved in the study of a drug in early development. These risks are not felt to be acceptable for children. Partial seizures are chosen because they represent the majority of seizures seen in adults. The population with intractable seizures is used because these patients are the most willing to participate in a phase II study, with an as yet unproven drug. Other populations are explored in phase III or postmarketing studies.

Seizure/Epilepsy Type

The classification of epilepsy and epileptic seizures is complex, and some aspects are still controversial. A modified representation of the international classification scheme is available in Table 1. The classification scheme distinguishes epilepsy syndromes, within which several seizure types can occur. It is considered more appropriate to choose drug study populations based on syndromes rather than seizure types, as patients with a certain syndrome are more homogeneous in terms of seizure etiology. Also, response to specific drugs is determined in most instances by seizure syndrome rather than by seizure type. This is illustrated by patients with generalized tonic-clonic convulsions (GTCC). This seizure type may occur in patients with partial, primary generalized, or secondary generalized syndromes. GTCC associated with partial epilepsy are likely to respond to carbamazepine, valproic acid, or phenytoin, and also to many emerging antiepileptic drugs (1,2). GTCC associated with primary generalized epilepsy may respond only to valproic acid or lamotrigine (3,4,5). GTCC associated with secondary generalized epilepsy are treatment-resistant and may not respond to any antiepileptic drug (2). If an antiepileptic drug with a narrow spectrum of activity is tested against GTCC without regard to syndrome, efficacy may be diluted out and the drug may appear ineffective.

Phase II and frequently phase III trials are performed in patients with partial epilepsy. If a drug appears to have a broad spectrum of activity based on preclinical or open trial data, it may be useful to demonstrate efficacy in other epilepsy syndromes. As the two other common syndromes, primary generalized epilepsy and secondary generalized epilepsy, are more common in children than in adults, such testing may also be useful in acquiring a pediatric indication. However, substantial problems are encountered in performing these trials.

Primary generalized epilepsy is a highly treatable condition. This leaves patients who have the condition little incentive to try an investigational drug. In treated patients, residual seizures may not be frequent enough for the purpose of demonstrating efficacy. Trials may be performed in patients with "refractory" primary generalized epilepsy, but these patients may in fact have a different underlying condition and may not be representative of the population as a whole. For these reasons, performing trials in this population is extremely difficult.

Complicating matters even further, seizure types are more variable than in patients with partial epilepsy and may be selectively responsive to therapy. Patients with primary generalized epilepsy have a combination of three seizure types—namely, absence (*petit mal*), myoclonus, and GTCC (*grand mal*). The primary generalized epilepsies are subdivided into syndromes based on seizure type and age at presentation. Long-term prognosis for remission of epilepsy may depend on syndromic classification. For example, pediatric absence epilepsy is first manifested in children of elementary school age. As the name suggests, absence seizures are usually the predominant seizure type, although some children eventually have GTCC as well. This syndrome frequently remits by adulthood. In contrast, juvenile myoclonic epilepsy typically presents in children near puberty, and seizure types, along with characteristic myoclonus, may include absence and GTCC. Although seizures are usually easily treated by the appropriate medications, the syndrome does not remit, and treatment must be lifelong. Trials in primary generalized epilepsy may recruit patients with a variety of syndromes, or may be limited to a single syndrome or seizure type. Clearly, this decision will in part be driven by the desired claim for labeling. Although recruitment from a wider population will result in a broader claim, there is a potential that it will be more difficult to demonstrate efficacy if the drug does not treat all generalized seizure types equally well. In some cases, pilot studies may be needed to determine the most appropriate population.

Recently, there has been renewed interest in using video-electroencephalographic (video-EEG) monitoring to count absence seizures. Absence seizures are brief, lasting 1 to 30 seconds, and consist primarily of staring and minor automatisms, such as eye blinking. They may occur up to hundreds of times a day. The patient is frequently unaware of the event. These factors may make absences difficult or impossible to track clinically. On the other hand, they show up exquisitely on EEG as generalized spike-and-wave bursts. Studies of valproic acid and ethosuximide in the 1960s and 1970s used video-EEG monitoring to demonstrate efficacy (6,7). A child with new-onset absence seizures can have a dramatic and easily demonstrable reduction in spike-and-wave discharges when appropriate medication is introduced. An ideal and rapid way to test new antiepileptic drugs for efficacy against absence seizures would be to admit such patients for 48 to 72 hours to a monitoring unit and perform a placebo-controlled trial. Unfortunately, such patients are difficult to recruit. Because they are treated easily with standard drugs, they are rarely seen at specialized epilepsy centers and are not interested in investigational treatments.

The secondary generalized epilepsies, exemplified by the Lennox-Gastaut syndrome, also produce significant problems for protocol design and implementation. This type of epilepsy is invariably associated with mental retardation, and seizures occur very frequently. Daily seizure counts may reach 100 or more. In patients who are profoundly retarded, it may be difficult to distinguish small seizures from tics and other behavioral disturbances; therefore, accurate seizure counts are difficult to obtain. One strategy that has been used to surmount this problem has been to obtain a video-EEG-correlated seizure count during 4 to 24 hours. The videotape can be used to train parents and caregivers to identify seizures correctly. In addition, a single, easily identified seizure type (usually tonic seizures) can be selected and tracked for the primary outcome variable. Other seizure types are also counted but have less impact on the success or failure of the trial. These strategies were used successfully in a felbamate trial, the first to demonstrate efficacy in the Lennox-Gastaut syndrome (8).

Age

Initial phase III trials are typically be performed in adults. Children and elderly patients are tested at a later stage. The Food and Drug Administration has recently encouraged early pediatric testing for drugs that are likely to be used in children. This often means concurrent pediatric and adult phase III trials. Trial designs and concerns in infants, older children, and the elderly are discussed in Chapters 15 and 16 and are not further discussed here.

Level of Intractability

The spectrum of severity of epilepsy ranges from new-onset cases in drug-naïve patients to intractable disease in patients who continue to have frequent seizures despite trials with all or most standard drugs.

Early trials are performed in patients with intractable epilepsy. This population is chosen because the patients have a sufficient number of seizures to make possible the demonstration of a statistical reduction in a reasonable period of time (usually 8 to 12 weeks); additionally, such patients are more willing to take the risk of receiving an unproven therapy and accept the inconveniences that accompany a trial situation. However, patients with intractable epilepsy do not constitute an ideal study population, for several reasons. The fact that they have failed many other drugs increases the likelihood that they will be resistant to a new drug as well. This is becoming increasingly obvious as more drugs with varied mechanisms of action are introduced. A new drug that overlaps substantially in the efficacy spectrum with existing antiepileptic drugs may appear ineffective when tested in an intractable population. In addition, because these patients are having frequent, uncontrolled seizures, they require treatment at all times. This precludes the option of performing true placebo-controlled trials.

Clearly, the ability to perform trials in patients with less intractable or even new-onset epilepsy is directly related to the amount of information available about the safety and efficacy of the intended treatment. Trials in patients with new-onset epilepsy are usually undertaken during phase IV. This population presents the advantage of being treatment-naïve. Therefore, monotherapy trials are more easily performed, with either active control or even placebo control.

A group that has not been well studied comprises patients who have sustained an injury that may put them at high risk for development of epilepsy but who have not had a seizure. Potentially, the ability of a drug to prevent epilepsy could be assessed by enrolling these patients in a controlled trial. Few such trials have been performed, and so far no drug has been demonstrated to have antiepileptogenic potential (9). The advantage of such a trial is that it could be performed with patients on monotherapy and placebo control; other issues, such as safety and cognitive effects, could also be addressed. However, even in the populations most at risk, such as persons who have sustained serious head trauma or have had intracranial bleeds, epilepsy develops in <20% of patients and may not occur until years after the insult. This means that such trials would require large numbers of subjects followed for long periods of time. High cost and low feasibility have precluded such trials with new antiepileptic drugs.

SELECTION OF BASIC TRIAL DESIGN

Blinding

There are several types of controlled trial that have been deemed acceptable by the Food and Drug Administration (10). One of these is a historical control, in which patients are placed on treatment and their response is compared with pretreatment baselines. This method has not been accepted as appropriate for epilepsy trials, because these patients are highly subject to placebo effect. In other words, patients who have an expectation that they may improve will demonstrate improvement with or without new treatment. Physicians may have difficulty accepting the reality of the placebo effect in the population of patients with intractable epilepsy, who have been switched from treatment to treatment without benefit, yet time and again patients in the placebo arm of multicenter epilepsy studies demonstrate a substantial reduction in seizures. The degree of placebo effect varies from study to study for unclear reasons. In recent studies, 10% to 20% of patients in the placebo arm of blinded trials have shown a 50% or greater reduction in seizures (11,12). For this reason, only a blinded, controlled trial is acceptable for the purpose of demonstrating efficacy. Side effect profiles may also be affected when patients know that they are on a new therapy. Therefore, the most accurate assessment of side effects comes from blinded trials.

In several circumstances, open trials are the only way to obtain useful data. Some idiosyncratic side effects are too rare to be assessed in the relatively small populations used for blinded trials. Larger, open studies may be necessary to expose larger number of patients before drug approval. Open, nonblinded trials are also appropriately performed as pilot studies to assess efficacy in new populations and to determine whether a blinded, controlled trial will be worthwhile.

Active Versus Placebo Comparisons

When performing controlled clinical trials, one must select a control group against which the treatment group will be compared. The control will be either a placebo (placebo-controlled trial) or another method of treatment, usually a standard drug (active-controlled trial). Active-control trials may be extremely informative for clinical purposes, as they assess whether a new treatment is at least as good as, if not better than, existing treatment. The presence of an active control also makes monotherapy trial design much easier. However, these trials are usually not appropriate to determine the efficacy of a new drug. Many active-control trials are able to demonstrate equivalence between drugs. One of the best examples of this is the Veterans Administration Cooperative Study (1), which randomly assigned patients with newly diagnosed seizures to different antiepileptic drug therapies. This allowed direct comparison of the drugs in terms of both efficacy and safety.

The likelihood of seizure control was equal in all four treatment arms, in this case phenytoin, phenobarbital, carbamazepine, and primidone. For the Food and Drug Administration to accept a trial as proof of efficacy, superiority of the new drug must be demonstrated (13). This is extremely difficult, particularly in the population of patients with intractable epilepsy, who are frequently used for clinical trials. In Europe, active-control trials that demonstrate equivalence between a new and standard therapy are considered acceptable proof of efficacy.

Adjunctive Versus Monotherapy Trials

Adjunctive (add-on) trials are commonly performed during phase II/III testing of a new antiepileptic drug. In this type of trial, the patients remain on whatever therapy they have been taking. Usually, baseline therapy is limited to two antiepileptic drugs. In the treatment phase, the investigational drug is added to baseline therapy. Efficacy is compared with results in a control arm in which placebo is usually added. Adjunctive trials have disadvantages. It is more difficult to prove efficacy in a patient who is already partially treated. Also, side effects may be magnified by combining drugs, and pharmacokinetic interactions may alter baseline or experimental drug levels. Despite these drawbacks, many patients and physicians prefer adjunctive trials. Although side effects may be magnified, there is less concern that seizures will worsen, as baseline drugs are not removed. It may be easier to recruit patients for adjunctive trials than for monotherapy trials.

Recently, new trial designs have been developed to circumvent the ethical and practical road blocks associated with monotherapy trials. The two most popular designs were described by Pledger and Kramer (14) and have subsequently been successfully used to obtain a monotherapy indication from the Food and Drug Administration (15,16). In the first, known as a surgical withdrawal design, patients who are having medication withdrawn for the purpose of presurgical evaluation are used as subjects. When most or all medication has been withdrawn, the experimental antiepileptic drug or placebo is added in a randomized, blinded fashion. The trial ends after subjects have experienced a prespecified number of seizures ("failures") or after a certain amount of time has elapsed without the subjects having had prerequisite number of seizures ("completers"). Trials are analyzed according to how many completers there are in the placebo group versus the treatment group.

The second design is performed in an outpatient setting. Patients are randomized to experimental drug or placebo, and baseline therapy is withdrawn. Usually, a modified, or "ethical" placebo is utilized rather than a true placebo, to reduce the likelihood of status epilepticus or secondary generalization. This can consist of either a minimally effective dose of the same investigational drug or of any other therapy that is presumed to be less effective than the test drug. As in the previous study design, outcome is assessed in terms of "failures" and "completers." Failure is determined on the basis of escape criteria, such as doubling of seizure frequency or increase in seizure severity. If more patients taking the experimental drug at a therapeutic dose are able to complete the trial without meeting escape criteria than are patients on placebo, the treatment is considered effective in monotherapy.

Time to failure is another parameter that can be assessed in both these trial designs. These protocols are now in common use when a monotherapy indication is sought. Although they successfully circumvent some of the problems encountered in monotherapy trials, there are still significant ethical issues raised by these study designs, or by any design that measures outcome in terms of worsening rather than improvement (17).

Parallel Versus Crossover Designs

The last major decision in regard to trial design is a choice between parallel and crossover designs. In the United States, the choice is driven by the Food and Drug Administration, which historically has not favored crossover designs because of potential unblinding as patients move from one treatment phase to the next. There is also concern that some antiepileptic drugs might cause a prolonged therapeutic effect that may persist even after the drug has been discontinued. Such a "carry-over" effect may endanger the outcome of the trial. Inserting a washout period between the two phases of the trial may protect against such an occurrence. Also, statistical methods are available to confirm that the treatment effect did not differ according to the order of the therapy (i.e., whether placebo or treatment came first) (18). Crossover trials tend to be long, and excessive dropouts can be a problem.

Crossover designs offer some advantages, and they have been accepted in some circumstances as proof of efficacy by the Food and Drug Administration (19). They require fewer patients to demonstrate efficacy, as all patients receive drug. They allow patients to determine a preference for a given treatment arm, as all subjects experience both. Also, these trials often provide the first indication that a new drug may produce a withdrawal effect, if patients worsen when crossing over from drug to placebo. For example, in several vigabatrin studies, possible withdrawal seizures were seen when vigabatrin was abruptly withdrawn in crossover trials. Tassinari et al. (20) reported 4 of 16 patients with "quasicontinuous seizures" after withdrawal, and Reynolds et al. (21) noted 2 of 10 patients with severe exacerbations of seizures, one of whom had status epilepticus. Exacerbations were not seen with conversion from placebo to vigabatrin (20,21,22).

INCLUSION/EXCLUSION CRITERIA

Inclusion/exclusion criteria for antiepileptic drug clinical trials have been the subject of a great deal of discussion and controversy. On the one hand, it is critical to exclude patients who are less likely to respond to a drug, are more likely to have adverse events, or are more likely to drop out. On the other hand, if the exclusion criteria are too narrow, investigators will have problems recruiting for the trial. A typical list of inclusion/exclusion criteria can be seen in Table 1. Some criteria are self-evident and need little explanation or defense. Others are more controversial and often serve as topics of debate as protocols are finalized.

Seizure Frequency/Type

Patients with relatively low seizure frequencies, such as one to two seizures per month, may be less likely to demonstrate a statistically significant seizure reduction in the 8- to 12-week treatment period. Therefore, patients are usually required to have an average of either three or four seizures per month to enter a trial. The higher the required seizure frequency, the more difficult recruitment becomes. Even the seemingly small difference between a requirement for three seizures per month versus four seizures per month may make a substantial difference. If a drug is potent, fewer seizures per month will be required to demonstrate efficacy. It may make sense to perform an early trial, when less is known about drug potency, with a higher seizure frequency requirement. However, as more becomes known, a lower seizure frequency requirement will speed recruitment. Several successful controlled trials have been performed with a requirement of three seizures per month. Patients are also frequently excluded from trials if they historically have long seizure-free intervals, to prevent an inaccurate picture of seizure frequency during the relatively short baseline and treatment periods. Many epileptic patients have seizures that cluster. The shorter the seizure-free interval allowed, the more patients will be ineligible for the trial. A typical criterion will exclude patients with seizure-free intervals of 28 days or longer.

Patients with partial epilepsy may experience simple partial, complex partial, or secondarily generalized tonic-clonic seizures. Complex partial seizures and generalized tonic-clonic seizures are usually easy to recognize and easily counted. Simple partial seizures are somewhat different. These seizures are not accompanied by alteration of awareness. They may simply consist of a sensation, thought, or emotion, without physical alteration. They frequently do not cause an alteration of the EEG. Therefore, at times it may be difficult to state definitively whether one has occurred or not. Historically, simple partial seizures are not always diminished by a new antiepileptic drug. In fact, some antiepileptic drugs may act by preventing seizure spread and actually convert complex partial seizures and generalized tonic-clonic seizures into simple partial seizures, causing a rise in the simple partial seizure count. Very little disability is caused by simple partial seizures, so elimination of complex partial and generalized tonic-clonic seizures is considered an excellent outcome. For these reasons, simple partial seizures have traditionally been counted but not included in the analysis for determination of seizure reduction. Similarly, patients with exclusively simple partial seizures have not been candidates for studies. Lately, there has been some softening of this position, and clinically observable simple partial seizures (i.e., motor manifestations or aphasia) are frequently counted with and given the same weight as complex partial and generalized tonic-clonic seizures. This again increases the pool of patients eligible for trials and speeds enrollment. As yet, it is too soon to determine whether inclusion of these patients has had a negative effect on determination of efficacy.

Psychiatric Disturbance

Another controversial issue has been whether to permit enrollment of patients with a history of psychiatric problems. The most conservative approach would be to eliminate all patients with any current or previous depression or psychosis. Epileptic patients have a greatly increased incidence of depression, and again, enrollment would suffer from such a strict policy. A more reasonable approach would be to exclude only patients with current psychiatric problems. Some patients may be psychiatrically stable but taking antidepressants or other drugs for psychiatric illness. Again, enrollment will be facilitated if these patients are permitted to be enrolled. In addition, interactions between the study drug and frequently used psychiatric medications can be assessed on a preliminary basis.

Use of Benzodiazepines

Many patients with severe, intractable epilepsy, such as those eligible for antiepileptic drug trials, experience seizure flurries. It is a relatively common practice to administer short-acting benzodiazepines to abort the flurry, thereby returning the patient to a functional state more rapidly and perhaps avoiding the necessity for emergency room intervention. Some protocols exclude all patients who have recently received "rescue" benzodiazepines. The concern is that a patient may receive such a compound during the baseline but not the treatment phase, thereby falsely lowering the relative baseline seizure frequency, or that more patients may receive benzodiazepines in the treatment than in the placebo group. Many protocols have permitted inclusion of these patients, and at present there is no indication that efficacy evaluation has suffered. Presumably, randomization prevents all such patients from landing in any one group or phase of the study. The impact on study outcome of including or excluding these patients has not been definitively determined.

TRIAL DURATION

Trial duration includes screen, baseline, titration, and treatment phases. The impact of baseline and treatment duration on trial outcome is discussed in Chapter 11. Shorter durations are preferred by patients, particularly when there is a possibility of receiving placebo during the treatment phase. Therefore, recruitment may be easier for a shorter trial. Also, longer trials may have a higher dropout rate. However, lengthening the baseline phase may permit enrollment of patients with fewer seizures per month. There are also sound reasons to extend the treatment phase. There is a possibility that some antiepileptic drugs may take time to demonstrate an effect, and that others may lose efficacy over time. Therefore, longer treatment phases may give a more fair representation of drug efficacy. Typically, baseline lasts 6 to 8 weeks and the treatment phase lasts 8 to 12 weeks. The duration of titration varies depending on the investigational drug.

CONVERSION TO OPEN EXTENSION

Conversion from the blinded portion of a controlled trial to the open extension is one aspect of trial design that typically causes problems. The simplest method of conversion would be to unblind the treatment regimen immediately after the patient had completed the blinded segment. Patients on active treatment could elect either to withdraw or remain on therapy, and patients on placebo could be titrated up to a therapeutic dose. Unfortunately, this method has the potential of producing investigator bias. For example, if the first two patients who completed had fatigue and had been on active treatment, the investigator might assume that the treatment causes fatigue and would look particularly for that particular adverse event or presume that all patients with fatigue were on active treatment. Therefore, the trial might become a single-blinded rather than a double-blinded trial. To date, in essentially all cases trials have remained blinded until the completion of conversion to open label. When only one treatment arm is being compared with placebo, this process is relatively simple. Titration kits can be created, based on patient treatment assignment, that convert patients on placebo to active drug in a blinded fashion. When the blind is broken, all patients are taking the same therapy. This method lengthens the time that patients are in a blinded condition by 1 to 6 weeks, depending on the rate of titration. Patients tolerate this relatively well, as they know that they all are receiving active treatment.

When there is more than one active treatment arm, blinded conversion becomes much more difficult. One example is the dose-ranging study, with low, medium, and high doses. The blind must be broken only when all patients are titrated to the same dose. There are potential ethical constraints. If the high dose is chosen as the ending dose, then patients who were doing well, or possibly were seizure-free on the intermediate or low dose, are "forced" to titrate to a higher dose unnecessarily. Conversely, if a low dose is chosen as the ending dose, patients who are doing well at the higher range are forced to titrate down, and seizure control may be jeopardized. Although there is no ideal solution, the commonly accepted practice is to have all patients titrate to an intermediate therapeutic dose. When the blind is broken, their physicians have the option of increasing the dose at will. Choosing the intermediate therapeutic dose lessens the potential that patients will be maintained on too high a dose simply because they were randomized to it in a clinical trial, when a lower dose would have been equally as effective and better tolerated.

The most difficult dilemma arises when there are two active treatment arms with different antiepileptic drugs. This may occur in an active-control comparison, or when a monotherapy outpatient trial is performed and the "ethical placebo" is another drug at a relatively low dose. This was the case in a felbamate trial in which low-dose valproate was used as a comparison (23). Once the trial has been completed, it is impossible to convert to open label without breaking the blind unless all patients are converted to one or the other therapy. Usually, the investigational drug at a therapeutic dose is chosen as the "optimal" therapy and patients are all converted to that therapy, as it is too burdensome to maintain the blind until all patients have completed the study, which frequently lasts for a period of 1 to 2 years. An alternative would be to allow conversion for patients who are not seizure-free or are dissatisfied with therapy and maintain the blind only for patients who are seizure-free and doing well. This would prevent patients from being converted from an effective therapy, possibly to a less effective one.

EFFECT OF DRUG CHARACTERISTICS ON TRIAL DESIGN

Trial design is far from "one size fits all." Every new investigational drug has different characteristics, which must be taken into account when a protocol is being written. The more that can be known about a new drug before designing a pivotal trial, the more likely it will be that the trial will be successful.

Pharmacokinetic Drug Interactions

Pharmacokinetic drug interactions must be thoroughly understood and taken into account when a phase II adjunctive efficacy/toxicity trial is undertaken. The majority of antiepileptic drugs, including newer agents, are hepatically metabolized. Two drugs that are metabolized in the liver are very likely to interact. Interactions can occur in one or two directions. The easiest interaction to deal with occurs when the investigational drug does not induce or inhibit hepatic metabolism but is itself subject to induction or inhibition. Topiramate and lamotrigine are examples. Both of these new drugs are subject to metabolic induction by commonly used antiepileptic drugs such as carbamazepine, phenytoin, and phenobarbital (24,25). In addition, the metabolism of lamotrigine is significantly inhibited by valproic acid. This effect has the potential to cause a wide distribution of blood levels in an adjunctive trial if patients on all types of baseline antiepileptic drugs are included, causing inadequate dosing in some and toxicity in others. This can easily be prevented by allowing only patients on enzyme-inducing baseline antiepileptic drugs to be enrolled and, if necessary, excluding patients on enzyme inhibitors. Of course, the enzyme induction must be taken into account when selecting an effective dose.

It is more problematic when the investigational drug itself causes enzyme induction or inhibition, as is the case with felbamate and remacemide (26,27). If the concomitant antiepileptic drug concentration is lowered, the seizure control of patients in the treatment group may deteriorate. If, on the other hand, levels increase, any seizure reduction in the treatment arm can be attributed to a change in baseline antiepileptic drugs rather than to the investigational antiepileptic drug. In a blinded trial, these problems may be difficult to solve. Often, an unblinded pharmacist will be required to maintain plasma levels of concomitant medications at baseline levels.

Pharmacodynamic interactions may also occur and are much more difficult to control for. In most instances, these interactions produce increased side effects but do not interfere with efficacy assessment.

Dosing Schedule

Dosing schedules should be determined by the pharmacokinetic or phamacodynamic half-life of the drug. Dosing four times or twice daily improves compliance and is easier for patients. Multiple doses per day are required for antiepileptic drugs with short half-lives. A lower apparent efficacy may be the consequence of choosing an interdose interval that is too long, as the serum concentration may fall below the therapeutic range.

Titration Schedule

Choosing an appropriate schedule for titrating an antiepileptic drug at the onset of a trial appears deceptively straightforward. Clinicians and pharmaceutical companies prefer titration to take as short a time as possible. This frequently leads to the error of selecting an overly rapid titration schedule. Rapid titration can lead to many adverse consequences. In the case of lamotrigine, it was discovered that rapid titration increased the incidence of rash (28). For felbamate and topiramate, the consequence was worsening of side effects, causing the drugs to appear more toxic than they actually were (29,30). Titration rate is such a critical issue that it may be worthwhile to do a short open-label titration study before initiating a phase II trial.

CONCLUSION

Trial design is critical for obtaining registration of drugs, thereby making them available to patients with epilepsy. It is also crucial in that everything that will be known about a compound at the time of approval will derive from clinical trials of one sort or another. It is difficult to reconcile the requirements of registering bodies such as the Food and Drug Administration, which demand a strictly controlled trial environment, with the need of clinicians to know how a drug will act in an imperfect "real world" setting. To many, the rigors of trial design seem like a contrivance, and the results may appear to have no value. Nevertheless, controlled clinical trials represent a vast improvement over the days when drug efficacy was taken at face value and patients were subjected to ineffective treatments with unknown risks. By the time that antiepileptic drugs are released, a great deal is known about them. This knowledge serves as a platform from which further knowledge can and should be obtained through experience and further investigation.

REFERENCES

1. Mattson RH, Cramer JA, Collins JF, et al. Comparison of carbamazepine, phenobarbital, phenytoin, and primidone in partial and secondary generalized tonic-clonic seizures. *N Engl J Med* 1985;313:145–151.
2. Mattson RH. Selection of antiepileptic drug therapy. In: Levy RH, Mattson RH, Meldrum BS, eds. *Antiepileptic Drugs*. 4th ed. New York: Raven Press; 1995:123–135.
3. Mattson RH, Cramer JA. Crossover from polytherapy to monotherapy in primary generalized epilepsy. *Am J Med* 1988;84:23–28.
4. Stewart J, Hughes E, Reynolds EH. Lamotrigine in primary generalized epilepsy. *Seizure* 1992; (Suppl A): 13–39.
5. Timmings PL, Richens A. Lamotrigine in primary generalized epilepsy. *Lancet* 1992;339:1300–1301.
6. Browne TR, Dreifuss FE, Dyken PR, Goode FG, Penry JK, Porter RJ, White BG, White PT. Ethosuximide in the treatment of absence (*petit mal*) seizures. *Neurology (Minneapolis)* 1975;25:515–524.
7. Penry JK, Porter RJ, Dreifuss FE. Quantification of paroxysmal abnormal discharge in the EEGs of patients with absence (*petit mal*) seizures for evaluation of antiepileptic drugs. *Epilepsia* 1971;12:278–279.
8. Felbamate Study Group in the Lennox-Gastaut Syndrome. Efficacy of felbamate in childhood epileptic encephalopathy (Lennox-Gastaut syndrome). *N Engl J Med* 1993;328:29–33.
9. Temkin NR, Dilkmen SS, Wilensky AJ, Keihm J, Chabal S, Winn HR. A randomized, double-blind study of phenytoin for the prevention of post-traumatic seizures. *N Engl J Med* 1990;323:497–502.
10. Katz R. The domestic drug-regulatory process: why time is of the essence. *Epilepsy Res Suppl* 1993;10: 91–106 (French JA, Dichter MA, Leppik IE, eds. *New Antiepileptic Drug Development: Preclinical and Clinical Aspects*).
11. French J, Pellock J, Ferendelli J, et al. Results of a multicenter, placebo-controlled, parallel study of vigabatrin in patients with focal epilepsy whose seizures are difficult to control. *Neurology* 1993;43(Suppl 2):A307.
12. Matsuo F, Bergen D, Faught E, et al. Placebo-controlled study of the efficacy and safety of lamotrigine in patients with partial seizures. *Neurology* 1993;43: 2284–2291.
13. Leber P. Hazards of interference: the active-control investigation. *Epilepsia* 1989;30(Suppl 1):S57–S63.
14. Pledger GW, Kramer LD. Clinical trials of investigational antiepileptic drugs: monotherapy designs. *Epilepsia* 1991;32:716–721.
15. Beourgeois BFD, Leppik IE, Sackellares JC, et al. Felbamate double-blind efficacy trial following presurgical monitoring. *Epilepsia* 1991;32(Suppl 3):18(abst).
16. Faught RE, Sachdeo RC, Remler MP, et al. Felbamate monotherapy for partial-onset seizures: an active-control trial. *Neurology* 1993;43:688–692.
17. French J. Which trials, what designs? *Epilepsia* (*in press*).
18. Hills M, Armitage P. The two-period crossover clinical trial. *Br J Clin Pharmacol* 1979;8:7–20.
19. Messenheimer J, Ramsay RE, Willmore LJ, Leroy RF, Zielinski JJ, Mattson R, Pellock JM, Valakas AM, Womble G, Risner M. Lamotrigine therapy for partial seizures: a multicentered, placebo-controlled, double-blind, crossover trial. *Epilepsia* 1994;35:113–121.
20. Tassinari CA, Michelucci R, Ambrosetto G, Fabrizio S. Double-blind study of vigabatrin in the treatment of drug-resistant epilepsy. *Arch Neurol* 1987;44:907–910.
21. Reynolds EH, Ring HA, Farr IN, Heller AJ, Elwes RDC. Open, double-blind, and long-term study of vigabatrin in chronic epilepsy. *Epilepsia* 1991;32: 530–538.
22. Loiseau P, Hardenberg P, Pestre M, Guyot M, Schecter PJ, Tell GP. Double-blind, placebo-controlled study of vigabatrin (gamma-vinyl GABA) in drug-resistant epilepsy. *Epilepsia* 1986;27:115–120.
23. Commission on Classification and Terminology of the International League Against Epilepsy. Proposal for revised clinical and electoencephalographic classification of epileptic seizures. *Epilepsia* 1981;22:489–501.
24. Yuen AWC. Lamotrigine: interactions with other drugs. In: Levy RH, Mattson RH, Meldrum BS, eds. *Antiepileptic Drugs*. 4th ed. New York: Raven Press; 1995:883–887.
25. Ben-Menachem E. Potential antiepileptic drugs: topiramate. In: Levy RH, Mattson RH, Meldrum BS, eds. *Antiepileptic Drugs*. 4th ed. New York: Raven Press; 1995:1063–1070.
26. Clark B, Hutchison JB, Jamieson V, Jones T, Palmer GC, Scheyer RD. Potential antiepileptic drugs: remacemide hydrochloride. In: Levy RH, Mattson RH,

Meldrum BS, eds. *Antiepileptic Drugs*. 4th ed. New York: Raven Press; 1995:1035–1044.

27. Fuerst RH, Graves NM, Leppik IE, Brundage RC, Holmes GB, Remmel RP. Felbamate increases phenytoin but decreases carbamazepine concentrations. *Epilepsia* 1988;29:488–491.
28. Yuen AWC. Safety issues. In: Richens A, ed. *Clinical Update on Lamotrigine: a Novel Antiepileptic Agent*. Tunbridge Wells: Wells Medical Ltd; 1992:69–75 (*International Clinical Practice Series*).
29. Faught E. Felbamate. In: Wyllie E, ed. *The Treatment of Epilepsy: Principles and Practice*. 2nd ed. Baltimore: Williams & Wilkins; 1996:913–919.
30. Privatera M, Fincham R, Penry JK, et al. Topiramate dose-ranging trial in refractory partial epilepsy. *Epilepsia* 1995;36(Suppl 4):533.

Antiepileptic Drug Development.
Advances in Neurology, Vol. 76,
edited by J. French, I. Leppik, and M. A. Dichter.
Lippincott–Raven Publishers, Philadelphia © 1998.

11

Reanalysis of Existing Trial Data: What Can Be Learned

J. Todd Sahlroot and Gordon W. Pledger

Division of Biometrics, Food and Drug Administration, Rockville, Maryland 20857 and Department of Biostatistics, R. W. Johnson Pharmaceutical Research Institute, Raritan, New Jersey 08869.

THE STANDARD ADD-ON TRIAL DESIGN

Add-on trials of antiepileptic drugs compare an investigational compound with a control treatment, usually placebo, in the presence of concomitant antiepileptic therapy. The design structure may be either parallel groups or crossover. Patients whose seizures are not controlled enter a pretreatment seizure-counting period, usually called baseline, during which the pre-existing antiepileptic therapy is continued without change. Baseline periods are normally 8 to 12 weeks in duration. Patients who have "enough seizures" during the baseline period, usually at least three or four per month on average, are then randomly assigned to receive either placebo or the investigational agent (or both in random order if the design is crossover). During the ensuing double-blind treatment period, ideally the concomitant antiepileptic therapy is still maintained as during the baseline period. The duration of the double-blind period is often similar to that of the baseline period, 8 to 12 weeks, but in some trials it has been as long as 6 months (1).

The views expressed are those of the author and not necessarily those of the FDA.

BASIS FOR CURRENT DESIGN FEATURES

Entry Criterion Requiring a Specified Seizure Rate

During an add-on, trial pre-existing antiepileptic therapy is continued. Thus, the trial population, regardless of treatment assignment, should not experience an increase in seizure activity in regard to either rate or severity. The only way that an experimental drug can be shown superior to a control, then, is for the group randomized to the test drug to demonstrate a measurable improvement in seizures, compared with the group receiving placebo. It follows that the successful demonstration of test drug efficacy requires that at least a substantial portion of the study subjects have a degree of seizure activity that allows room for improvement.

Baseline Period of Specified Duration

The baseline period serves two primary functions: (a) to confirm that subjects who are randomly assigned to a treatment arm have seizures at the level required for trial eligibility (see preceding paragraph), and (b) to estimate subjects' seizure rates and characterize their seizure types and severity while they are receiving fixed antiepileptic therapy. Strictly speaking, neither determination is necessary for clinical trial validity. Suppose, for example, that patients have been enrolled on the basis of retrospective information, perhaps just that they recall having experienced several seizures per month while receiving antiepileptic drug treatment. Suppose further that during the double-blind treatment period patients assigned to the test drug group report statistically significantly fewer seizures than do patients assigned to the placebo group (and there is no change in seizure type or severity for the seizures that occur). Such a trial result would constitute a valid demonstration of antiepileptic efficacy for the test drug under the (adjunctive therapy) conditions of the trial design.

The problem with the above scenario, of course, is that it is unlikely. Given the magnitude of the treatment effect that can be reasonably expected in patients with refractory epilepsy, and given the large variability of seizure patterns in these subjects, the statistical power of a trial conducted in such a fashion to show a significant difference between treatments, with what is usually considered a feasible sample size, would be low. The statistical power of a clinical trial to detect a between-treatment difference of D is the probability, given that the "true difference" is D, of observing a statistically significant result. Power can be increased in several ways: by increasing sample size, reducing variability, or choosing trial subjects who are likely to respond to the test drug.

The dual functions of the baseline period, as described above, are intended to increase the statistical power of the trial. It is reasonable to expect that a period of seizure counting under conditions like those of the double-blind treatment period will yield a more accurate estimate of a patient's current seizure rate than would be obtained on the basis of retrospective information. This improved estimate should increase the likelihood of enrolling only patients with the requisite number of seizures; it also provides, for each patient randomized, a seizure rate from which to measure the patient's change during the treatment period.

A frequently used efficacy endpoint is percentage reduction from baseline seizure rate. This endpoint equates the improvement reported for a patient who goes from a baseline rate of 100 seizures per month to a treatment period rate of 50 seizures per month with the improvement of a patient whose baseline rate is 10 seizures per month and whose on-treatment rate is five seizures per month. Both patients had a 50% reduction in seizure rate. In the absence of baseline seizure information, the patient with five seizures per month during treatment would be considered to have a better outcome, perhaps much better, depending on the method of statistical analysis.

The reduced statistical power resulting from the lack of baseline seizures rate estimates can be seen in the following simplified example. Suppose that the population entering a clinical trial consists of two 10-patient subgroups. One subgroup barely meets the entry criterion of four seizures per month immediately before randomization, whereas members of the other subgroup have a pretreatment seizure rate of 30 seizures per month. Assume that the effect of the test drug is a 50% reduction in seizure rate for patients in either subgroup, and that placebo-treated patients have no change in their seizure rate. Suppose further that the randomization process fortuitously assigns five patients in each subgroup to the test drug and five to placebo.

If baseline seizure rates are unknown, then the results of the trial might be given in terms of treatment period monthly seizure rates as follows:

	Placebo	Test drug
Subgroup No. 1	4	2
	4	2
	4	2
	4	2
	4	2
Subgroup No. 2	30	15
	30	15
	30	15
	30	15
	30	15
Mean	17	8.5
Standard deviation	13.70	6.85

If baseline seizure rate data are available, the results of the trial in terms of percentage reduction from baseline are as follows:

	Placebo	Test drug
Subgroup No. 1	0%	50%
	0%	50%
	0%	50%
	0%	50%
	0%	50%
Subgroup No. 2	0%	50%
	0%	50%
	0%	50%
	0%	50%
	0%	50%
Mean	0%	50%
Standard deviation	0%	0%

The treatment effect will be demonstrable under both scenarios. The most notable difference is that in the absence of baseline data the variation is increased, and therefore a larger sample size will be required to achieve statistical significance.

If it is accepted that good estimates of baseline seizure rates will increase power, then it would seem to follow that better estimates of baseline seizure rates will increase power further. Within limits, longer baseline periods should result in more precise estimates of baseline seizure rates.

Treatment Period of Specified Duration

As discussed in connection with the baseline period, the precision of the estimate of the on-treatment seizure rate should improve as the duration of the treatment period increases. Typically, during the first portion of the double-blind treatment period, the test drug is titrated to the planned steady-state dosage. The titration period itself may be several weeks, and the planned analysis may or may not include that portion of the treatment period. Thus, in a typical trial, the duration of the double-blind treatment period excluding the initial titration portion is at least as long as the baseline period; it is sometimes considerably longer (1).

PROBLEMS WITH CURRENT DESIGN FEATURES

As discussed above, longer baseline and treatment periods lead to better estimates, so why aren't the periods becoming longer and longer? The disadvantages are clear. Long baseline periods represent long delays before a patient can have the opportunity for pharmacologically induced improvement in seizures. The same is true for long double-blind treatment periods, in that a patient may be receiving placebo. Thus, trial designs with too-long periods are unattractive to potential trial subjects. A trial with a wonderful design but no actual patients enrolled is often considered less than optimal.

In addition to patient acceptability problems, trial designs with lengthy treatment periods can give rise to issues regarding analysis and interpretation of results. As the duration of the treatment period increases, the loss of patients to follow-up also increases. Dropouts resulting from such causes as intercurrent illness, geographic moves, and normal fluctuations of seizure patterns that may be interpreted as loss of efficacy complicate the interpretation of trial results. Normally, the statistical analysis should include all subjects randomized (intent-to-treat analysis) (2,3), but this type of analysis is not a panacea. Although generally less subject to bias than other approaches (so-called "evaluable patient" or "per protocol" analyses), the intent-to-treat analysis cannot work miracles. If the goal of a long treatment period is to show sustained efficacy but 40% of the subjects have been lost to follow-up before the time point of interest, then the analysis may not be representative of the effect of the test drug.

Another issue involving the duration of the treatment period is that often it is unrelated to how the patient is doing. A patient who is suddenly having far fewer seizures than during the baseline period will likely have no problem completing the planned duration, but a patient who has seen no improvement at all may be eager to try something else. Response-dependent treatment period durations have been proposed (e.g., time-to-*K*th-seizure; see ref. 4) and could be examined through reanalysis of existing trial data.

METHODS USED TO EXAMINE POTENTIAL EFFECTS OF DESIGN CHANGES

To examine the potential effects of changes in baseline and double-blind treatment durations, we retrospectively analyzed data from seven randomized, placebo-controlled, add-on clinical trials using one of three antiepileptic drugs, denoted A, B, and C. Drug A was used in four trials (sample sizes ranging from 28 to 45 subjects per group), drug B in one trial (approximately 70 subjects per group), and drug C in two trials (approximately 100 subjects per group). Four trials had designs with three or more treatment groups, that is, two or more different doses or regimens of the active drug. Two of these trials, using drug A, had four treatment groups (including placebo), and the other two trials used drug C in designs with three and four treatment groups (including placebo). For these multiple-arm trials, one dose of the active drug was selected for pair-wise comparison with placebo, so that these trials would be more closely comparable in regard to design and analysis with trials having just one active treatment group.

Baseline durations for the trials ranged from 8 to 12 weeks and double-blind durations from 12 to 16 weeks. Double-blind treatment periods started with titration periods 4 to 5 weeks long. To examine the effect of shortening baseline or double-blind treatment periods, portions of the baseline and double-blind treatment periods were selected for analysis. Only seizures occurring during these selected portions were used to compute seizure rates. As shown in Fig. 1, we selected the portion of the baseline period immediately preceding the double-blind period (i.e., immediately preceding randomization), and the portion of the double-blind treatment period immediately after baseline (i.e., immediately after randomization).

To qualify for randomization, subjects had to experience minimum seizure rates during baseline. (There were no restrictions on maximum seizure rates.) Entry criteria requiring a specified baseline seizure rate were relatively consistent from trial to trial. Five trials, those

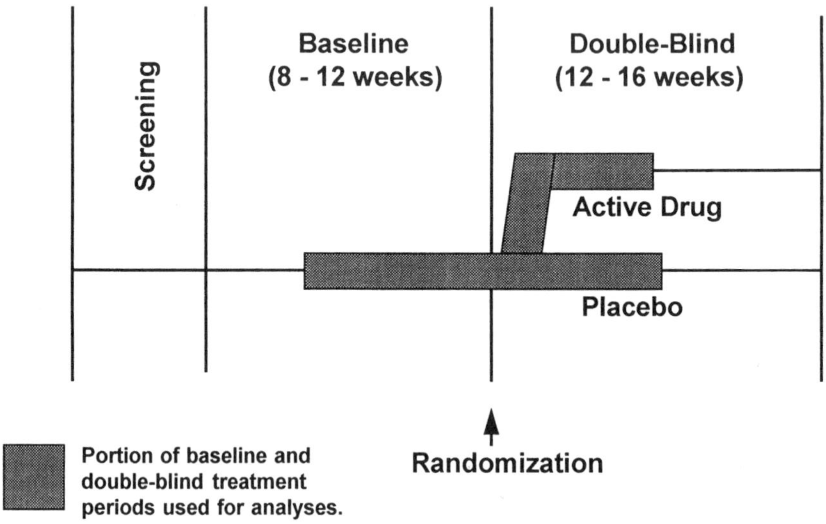

FIG. 1. Schematic of clinical trial design.

involving drugs A and B, required subjects to experience (on average) at least one seizure per week of baseline. Additionally, subjects using drug A could experience no more than 20 consecutive seizure-free days. Subjects using drug B were also required to have at least two seizures during both 4-week blocks. One trial with drug C required at least eight seizures per 12-week baseline and at least one seizure in two of three 4-week blocks. The other trial with drug C required at least six seizures per 8-week baseline and at least one seizure in both 4-week blocks.

We used the sponsor's protocol-defined primary endpoint to analyze individual trial results. All sponsors used one of two primary endpoints: percentage reduction in seizure rate from baseline (drug A) or change in seizure rate from baseline (drugs B and C). The seizure rate was defined as the number of seizures during a fixed period divided by the number of days in the period. Change in seizure rate from baseline was defined as the baseline period seizure rate minus the double-blind treatment period seizure rate. Percentage seizure rate reduction from baseline was defined as follows:

(Change in Seizure Rate from Baseline/
Baseline Seizure Rate) x 100

Our statistical model was the analysis of variance (ANOVA), with treatment, center, and treatment-by-center interaction as fixed effects. The ANOVA, which assumes errors are normally distributed with constant variance, is robust to modest departures from normality or homoscedasticity (constant variance). However, because seizure data are often severely skewed, nonparametric procedures based on ranks are often used. We chose the rank-transform method of Conover and Iman (5) which applies a parametric model, in this case the ANOVA, to the ranks of the data instead of the raw data themselves. The rank-transform approach is particularly appealing because well-known parametric procedures can be relied on, and these procedures, when applied to ranks, are closely related to nonparametric procedures.

Not all sponsors shared our analysis methodology. We chose a single model and statistical method across trials so that different methodologies could not introduce additional variability into the results. We did, as already discussed, use the sponsor's designated primary endpoint. Our decision to do so was based on the conviction that the endpoint is an intrinsic part of the basic trial design, and as such should not be subject to change.

RESULTS

Tables 1 through 7 (one table per clinical trial) display *p*-values for the different analyses. Trials are labeled alphanumerically, the first character (letter) indicating the drug, the

TABLE 1. *Trial A1: p-values for percentage reduction in seizure rate from baseline*

Baseline duration (wk)	Double-blind duration (wk)			
	16 (full)	8	4	2
12 (full)	<.001	<.001	.001	.023
6	.005	.005	.010	.046
4	.022	.030	.045	.17
2	.081	.092	.051	.17

TABLE 2. *Trial A2: p-values for percentage reduction in seizure rate from baseline*

Baseline duration (wk)	Double-blind duration (wk)			
	16 (full)	8	4	2
12 (full)	<.001	.002	<.001	.020
6	<.001	.002	<.001	.007
4	.002	.003	<.001	.013
2	.018	.022	.009	.073

TABLE 3. *Trial A3: p-values for percentage reduction in seizure rate from baseline*

Baseline duration (wk)	Double-blind duration (wk)			
	16 (full)	8	4	2
8 (full)	.004	.004	.006	.023
6	.011	.019	.015	.048
4	.023	.028	.026	.14
2	.059	.11	.052	.34

TABLE 4. *Trial A4: p-values for percentage reduction in seizure rate from baseline*

Baseline duration (wk)	Double-blind duration (wk)			
	13 (full)	8	4	2
8 (full)	<.001	.004	.038	.055
6	<.001	<.001	.008	.020
4	.001	.006	.023	.061
2	.003	.012	.021	.029

TABLE 5. *Trial B1: p-values for change in seizure rate from baseline*

Baseline duration (wk)	Double-blind duration (wk)			
	16 (full)	8	4	2
8 (full)	.052	.17	.16	.34
6	.079	.24	.17	.49
4	.076	.24	.21	.38
2	.024	.037	.056	.25

TABLE 6. *Trial C1: p-values for change in seizure rate from baseline*

Baseline duration (wk)	Double-blind duration (wk)			
	16 (full)	8	4	2
12 (full)	.004	.015	.003	.006
6	.001	.004	.002	.013
4	.17	.18	.024	.10
2	.22	.13	.011	.10

TABLE 7. *Trial C2: p-values for change in seizure rate from baseline*

Baseline duration (wk)	Double-blind duration (wk)			
	12 (full)	8	4	2
8 (full)	.020	.11	.061	.043
6	.097	.45	.39	.79
4	.11	.38	.35	.83
2	.067	.33	.36	.83

second character (number) indicating one of the clinical trials with that drug. (Trials using the same drug are not sequenced in any particular order.) Each table consists of 16 cells, each of which represents an analysis conducted using various baseline and double-blind treatment durations. For example, in

TABLE 8. *Number of trials (among seven) with significant p-values**

Baseline duration (wk)	Double-blind duration (wk)			
	12 to 16 (full)	8	4	2
8 to 12 (full)	7	5	5	4
6	5	5	5	5
4	4	4	5	1
2	3	3	4	1

*$p \leq .054$.

Table 1 (drug A, trial 1), the upper left cell, denoted (1,1), shows $p < .001$ for the analysis using the "full" data, 12 weeks of baseline and 16 weeks of double-blind treatment. Cell (3,3) shows $p = .030$ for the analysis using seizure data from the last 4 weeks of baseline and the first 8 weeks of double-blind treatment. Four analyses in Table 1, all with 2-week baseline or 2-week double-blind treatment durations, produced *p*-values >.054.[1] This pattern, in which shorter baseline or double-blind treatment durations produced generally higher *p*-values, is replicated in the other tables. This should not be surprising; we expect higher within-patient variability in seizure rates during shorter periods, variability that in turn works to obscure treatment differences.

The tables also illustrate the notion of sampling variability. For example, in Table 2, consider columns 2 and 3, corresponding to 8- and 4-week double-blind treatment durations, respectively. The *p*-values in the same row represent results for baseline periods of equal duration. Each *p*-value in column 3 is smaller than its same-row *p*-value in column 2. Thus, the observed trend that shortened periods produce larger *p*-values can be disrupted for individual samples.

Table 8 combines results across Tables 1 through 7. The table shows, for each combination of baseline and double-blind treatment durations, the number of trials among the seven with statistically significant results. Dividing each number in each cell by 7 gives a rudimentary estimate of power. For example,

[1]The value of .054 is a convenient cutoff that arises within the context of these examples; it does not represent a standard criterion that the Food and Drug Administration relies on.

five of seven trials (71%) in the (3,3) cell (4-week baseline and double-blind treatment durations) had statistically significant results. (We usually strive for at least 80% power.) This estimate, however, is surely too high because of selection bias; trials were chosen in part because they were statistically significant when the full data were used.

DISCUSSION AND CONCLUSIONS

We retrospectively analyzed data from seven randomized, placebo-controlled, add-on clinical trials of three antiepileptic drugs. Our results indicate that use of shortened baseline or double-blind treatment periods produced generally higher p-values than use of the full data. Still, many analyses produced significant p-values for durations as short as 2 to 4 weeks. For any baseline duration, more than one third (39%) of analyses with 2-week double-blind treatment durations and two thirds (68%) of analyses with 4-week durations produced statistically significant results. These analyses involved double-blind treatment data *from drug titration periods only*, precisely the data that many sponsors exclude from analysis. Our results suggest that these data often convey important information about treatment effects. Furthermore, these data allow a straightforward analysis of all randomized patients (intent-to-treat analysis).

A surprising aspect of the data is that the quantity of baseline seizure information is no less important than the quantity of double-blind treatment information in delineating treatment effects. One week of baseline data appears to be just as informative as a week of double-blind treatment data. If, in fact, data from baseline and double-blind treatment periods carry roughly "equal" seizure information, this consideration, together with others, can help us determine the optimal durations of these periods when designing clinical trials.

Future work will involve looking at other trial designs (e.g., crossover designs), different endpoints (time-to-Kth-seizure) and entry criteria (changes in required baseline seizure rates). Retrospective analyses of seizure rate data from these seven parallel group trials suggest the feasibility of conducting antiepileptic drug trials of shorter durations capable of detecting treatment differences.

REFERENCES

1. Pledger GP, Sackellares JC, Treiman DM, et al. Flunarizine for treatment of partial seizures: results of a concentration-controlled trial. *Neurology* 1994;44: 1830–1836.
2. Friedman LN, Furberg CD, DeMets DL. *Fundamentals of Clinical Trials*. Boston: John Wright-PSG; 1981: 156–165.
3. Pledger GW, Sahlroot JT. Alternative analyses for antiepileptic drug trials. In: French JA, Dichter MA, Leppik IE, eds. *New Antiepileptic Drug Development: Preclinical and Clinical Aspects*. Amsterdam: Elsevier; 1993;167–174.
4. Shafer JB, Tempkin NR. Comparison of alternative outcome measures for antiepileptic drug trials. *Arch Neurol* 1986;43:877–881.
5. Conover WJ, Iman RL. Rank transformation as a bridge between parametric and nonparametric statistics. *Am Statistician* 1981;35:124–133.

Antiepileptic Drug Development.
Advances in Neurology, Vol. 76,
edited by J. French, I. Leppik, and M. A. Dichter.
Lippincott–Raven Publishers, Philadelphia © 1998.

12

Monotherapy Trials

Elizabeth A. Garofalo

Department of Clinical Research, CNS Parke-Davis Pharmaceutical Research Division, Warner-Lambert Co., Ann Arbor, Michigan 48105.

INTRODUCTION

Antiepileptic drugs have been studied in controlled clinical trials to establish their efficacy and safety. Optimally, these trials are designed to provide information that is clinically relevant and supports a regulatory submission. In recent years, there has been a trend toward studying antiepileptic drugs in monotherapy earlier in development (1). This has led to the development of new trial designs that can provide evidence of the efficacy of a new antiepileptic drug in monotherapy. The following aspects of monotherapy trials of investigational antiepileptic drugs are discussed in this chapter: the historical setting for the design of these trials, the epilepsy populations available for study, current monotherapy study designs, efficacy results from recent monotherapy trials, and future possibilities in trial design.

HISTORICAL SETTING

Guidelines have been formulated for the important elements in the design of any clinical trial (2). A clear statement of the objective of the trial must be offered, and a summary of the analysis method must be provided. The design must permit a valid comparison with a control. Placebo control is considered the optimal choice; other options include dose-comparison control, concurrent control, and no-treatment control. An active-treatment concurrent control or historical control is also considered acceptable if appropriate arguments are made to substantiate that choice. Standard trials to determine the clinical efficacy and safety of antiepileptic drugs have a placebo-controlled, add-on design (3). In trials with this design, pharmacokinetic and pharmacodynamic interactions may occur when the compound under study is added to baseline antiepileptic drugs, sometimes confounding the results. Additionally, the epilepsy of the medically refractory patient population studied in these trials may be too severe to expect any improvement in seizure control when the new agent is added to the baseline antiepileptic drugs (4,5). For these reasons, monotherapy trials are desirable (6). The most commonly performed and published monotherapy trials have been active-control equivalence trials (7,8). The interpretation of these trials is complicated by a number of inherent problems (9,10,11). Therefore, there has been a movement toward exploring new clinical trial designs in monotherapy that can be undertaken earlier in the development of a new antiepileptic drug and provide controlled efficacy information without placing the patient at an unacceptable risk. To this end, the Epilepsy Branch of the National Institutes of Health in 1988 held a workshop on design issues in controlled clinical trials of investigational antiepileptic drugs. A part of the discussion centered on monotherapy studies. Since then, a number of monotherapy trials with several antiepileptic drugs have been concluded, and accumulated experience with monotherapy trial designs is growing.

EPILEPSY POPULATION

An initial consideration in designing a monotherapy trial is the epileptic patient population intended for study. Within this population, patients with different seizure types and epileptic syndromes are represented and may be selected for study. These patients, available for monotherapy trials, represent a continuum that can be broken down into three large categories. First are patients with new-onset epilepsy, including patients who present following a single seizure (12) or who have had a minimum of two seizures before entrance into a monotherapy trial. Next are patients currently under treatment with antiepileptic drugs. Some patients respond to initial treatment with complete seizure control but are considered drug failures because of intolerable side effects. A separate group consists of patients who do not achieve complete seizure control on the initial agent. Medically refractory patients, including those who have failed multiple drugs, may also be targeted for monotherapy study designs. A final group of patients who may be considered for trials are those who have been treated on a long-term basis and have been seizure-free for a period of time before entering a study (13).

CURRENT MONOTHERAPY TRIAL DESIGNS

Three basic study designs are currently in use. The fundamental differences between designs include the patient population under study, the choice of control, the way in which monotherapy is initiated, and the efficacy analyses. Beyond these fundamental components of the trial design, many other variables exist and may be important. Some of the differences include length of baseline and double-blind phases, inclusion and exclusion criteria, and rules for determining an exit from the study.

Outpatient Withdrawal Design

The first trial is designed to study patients with medically refractory epilepsy on one or several baseline concomitant antiepileptic drugs (Fig. 1). Following a fixed-length baseline phase, during which seizure frequency is

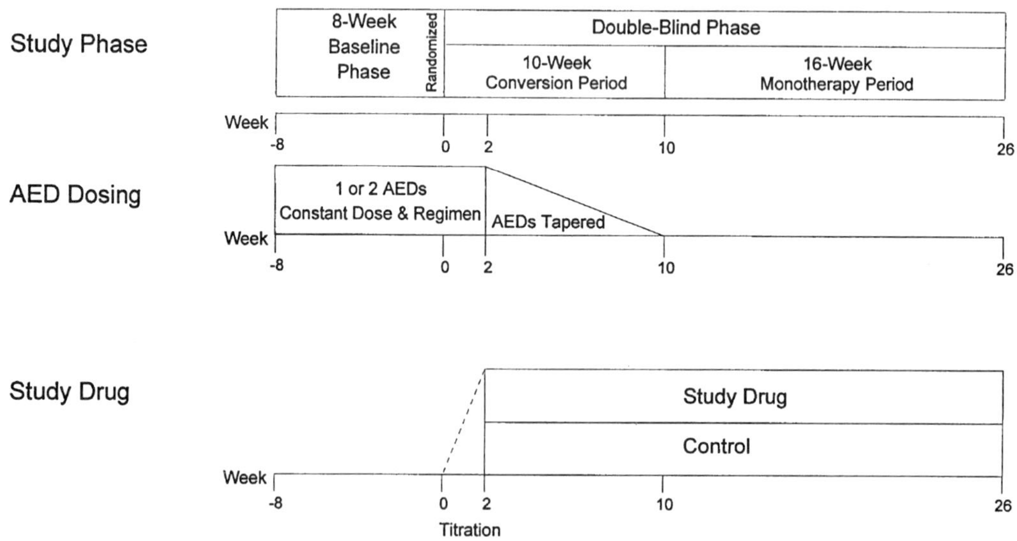

FIG. 1. Example schematic of a monotherapy outpatient withdrawal design. The study is divided into the baseline and double-blind phases.

determined, patients are randomized and titrated in a blinded fashion onto the drug (and control agent) under study. Following or during this conversion period, the patient's baseline antiepileptic drugs are withdrawn and the patient remains in the monotherapy period of the double-blind phase for a set period of time, generally 4 to 6 months. Because this trial occurs in an outpatient setting, placebo control is not feasible because of the possibility of unacceptable seizure exacerbations. Therefore, dose-control, low-dose active-control, and concentration-control designs have been used to show a statistically significant difference between the treatment arms. The efficacy endpoint, which is predetermined, includes individualized exit criteria based on each patient's seizure frequency, quantified during a baseline phase. Therefore, patients are not continued in the trial if they exceed this limit. The design of this trial lends itself to an analysis of time-to-exit from the trial or of the percentage of patients able to complete the trial. The analysis of time-to-exit uses all the data available for each patient, allowing for a more complete picture of retention in the trial than does simply looking at the percentage of completers in each group. Additionally, seizure frequency during the (variable-length) treatment phase may be analyzed in comparison with baseline. However, the analysis of seizure frequency may be subject to bias because of the need to impute seizure frequency data from patients who exited at early time points or to exclude patients from the analysis if they were not retained in the study for an arbitrary length of time (6).

This particular study design has the advantage of mimicking clinical practice, in that some patients in the outpatient setting may be converted to monotherapy in a similar fashion. The refractory patient population under study is easily recruited into trials, because these patients are highly represented at tertiary care medical centers, where studies are performed. Such patients are highly motivated to seek out new therapies and therefore are willing to accept the risks involved in withdrawing from their baseline antiepileptic drugs.

The disadvantages are that the study itself becomes long and complicated because of the taper off of the baseline antiepileptic drugs and continued treatment on monotherapy. During the taper off phase, patients may experience withdrawal seizures (14,15,16) that may not be amenable to treatment with the antiepileptic drug under study. In addition, exit events may be difficult to mandate. Therefore, patients must be given the option to exit from the trial even if seizure frequency does not exceed the protocol-specified rate but does represent an intensification or prolongation of seizures. If more patients exit from the trial because of seizure intensification or adverse events than anticipated, the power for the trial may be significantly decreased. The final disadvantage of this trial design is that the safety profile contains data from both monotherapy and polytherapy exposure. Therefore, it is difficult to attribute adverse events to a single agent, and the adverse event profile in monotherapy cannot be determined.

Inpatient Withdrawal Design

A second type of monotherapy study design again includes medically refractory patients who are withdrawn from their baseline antiepileptic drugs during hospitalization and before randomization in the trial (prestudy phase) (Fig. 2). These patients often are candidates for epilepsy surgery. In this type of study, low-dose active control, dose control, or placebo control can be considered to show a difference between the variable-length treatment regimens. Patients are randomized into the trial after experiencing a specified number of seizures in the prestudy phase and exit from the trial after experiencing a predetermined number of seizures (variable time point) or after a set period of time during the treatment phase. The efficacy endpoint may be the time-to-exit, the percentage of completers, or seizure frequency. These trials can

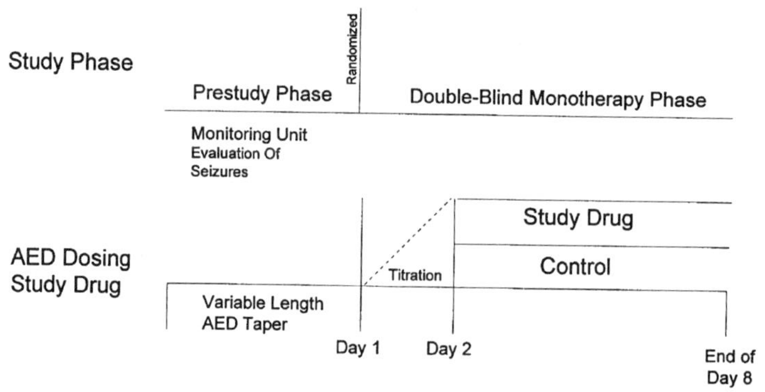

FIG. 2. Example schematic of a monotherapy inpatient withdrawal design. The study is divided into two phases: the variable-length prestudy phase and the double-blind monotherapy phase.

be brief in duration, lasting on the order of 1 to 2 weeks.

There are several advantages to this trial design. The drug under study can be administered as monotherapy from the onset of the study. The trial is of short duration, which is advantageous to patients. It is easier to mandate exit events in a hospital environment. Several choices are available for the control agent. And finally, the safety profile is one in which pure monotherapy data can be obtained. Disadvantages, however, include a short duration of therapy, which may be difficult to extrapolate to prolonged seizure control in monotherapy in the outpatient setting. Secondly, these study protocols are complicated because of the need to observe a set number of seizures within a brief period of time before entry into the study. Simultaneously, antiepileptic drugs are being withdrawn and antiepileptic drug concentrations are being monitored to determine the point of monotherapy. In many cases, patients may experience the requisite number of seizures for entry into and exit from the study in a few days; therefore, adverse events may reflect both frequent seizures and drug effect. The other very limiting aspect of this type of trial is the need for rapid initiation or titration of the study drug. If a drug cannot be titrated to full efficacy rapidly, the study becomes untenable because of safety issues. The use of short-acting benzodiazepines may alleviate some of these concerns (6). However, if the antiepileptic drug under study must be titrated during many days, the study feasibility decreases because of the need for a long hospitalization. Finally, the safety profile reflects monotherapy exposure of a short duration and may not be predictive of adverse events seen in the outpatient setting.

Initial Monotherapy Design

Finally, patients with new-onset epilepsy may be studied in initial monotherapy (Fig. 3). Placebo-control, dose-control, or low-dose active-control study designs may be possible. As previously discussed, time-to-exit criteria analysis, percentage completion, or seizure frequency may be studied as the efficacy endpoint. In this patient population, placebo control may be an option and would maximize the ability to show a difference between placebo and the compound under study.

This study has the advantage of initial treatment of patients with monotherapy, as in clinic practice. Protocols may be simpler in design. The safety profile in this case is representative of initial use in an outpatient setting.

Disadvantages include long duration of the trial because of the low frequency of seizures in this study population. More patients may be lost to follow-up during the study. Recruitment is complicated by the need to identify patients shortly after the diagnosis of epilepsy is

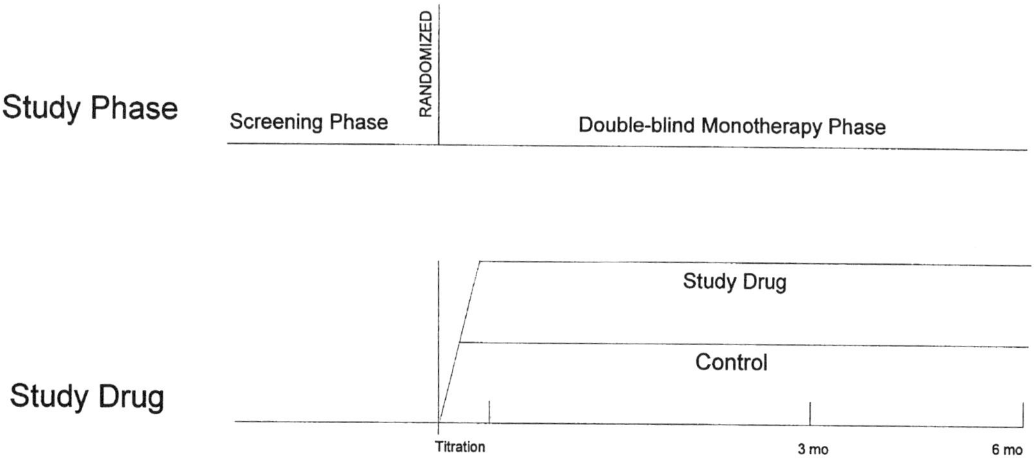

FIG. 3. Example schematic of an initial monotherapy design. The study phases include screening and the double-blind monotherapy phase.

established and recommend that they be entered into a clinical trial as the first option for therapy. For this type of study to proceed, well-established evidence of anticonvulsant activity for the new compound must be available.

MONOTHERAPY TRIAL RESULTS

Eight monotherapy trials have been published in abstract or manuscript form. In each case, the patient population studied had a diagnosis of refractory partial epilepsy. Emphasis here is on the basic design of the trials, outcome parameters, and efficacy outcomes.

Felbamate

Two outpatient double-blind trials have been reported in full (17,18). Both trials were conducted according to an identical study design, one at a single center and one at multiple centers. Felbamate (3600 mg/d given four times daily) was compared with a low dose of valproate (15 mg/kg per day). During a 56-day baseline period, patients were required to have at least four partial-onset seizures per 28 days and were receiving one antiepileptic drug at a therapeutic level. Patients were converted to felbamate or low-dose valproate during the first 28 days of the monotherapy treatment phase. Monotherapy was maintained for an additional 84 days. Study endpoints were completion of the study or fulfillment of an exit event. Patients were exited from the study for the following reasons: (a) a twofold increase in monthly seizure frequency, (b) a twofold increase in highest 2-day seizure frequency, (c) occurrence of a single generalized tonic-clonic seizures if there had been none during baseline, and (d) significant prolongation of generalized tonic-clonic seizures. The primary efficacy variable was the number of patients who exited the study in each treatment group.

In the multicenter trial, the number of patients who met exit criteria was 40% (18/45) in the felbamate group and 78% (39/50) in the low-dose valproate group. In the single-center trial, 14% (3/21) of patients in the felbamate group met the exit criteria, whereas 90% (19/21) did so in the low-dose valproate group. In these trials, the difference in the percentage of patients meeting the exit criteria is statistically significant in favor of felbamate (p = .039 and p <.001, respectively) (Table 1).

Two inpatient trials have been reported (19,20). The first, a single-center, 18-day trial, compared felbamate (3600 mg/d) with placebo in 40 patients who had refractory partial

TABLE 1. *The four published felbamate monotherapy trials*[a]

Design	Centers, No.	Patients enrolled, No.	Analysis and results	Reference
Outpatient Active control	S	44	Time to exit $p < .001$	Sachdeo et al. 1992 (18)
Outpatient Active control	M	111	Time to exit $p = .039$	Faught et al. 1993 (17)
Inpatient Placebo control	S	40	Seizure frequency $p = .008$	Theodore et al. 1995 (20)
Inpatient Placebo control	M	52	Seizure frequency $p = .065$	Devinsky et al. 1995 (19)

S, single center; M, multicenter.
[a]Included are all the study designs, number of study centers, number of patients enrolled, reported analysis and results, and reference article.

seizures. Patients were tapered off their baseline antiepileptic drugs for at least 48 hours and had undeterminable antiepileptic drug concentrations for least 24 hours before randomization. No more than five generalized tonic-clonic seizures were allowed in baseline. Following randomization, felbamate was titrated during 4 days, after which seizure counting began and continued for 14 days. Patients were exited from the trial if they experienced more than five generalized tonic-clonic seizures in a week, partial status epilepticus, or unacceptable drug toxicity. The primary efficacy variable was the average frequency of all seizure types among completers of the 14-day evaluation period. The analyses were also performed for complex partial, simple partial, and generalized tonic-clonic seizure. The study was terminated early following regulatory approval of the drug. Eight of 19 patients receiving placebo and 13 of 21 patients receiving felbamate completed the 18-day study. Among study completers, there was a significant decrease in mean daily seizure rate in favor of felbamate (0.473 placebo, n = 8; 0.083 felbamate, n = 13; $p = .008$). However, the same analysis of complex partial seizures and generalized tonic-clonic seizures revealed only a trend toward improvement. The comparison of time-to-exit from the trial showed a trend towards a difference between the two treatment groups.

In the second inpatient trial, 52 patients were enrolled in a double-blind, placebo-controlled, multicenter study. Patients had to experience two to 10 simple partial or complex partial seizures or two generalized tonic-clonic seizures in the 2 days before randomization and be off of baseline antiepileptic drugs for 24 hours. Patients were randomized to 3600 mg titrated during 2 days or to placebo during a 10-day inpatient trial. Patients were exited from the trial if they had four seizures beginning on day 2 exactly 24 hours after initiation of study medication. In the primary analysis of all 52 patients, the mean rank of the daily seizure frequency showed a trend toward statistical significance in favor of felbamate ($p = .065$). The median time-to-exit (after the fourth seizure) also show a trend towards statistical significance in favor of felbamate ($p = .068$) (Table 1).

Gabapentin

One multicenter, outpatient, double-blind, dose-controlled trial has been reported in abstract form (21). Three doses of gabapentin (600 mg/d, 1200 mg/d, 2400/d mg given three times daily) were compared. During an 8-week baseline, patients were required to have at least four complex partial or secondarily generalized tonic-clonic seizures (called study seizures) while being treated with one or two antiepileptic drugs at a therapeutic level. Patients were converted to blinded gabapentin during the first 70 days of the monotherapy phase. Monotherapy was maintained for an additional 120 days. Patients were required to exit the study if they experienced any of the following events: (a) greater than twofold increase in 28-day study seizure rate, (b) greater than twofold increase in highest 2-day seizure rate, (c) single generalized tonic-clonic seizure if there had been none in the past 2 years, (d) status epilepticus, (e) unacceptable increase in the frequency or intensity of seizure activity. The primary efficacy variable was time to exit from the double-blind phase of the study. In this trial, no significant differences among dosage groups were detected in time-to-exit from the study (Table 2).

One multicenter, inpatient, double-blind, dose-controlled trial has been reported (22). This 8-day trial compared two doses of gabapentin (300 mg/d, 3600 mg/d given three times daily) in 82 hospitalized patients whose antiepileptic medications had been discontinued for seizure monitoring. At randomization, all concomitant antiepileptic drugs were discontinued and antiepileptic drug levels were documented to be as follows: phenytoin ≤7 μ/mL, carbamazepine ≤4 μg/mL, and valproic acid ≤25 μg/mL. Patients were required to have had at least three complex partial or secondarily generalized tonic-clonic seizures (study seizures) within the 72 hours or four seizures within the 120 hours before randomization. Study drug was initiated at full dose on study day 1. All patients received a single dose of oral lorazepam (1 to 4 mg depending on weight) with the first dose of gabapentin.

Patients were exited from the trial beginning on study day 1 if they experienced any of the following: (a) four study seizures, (b) single generalized tonic-clonic seizure if no history, (c) status epilepticus, (d) prolongation or intensification of seizures. The primary efficacy variable was time-to-exit, which was significantly longer ($p = .0001$) in the 3600-mg group (Table 2).

Topiramate

Topiramate has been studied in a single-center, outpatient, monotherapy, dose-controlled trial of 48 patients with refractory partial seizures (23). The study consisted of an 8-week baseline phase in which patients were required to have four partial seizures. Patients received 1 to 2 weeks of open treatment of 100 mg of topiramate as add-on therapy, followed by a 5-week, double-blind conversion phase. During conversion, patients were tapered off their baseline antiepileptic drugs while being titrated to either low-dose (100 mg/d) or high-dose (1000 mg/d) topiramate or the maximal tolerated dose. The primary outcome was time

TABLE 2. *The four published abstracts of monotherapy trials*[a]

Design	Centers, No.	Patients enrolled, No.	Analysis and results	Reference
Gabapentin				
Outpatient	M	275	Time to exit	Hayes et al.
Dose control			$p = .836$	1995 (21)
Inpatient	M	82	Time to exit	Bergey et al.
Dose control			$p = .0001$	1995 (22)
Topiramate				
Outpatient	S	48	Time to exit	Sachdeo
Dose control			$p = .002$	1995 (23)
Valproate				
Outpatient	M	264	Seizure frequency	Sackellares
Concentration control			$p < .05$	1995 (24)

S, single center; M, multicenter.
[a]Studies of gabapentin, topiramate, and valproate. Included are the study design, number of study centers, number of patients enrolled, reported analysis and results, and reference abstract.

to one of the following exit events: doubling of 28-day seizure frequency, single generalized tonic-clonic seizure if none during baseline, or prolongation of seizure duration requiring intervention. Fifty-one patients entered into baseline and 48 were randomized, 24 in each group. Time-to-exit was statistically significantly longer in the high-dose group than in the low-dose group ($p = .002$) (Table 2).

Valproate

Valproate in high-trough (80 to 150 μg/mL) concentration and valproate in low-trough concentration (25 to 50 μg/mL) were compared in a multicenter, double-blind efficacy trial of patients with partial epilepsy (24). An 8- to 12-week baseline period was followed by a 24-week double-blind phase. Following randomization into the trial, patients were titrated to the high- or low-concentration range and their baseline antiepileptic drugs were discontinued. Outcome parameters included a comparison of the median reduction in seizure frequency between the two groups. In the high-concentration group, 130 patients experienced a median reduction of 2.0 complex partial seizures in 8 weeks (baseline rate of 13.1 complex partial seizures in 8 weeks), in comparison with a median reduction of 1.1 complex partial seizures in 8 weeks (baseline rate of 14.2 complex partial seizures in 8 weeks) in the 134 patients in the low-concentration group ($p < .05$) (Table 2).

ALTERNATE TRIAL DESIGNS AND PATIENT POPULATIONS

The current study designs provide a basis for testing anticonvulsants in monotherapy. Limitations exist, and study designs may be amenable to modification to simplify the studies and measure anticonvulsant effect more reliably. Current experience points to possible changes in study design. First, the inclusion of patients with refractory epilepsy necessitates withdrawal from anticonvulsants. The optimal length of this phase is not clear, and the use of short-acting antiepileptic drugs might be considered to retain patients in a trial until they are on monotherapy with the agent under study. Ways to enrich, for patients more likely to be converted to monotherapy, need to be studied. A lead-in phase of conversion to monotherapy on the study drug followed by randomization to a double-blind, dose-controlled phase would enrich for patients who successfully attained monotherapy. Other factors to consider include number of antiepileptic drugs tried previously and number of antiepileptic drugs at baseline. Enrollment of patients who are being treated with the same single antiepileptic drug at baseline may eliminate differential effects of withdrawal from various antiepileptic drugs. Targeting other study populations should be considered. Patients who have been seizure-free for 2 years and are being tapered off antiepileptic drugs could be considered for a monotherapy trial.

A move to study less refractory patients, even patients with new-onset epilepsy, is desirable. Within the group of new-onset patients are those with epilepsy syndromes, providing a homogeneous group for study. Finally, further study of completed trials may serve to indicate other possible sensitive efficacy endpoints, such as time-to-first-seizure, or a novel analysis of seizure frequency (25).

CONCLUSIONS

In conclusion, a number of monotherapy trials have been implemented and completed in recent years. This has lead to at least three prototypic designs that each have a number of advantages and disadvantages. As we have gained more experience, it is clear that these study designs appear to be useful and successful in determining the efficacy of antiepileptic drugs in monotherapy. It is also clear that further refinement would be advantageous and that we have not maximized the trial designs or the patient populations under study. Finally, further studies are under way that will continue to add to our knowledge of monotherapy trial designs for new antiepileptic drugs.

REFERENCES

1. Kramer LD, Pledger GW, Kamin M. Prototype antiepileptic drug clinical development plan. *Epilepsia* 1993;34:1075–1084.
2. Federal Food, Drug, and Cosmetic, as amended. Washington, DC: US Government Printing Office; 1976:50.
3. Commission on Antiepileptic Drugs of the International League Against Epilepsy. Guidelines for clinical evaluation of antiepileptic drugs. *Epilepsia* 1989;30: 400–408.
4. Temkin NR, Wilensky AJ. New AEDs: are the compounds or the studies ineffective? *Epilepsia* 1986;27: 644–645.
5. Wilensky AJ. Antiepileptic drug trials—are present methodologies satisfactory? *Epilepsia* 1990;31: 645–646.
6. Pledger GW, Kramer LD. Clinical trials of investigational antiepileptic drugs: monotherapy designs. *Epilepsia* 1991;32:716–721.
7. Ramsay RE, Wilder BJ, Berger JR, Bruni J. A double-blind study comparing carbamazepine with phenytoin as initial seizure therapy in adults. *Neurology* 1983;33: 905–910.
8. Wilder BJ, Ramsay RE, Murphy JV, Karas BJ, Marquardt K, Hammond EJ. Comparison of valproic acid and phenytoin in newly diagnosed tonic-clonic seizures. *Neurology* 1983;33:1474–1476.
9. Temple R. Government viewpoint of clinical trials. *Drug Inform J* 1982;1:10–17.
10. Leber PD. Hazards of inference: the active-control investigation. *Epilepsia* 1989;30(Suppl 1):S57–S63.
11. Katz R. Perspective of the Food and Drug Administration. In: Porter RJ, Schoenberg BS, eds. *Controlled Trials in Neurological Disease*. Boston: Kluwer Academic Publishers; 1990:97–104.
12. First Seizure Trial Group (FIR.S.T. Group). Randomized clinical trial on the efficacy of antiepileptic drugs in reducing the risk of relapse after a first unprovoked tonic-clonic seizure. *Neurology* 1993;43:478–483.
13. Medical Research Council Antiepileptic Drug Withdrawal Study Group. Randomised study of antiepileptic drug withdrawal in patients in remission. *Lancet* 1991; 337:1175–1180.
14. Theodore WH, Porter RJ, Raubertas RF. Seizures during barbiturate withdrawal: relation to blood level. *Ann Neurol* 1987;22:644–647.
15. Bromfield EB, Devinsky O, Reeves P, Nice FJ, Theodore WH. Phenytoin withdrawal and seizure frequency. *Neurology* 1989;39:905–909.
16. Malow BA, Blaxton TA, Stertz B, Theodore WH. Carbamazepine withdrawal: effects of taper rate on seizure frequency. *Neurology* 1993;43:2280–2284.
17. Faught E, Sachdeo RC, Remler MP, et al. Felbamate monotherapy for partial-onset seizures: an active control. *Neurology* 1993;43:688–692.
18. Sachdeo R, Kramer LD, Rosenberg A, Sachdeo S. Felbamate monotherapy: controlled trial in patients with partial-onset seizures. *Ann Neurol* 1992;32:386–392.
19. Devinsky O, Faught RE, Wilder BJ, Kanner AM, Kamin M, Kramer LD, Rosenberg A. Efficacy of felbamate monotherapy in patients undergoing presurgical evaluation of partial seizures. *Epilepsy Res* 1995;20:241–246.
20. Theodore WH, Albert P, Stertz B, et al. Felbamate monotherapy: implications for antiepileptic drug development. *Epilepsia* 1995;36:1105–1110.
21. Hayes AG, Garofalo EA, Greeley CA, et al. A double-blind multicenter study of gabapentin (GBP; Neurontin) monotherapy in patients with medically refractory partial seizures. *Epilepsia* 1995;36(Suppl 4):S89.
22. Bergey GK, Crockatt JG, Leiderman DB, Malicsi MJR, Garofalo EA, and the US Gabapentin Study Group 88/89. Multicenter, double-blind study of gabapentin monotherapy in hospitalized patients with refractory epilepsy. *Epilepsia* 1995;36(Suppl 4):S68.
23. Sachdeo R. 21st IEC proceedings: single-center topiramate monotherapy trial. *Epilepsia* 1995;36(Suppl 3): S151.
24. Sackellares C. 21st IEC proceedings: Depakote monotherapy in the treatment of complex partial seizures. *Epilepsia* 1995;36(Suppl 3):S66.
25. Shofer JB, Temkin NR. Comparison of alternative-outcome measures for antiepileptic drug trials. *Arch Neurol* 1986;43:877–881.

Antiepileptic Drug Development.
Advances in Neurology, Vol. 76,
edited by J. French, I. Leppik, and M. A. Dichter.
Lippincott–Raven Publishers, Philadelphia © 1998.

13

The Impact of Foreign Data on a New Drug Application

Hal Galbraith and Steven D. Walker

Hoechst Marion Roussel, Kansas City, Missouri 64137 and
Parke-Davis Pharmaceutical Research Division, Warner-Lambert Co., Ann Arbor, Michigan 48105.

INTRODUCTION

Many, if not most, drug development programs in recent years have represented a global effort on the part of the sponsoring company. With the continuing consolidation of the pharmaceutical industry into large international organizations, this trend will likely increase. For this reason, the quantity of data being generated from preclinical and clinical trials conducted outside the United States is increasing. Efforts continue to be made to harmonize development programs in several therapeutic areas, so as to maximize the utility of data generated around the world (1). These efforts have met with a variety of challenges, including the need for regulatory agencies to agree on requirements for both preclinical and clinical testing. Just as importantly, sponsoring companies must work diligently within their own structure to coordinate their efforts to provide a consistent, global approach while accommodating any country- or region-specific requirements. A clear development plan established as early as possible in the process, including phase IIIb and IV studies, to guide future decisions about the use of foreign data will prove to be a most valuable expenditure of time as New Drug Applications (NDAs) are prepared and submitted to the Food and Drug Administration and when questions regarding databases must be answered.

For submissions to the Food and Drug Administration, it is important to decide as early as possible which data from outside the United States will be used and how they will be used. Data can be submitted to the Food and Drug Administration with an intent to

- demonstrate efficacy,
- supplement the U.S. patient exposure for safety, and/or
- support an already adequate U.S. data package.

In each case, the level of documentation and the guidelines under which data are generated will have an impact on the acceptability of the data. Proper planning and care in generating, documenting, compiling, and summarizing the data will minimize delays in review and approval of the NDA. In an ideal situation, all decisions about use of data, in regard to the points mentioned above, are made at the start of planning for the development program and subsequent submission.

The NDA for SABRIL (vigabatrin) was filed in May of 1994. A large portion of the safety data for the NDA came from European safety and efficacy studies that had taken place during a period of approximately 10 years. These studies formed the basis of submissions to European regulatory authorities, with initial approval for SABRIL occurring in

TABLE 1. *Database construction issues*

- Multiple languages
- Diversity in design of case report forms
- Individual site versus central laboratories
- Patient tracking across protocols
- Differences in adverse reporting practices
- Documentation of methods and decisions

the United Kingdom in November of 1989. The Food and Drug Administration responded in May of 1995 with a request to provide more verification of the data from the European studies, which had been presented in summary form. Much of the following discussion is based on lessons learned from this experience of attempting to reconstruct a database involving nearly 2000 patients from 99 European protocols. Of the 99 protocols, it was determined that data from 83 had to be completely rebuilt for incorporation into the overall database.

If the purpose of including data from foreign trials is to demonstrate efficacy, the Food and Drug Administration requires that the trials will have been conducted according to applicable GCP (Good Clinical Practice) regulations (2). This is also true if the data are to be used to build an adequate exposure cohort for safety verification. This means, of course, that all patients have provided informed consent, that adequately designed protocols have prospectively guided the clinical trial, that all information generated by the trial is reported in case report forms with adequate supporting documentation, that all treatment-emergent events have been recorded, and that study sites can be subjected to an Food and Drug Administration audit.

It is also critical that comprehensive databases can be constructed from the available study results that summarize individual protocols, groups of protocols, or the entire NDA. The integrated summary of safety is an example of how these databases play a critical role for the submission and the review of the submission. Several issues may arise as databases are constructed; these are listed in Table 1.

MULTIPLE LANGUAGES

When studies are performed in multiple countries, languages vary and English translations are required. This can involve all or part of the entries on the case report form. Even if the case report form is in English, supporting documentation (e.g., laboratory results, electroencephalographic and electrocardiographic findings) may require translation. It is critical in this situation to identify a reliable translation service. It is also advisable to do spot checks of translations with doctors or other health care professionals who work in the particular medical specialty and speak both English and the language involved.

About 75% of the SABRIL case report forms from Europe required some translation. Eight languages were involved, including Swedish, German, French, Italian, Finnish, Danish, Spanish, and Portuguese.

DIVERSITY IN CASE REPORT FORM DESIGN

If the drug development program did not incorporate design standards for case report forms to produce consistent collection formats, then the same core data will have been collected differently across protocols. This diversity of collection formatting, even though it may represent the same core data, can drastically affect the ability to design databases, enter data into the database, and pool data across protocols. For example, important data in comment fields can be difficult to integrate from study to study. Standardized modules and collection forms designed to capture these data improve the ease of subsequent integration.

With SABRIL, many of the European case report forms did not capture dosing and study information in a consistent fashion to allow easy integration. Standardized fields had to be set up for these data so that they could be entered into the reconstructed databases.

INDIVIDUAL SITE VERSUS CENTRAL LABORATORIES

The use of centralized laboratories greatly eases data collection and interpretation. Without the use of centralized laboratories, such problems as the following arise:

- differing unit conventions,
- multiple reference ranges or unavailability of reference ranges,
- need for conversion or standardization to allow summarization across protocols.

Conversion to single standardized units, either SI (*Système International*) or conventional, should be carried out. Data can then be summarized and reported across protocols, with outliers identified according to sponsor definitions.

The SABRIL database required identification and coding of parameters and associated units from each laboratory. The parameter code, numeric values, and units were then entered into a database. This eliminated the need to translate and standardize the order of each laboratory slip for data entry purposes.

PATIENT TRACKING ACROSS PROTOCOLS

Large development programs that take place over several years can result in the same patients participating in multiple protocols. The most common scenario involves patients who satisfactorily complete blinded protocols and choose to enter a long-term, open-label, follow-up protocol intended to continue to document safety and efficacy. These protocols often last until the drug is approved and is available by prescription in a given country. To minimize administrative problems, all patients entering a drug protocol should be assigned a unique identification number serving to link them across protocols throughout the entire development program. When this is not done, and especially if programs are lengthy and involve several open-label protocol changes, patient tracking can prove quite difficult. It is important to recognize that if patients are not uniquely identified, an artificial inflation of patient exposure can occur. If patients do not receive a unique identifier and therefore receive several numbers for identification, they can be tracked through the program, but only with a significant amount of work. This tracking procedure involves comparing demographics and other information derived from investigators to confirm identities.

In most cases, the European SABRIL program applied this discipline. In cross-checking demographics, a few discrepancies were noted and the unlinked patients were identified, preventing duplication in reporting of exposure.

ADVERSE EVENT REPORTING

Adverse event reporting practices have evolved extensively during the last 10 to 15 years. Typically, treatment-emergent events tend to be reported at a higher frequency in the United States than in Europe, and it is important to consider this when reviewing European case report forms, especially when these span a period of several years. Differences in reporting practices and the formats of adverse event reporting forms and changing policies over time can create difficulties when the safety database is built.

Older case report forms, whether from outside the United States or from U.S. studies, should be reviewed carefully for unreported findings that would be considered treatment-emergent events according to current standards. This type of information can be found in comments fields. It can also be gleaned by reviewing changes in concomitant medications and comparing the results of prestudy and poststudy physical and safety examinations. In cases of treatment-emergent events, it is always helpful when investigators can be consulted for details. The older the study, however, the more difficult this becomes—in terms of finding the investigator who was involved or expecting accurate recall of details. With SABRIL, board- certified and currently practicing clinical consultants were asked to evaluate changes in prestudy and poststudy neurologic and ophthalmologic examination findings to determine whether any unreported adverse events occurred.

When sponsors are confronted with the prospect of reconstructing a safety database that spans as much as a decade, a summary database of all events reported, appropriately coded and categorized for maximal consistency, should be constructed. Reporting of all events is necessary because of lack of first-hand investigator input on treatment causality.

DOCUMENTING METHODS AND DECISIONS

One thing that seems certain in today's environment is that change is inevitable. Possible changes that can affect a drug development program include the following:

- changes in sponsor project team members,
- changes in regulatory reviewers,
- changes in regulations or guidelines,
- changes in company control.

Obviously, the longer the development program, the greater the likelihood of a change occurring that will have a significant impact on the submission and review. To minimize the potential negative impact of changes on the program, certain steps should be taken along the way (Table 2). First, it is important to establish an overall set of rules for assessing study quality, to determine how studies will be utilized in an NDA (i.e., whether studies will be considered pivotal or supportive). Also, database construction methods should be set up ahead of time so that data can be handled efficiently and with a minimum of questions during NDA preparation. It may be appropriate to have a "Methods" section as part of the integrated safety summary. Finally, decisions that are made regarding the analysis, collection, assessment, or evaluation of data, both efficacy and safety, should be documented in a place easily referenced, so that changes in personnel or company control will not require reconstruction of past decisions or development of new procedures to be followed. This may have been the single most difficult challenge for the team associated with SABRIL. From the initiation of studies to the writing and filing of the NDA, a period of about 14 years, many significant changes took place. The company that initiated the development program was Merrell Dow, with headquarters in Cincinnati. In 1989, the merger with Marion Laboratories and subsequently Hoechst AG resulted in new headquarters and differences in priorities and standard operating procedures. The clinical and regulatory teams changed several times. As a result, many procedures had to be determined as the need arose to evaluate and reconstruct the European safety database.

TABLE 2. *Establishing and documenting procedures to minimize impact of change*

- Prospectively establish how study quality will be assessed, to determine whether it is pivotal or supportive
- Develop rules and methods for database construction
- Maintain a reference for these procedures and determinations
- Include a "Methods" section in the integrated safety summary

SUMMARY AND IMPORTANT LESSONS

The inclusion of foreign data in an NDA can provide critically important documentation that can favorably affect review of the submission. It is critical, however, to ensure that the data are of adequate quality, have supporting documentation, and can be reported in an integrated fashion.

To minimize problems that may arise late in the process of preparing an NDA or when questions from the Food and Drug Administration about databases are being answered, it is desirable to have a well-conceived global development plan, including phase IIIb and IV studies, drafted as early as possible. In addition, it is critical to establish methods and document decisions that determine how study quality will be assessed and how databases will be constructed. Foreign studies that will be used as pivotal efficacy and safety studies or that will be used to verify safety will need to be of GCP quality.

Constructing a database using foreign data can present challenges that arise from a variety of sources. If faced with the challenge of reconstructing databases from study results that were produced during several years without the luxury of a fully integrated global program, it is necessary to establish standards for dealing with multiple reporting languages, collecting information about adverse events that may not have been treated as treatment-emergent events, analyzing laboratory data from noncentralized sources, and tracking patients who may have been included in multiple protocols.

The experience with SABRIL confirms that every effort should be made to maintain the highest level of quality in study conduct, data collection, and database construction as global plans unfold. This will minimize problems as NDAs are written, submitted, and reviewed, regardless of the geographic origin of the study data and the length of time involved.

REFERENCES

1. International Conference on Harmonisation (ICH) of Technical Requirements for Registration of Pharmaceuticals for Human Use: Background Paper. ICH Steering Committee and International Federation of Pharmaceutical Manufacturers Associations; October 1995 revision.
2. 21 CFR, Part 312.120. Foreign Clinical Studies Not Conducted Under an IND.

Antiepileptic Drug Development.
Advances in Neurology, Vol. 76,
edited by J. French, I. Leppik, and M. A. Dichter.
Lippincott–Raven Publishers, Philadelphia © 1998.

14

Issues for Women in Antiepileptic Drug Development

Martha J. Morrell

Department of Neurology, Stanford University Medical School, Stanford, California 94305.

INTRODUCTION

The development process for a new antiepileptic drug should ideally address issues of importance to the women who will use the drug—many of which concern reproductive health. However, the drug development process is shaped not only by the desire for scientific knowledge, but also by sociopolitical beliefs and values that may not adequately represent the interests of all populations, including women. Two areas of potential concern to women with epilepsy are addressed in this chapter:

1. Are women of reproductive age with epilepsy able to gain appropriate access to clinical drug trials, and are adequate safeguards provided against harm to the women and to potential fetuses?
2. Are issues of concern to women of reproductive age adequately addressed during the drug development process?

Issues associated with the preclinical development of antiepileptic drugs (and other drugs) and issues arising in the postmarketing period are addressed separately. Particular attention is directed toward areas in which the drug development process is perceived to address the concerns of women inadequately.

PREMARKETING ISSUES

Access to Trials

Inclusion of Women of Childbearing Potential

The extent to which women have been involved in clinical drug trials has reflected societal beliefs concerning the status of women. These attitudes have shifted in response to historical events. In the 1950s through the 1980s, the prevailing regulatory tone was one of protectionism. This arose in response to revelations of research subject abuse (Tuskegee Syphilis Project) and in reaction to discoveries of adverse morphologic outcome in children exposed to certain drugs *in utero* (thalidomide). During the years following World War II, attitudes about the role of women in society and a woman's ability to make an informed choice also reinforced the belief that women of childbearing potential, and pregnant and lactating women, formed a vulnerable population in need of special protection.

These assumptions were evident in the 1977 guidelines of the Food and Drug Administration (FDA) directing that women of childbearing potential be excluded from phase I and early phase II trials (1). Once data had been obtained regarding the relative efficacy and safety of the pharmaceutical, and once preclinical data on fertility and teratogenesis in animals were available, then women of childbearing potential could participate in later phase II trials. In 1977, a woman of childbearing potential was narrowly defined as any woman physiologically capable of becoming pregnant, regardless of sexual activity, sexual practices, and contraceptive use. This policy did not address the manner in which safety and efficacy should be assessed to determine whether participation was appropriate, but left decisional authority to Institutional Review Boards (IRBs), investigators, and research subjects.

In the past two decades, attitudes have evolved. Consumers, investigators, and governmental agencies have expressed concerns that guidelines and regulations implemented to protect research subjects are overly restrictive and are, in fact, detrimental to the health of the groups denied access. This has led to a number of significant changes in regulatory policy, all of which are based on the assumption that patients included in clinical studies should reflect the population that will receive the drug (2).

In 1990, the National Institutes of Health (NIH) directed that women and minorities be included in clinical trials (3). The 1993 NIH Revitalization Act directed the NIH to establish guidelines for the inclusion of women and minorities in federally funded biomedical and behavioral research involving human subjects, except when specific criteria for the exclusion of these groups could be satisfied (4).

In 1994, the NIH released guidelines on the inclusion of women and minorities as subjects in clinical research (5). These guidelines mandate that women and minorities be included in phase II trials in sufficient numbers so that valid analysis of differences in intervention effect can be accomplished. Although the NIH acknowledged the concern of many investigators that the detection of significant gender-based differences in response might require large, time-consuming, and expensive clinical studies, the guidelines emphasize that cost is not an acceptable criterion for exclusion. Investigators are further required to initiate programs and support outreach efforts to recruit underrepresented groups.

In 1993, the FDA withdrew its restriction on participation of women of childbearing potential in early clinical trials (6). Three reasons were cited for reversing the 1977 FDA guidelines: the expectation that gender-specific data obtained early in a drug investigation would be used to make appropriate adjustments in larger clinical studies, the need to avoid unwarranted discrimination against women, and the desire not to perpetuate the view of male patients as the primary focus of drug development.

Inclusion of Pregnant or Lactating Women

Epilepsy is a chronic disease, and antiepileptic drugs are likely to be used in women while they are pregnant and lactating. Although regulations now support and even demand the inclusion in clinical trials of women of childbearing potential who are using effective contraception, controversy and discomfort still exist regarding the participation of pregnant and lactating women. One must consider how best to define the risks and benefits of a particular antiepileptic drug in this population.

Although federal statutes, regulations, guidelines, and policies have been enacted that encourage the inclusion of women of childbearing potential in clinical trials, no specific guidance has been provided concerning the inclusion of pregnant women. Federal policies and Health and Human Services regulations have generally assumed that pregnant women would be excluded (7). Constitutional, legislative, and tort law have failed to provide a clear framework in which to clarify the appropriateness of inclusion of pregnant women in clinical drug trials.

Federal regulations have largely restricted the access of pregnant and lactating women to clinical trials, but policies are being re-examined. In addition to the protections provided to volunteers in research studies (8), Department of Health and Human Services (DHHS) regulations also provide protections pertaining to research development and related activities involving pregnant women, fetuses, and human in vitro fertilization. A DHHS regulation (7) directs that pregnant women may not be research subjects except under two circumstances: if the purpose of the activity is to meet the health needs of the mother and the fetus will be placed at risk only to the minimal extent necessary to meet such needs, and if the risk to the fetus is minimal. This has been interpreted as supporting the inclusion of pregnant women in trials of antiviral agents and cancer chemotherapy after informed consent has been obtained.

Consent requirements for pregnant women are very stringent. The DHHS specifies that "... both mother and father (must give) ... informed consent. The father's consent is (not necessary) if the purpose of the activity is to meet the health needs of the mother, his identity or whereabouts cannot be reasonably ascertained, he is not reasonably available, or the pregnancy results from rape" (7).

The NIH and FDA directed the Institute of Medicine (IOM) to examine policies regarding inclusion of pregnant and lactating women in clinical trials. The IOM Committee on Women in Research made a controversial recommendation in 1994 that pregnant and lactating women be considered eligible to be subjects in clinical research (9). The IOM report stated that "... the prevailing presumption regarding the participation of pregnant women in clinical trials ... (should) be shifted from one of exclusion to one of inclusion." The IOM felt that women who are or may become pregnant during the course of a research study should be viewed like any other competent adult who is a potential research subject.

The justification for the IOM statement was as much ethical as medical, derived from principles of respect for the autonomy of women and their capacity to act as responsible moral agents. Two principles cited included distributive justice, which implies that "... the benefits as well as the burdens of clinical research ... should be equitably distributed among all individuals in society," and respect for humans, which implies that men and women should share equally in the opportunity to serve as subjects in clinical research.

The IOM indicated that investigators and IRBs have the responsibility of ensuring that pregnant and lactating women are provided with adequate information about the risks and benefits to themselves and their potential offspring. When risks are not known, the decision regarding acceptability of the risks to the fetus should be made by the woman as part of the consent process. Exclusion of women from the study by the IRB is warranted only if there is no prospect of benefit to the pregnant woman and if there is a known or plausibly inferred risk of fetal harm. According to the IOM, "Far from needing protection, the pregnant woman is the most motivated and in the best position to decide for the health of herself and the potential child."

Three levels of law—constitutional, legislative, and tort—are relevant to this discussion. The 14th Amendment is the equal protection clause of the United States Constitution. The 14th Amendment guarantees the protection of "life, liberty, and property" and has been interpreted to provide decisional privacy with respect to terminating life-sustaining treatment and obtaining an abortion. It also implies the right to assume the risk of experimental drugs. In addition, the 14th Amendment states that "... no state shall ... deny to any person within its jurisdiction equal protection of the laws." This could be interpreted as contradicting DHHS regulations that bar the inclusion of pregnant women in research. This amendment might be used as a constitutional challenge to consider the liberty and privacy interests of a woman versus state interests concerning fetal protection and protection of the woman's health.

Legislative laws also address the participation of pregnant women in clinical trials. The Pregnancy Discrimination Act of 1978 (10) bans discrimination on the basis of pregnancy, childbirth, or related conditions. Title VII of the Civil Rights Act of 1964 (11) forbids employers to discriminate on the basis of race, color, religion, sex, or national origin.

The Supreme Court interpretation of Title VII has been somewhat contradictory. The Supreme Court has written that differential treatment of pregnancy does not represent a suspect gender classification in the context of a state disability insurance program. In general, however, the Court has been consistent in its rulings that pregnant women cannot be discriminated against in the context of employment unless gender is a *bona fide* occupational qualification (12).

A Supreme Court case relevant to this issue is *United Automobile Workers v. Johnson Controls* (12,13). Johnson Controls, a manufacturer of batteries, established a fetal protection policy that excluded women capable of bearing children from jobs involving exposure to lead. This policy was established after eight women became pregnant while maintaining critically high blood lead levels as established by Occupational Safety and Health Administration (OSHA) guidelines. In 1984, a class action suit challenged the policy as a violation of Title VII. A federal district court and the United States Court of Appeals upheld Johnson on the basis of medical evidence of potential harm to the fetus. The Supreme Court reversed these decisions, stating that it was wrongfully discriminatory to exclude women from a benefit on the grounds of fetal protection. The Court felt that the bias in this policy was obvious, as "... fertile men but not fertile women are given a choice as to whether they wish to risk their reproductive health for a particular job." The Court went on to note that the company did not seek to protect all unconceived children, only those of its female employees. The Court also felt that the act was in violation of the Pregnancy Discrimination Act once the company had chosen to treat all its female employees as potentially pregnant—a policy that evinces discrimination. Whereas Johnson Controls argued that its policy was ethical, socially responsible, and medically defendable, the Court wrote, "It is no more appropriate for physicians to attempt to control women's opportunities . . . on the basis of their reproductive role than it is for the courts or individual employers to do so." The Court concluded, "Decisions about the welfare of future children must be left to the parents who conceive, bear, support, and raise them rather than to the employers who hire those parents." These decisions may be relevant to issues concerning the exclusion of pregnant women in clinical trials.

Tort law may also address the interests of woman and fetus. Tort liability is civil or private law that evolves from decisions made by judges to compensate individuals for injury resulting from the actions of a defendant. Tort law varies by state, and each state may have a different variation of tort law applying to whether a woman's informed consent can bar independent action by a child harmed as a fetus. Although state tort liability usually holds that warnings may preclude claims by injured *parties*, warnings may not preclude claims by injured *children*, because in general parents cannot waive action on behalf of their children and the parent's negligence cannot be imputed to the children.

Two legal theories might be asserted against manufacturers of pharmaceuticals in a tort action: negligence, and strict liability.[1] In a negligence action, the plaintiff must prove that the defendant (the manufacturer or investigator) had a legal duty toward the plaintiff, the defendant breached that duty, the plaintiff suffered an injury, and breech of duty by the defendant was the cause of the plaintiff's injury. For example, in a drug product liability case, the plaintiff would claim not to have been given the information that would permit a truly informed consent. Under strict liability, the manufacturer of a product that is "in a defective condition unreasonably dangerous to the . . . consumer" is subject to liability for injury caused to the consumer without proof of fault by the manufacturer. However, products deemed "unavoidably unsafe" are exempt from this rule if the manufacturer has given proper directions and warnings for the use of

[1]Flannery EJ. Confronting legal concerns in pregnancy research—the perspective of the company. Presented at the Regulated Products and Pregnant Women Workshop. Food and Drug Administration, Crystal City, Virginia, November 8, 1994.

their products. Therefore, a prescription drug is not considered unreasonably dangerous if it is accompanied by adequate warnings of potential side effects. In many states, prescription drugs, prescription medical devices, and vaccines are exempt from strict liability on a case-by-case basis. The manufacturer must bear the burden of proving that the benefits of their product outweigh the risks at the time of its release. Nevertheless, although these are realistic concerns regarding liability, manufacturers have not faced substantial litigation from participants in clinical trials.[2]

There are no case precedents to resolve the question of whether informed consent from a pregnant woman is relevant to determine the likelihood of a successful tort action for injuries to offspring that may have been caused by inclusion of the pregnant woman in a drug trial. The Supreme Court addressed tort liability for fetal injury in *United Automobile Workers v. Johnson Controls*. According to the Court, under Title VII liability for fetal injury is remote if an employer has followed federal guidelines and has fully informed its workers of the risks involved.

Other issues to consider concerning tort liability include the statute of limitations for research-related injury and the parties who would be liable in a negligence action. At present, the fetus can sue to the age of majority for any adverse consequences related to exposure to a pharmaceutical agent. Whether liability in such a suit applies only to pharmaceutical companies or involves health care providers as well has not been established. Excluding pregnant women from clinical trials has been viewed as a way to avoid liability for injuries, especially to potential offspring. However, liability may also be related to exclusion, particularly for drugs that will subsequently be used to treat pregnant women. Pharmaceutical companies and health care providers may be liable for injury to pregnant women and their fetuses that occurs after marketing if failure to test for a foreseeable risk can be proved. A pregnant woman or injured offspring might sue a manufacturer after a pharmaceutical is marketed because the pharmaceutical had not been tested in this population before release—particularly if pregnant women are expected users. Health care providers might also be liable for administering drugs to pregnant women before they have been tested in controlled trials of pregnant women.

If pregnant women are to be included in investigational drug trials, then investigators must ensure that an adequate number of pregnant women can be recruited and retained in the study to allow valid and meaningful scientific conclusions to be drawn. If insufficient numbers are recruited, then the manufacturer will not be allowed to provide any statement of the drug's appropriateness for use in this population. In this case, failure to include a sufficiently large number of pregnant women might be considered negligent.

Given these liability issues, inclusion of pregnant women will probably proceed only when adequate compensation mechanisms have been established. These compensation mechanisms could be contractual or legislative, as with the Vaccine Compensation Act. The IOM in 1994 (9) recommended that the NIH thoroughly review the area of compensation for research injury in general and that compensation mechanisms address prenatal and preconceptional injuries to children resulting from a parent's participation in a clinical study.

Although legal issues may appear to discourage the inclusion of vulnerable populations such as pregnant women and their fetuses in investigational drug trials, a rational and consistent application of legal and ethical principles can also be argued to prevent the arbitrary exclusion of any class of people from the benefits of research. The potential benefit of participating in the trial may be the most important factor in determining if participation is appropriate. Risk to the fetus may be acceptable if the study is likely to have im-

[2]Reisman EK. Products liability what is the current situation and will it change (and how) when more women are included in studies? Presented at the Women in Clinical Trials of FDA-Regulated Products Workshop. Food and Drug Law Institute, Washington, D.C., October 5, 1992.

portant medical benefits for the mother. Women with life-threatening conditions such as cancer and AIDS have typically been included in the earliest phases of drug testing. Whether sufficient benefit is derived from participation in an investigational drug trial of an antiepileptic drug might be argued, given that alternative pharmaceutical agents exist.

Inclusion of pregnant women is most appropriate when the woman is provided with sufficient information to allow informed consent. This includes information regarding potential mechanisms of teratogenesis of existing antiepileptic drugs and hypotheses regarding teratogenic effects of the tested agents. Such hypotheses would be drawn from knowledge of the pharmacokinetics of the new agent as well as animal studies of reproductive toxicology. This information would guide the design of appropriate trials to include pregnant and lactating women.

Clinical Issues: Contraceptive Use During Investigational Trials

The FDA 1977 guidelines on the participation of women of childbearing potential in phase I and early phase II trials excluded premenopausal women who were sexually active and using no contraception; it also excluded women using mechanical, oral, or injectable contraceptives, women whose partners had had vasectomies, women who were sexually inactive, and homosexual women (1). The revised FDA guidelines of 1993 state, "It is expected that, in accordance with good medical practice, appropriate precautions against becoming pregnant and exposing the fetus to a potentially dangerous agent during the course of a study will be taken by women participating in clinical trials" (6). The FDA in 1993 also indicated that it is expected that women will receive adequate counseling regarding the importance of taking precautions against becoming pregnant and that efforts will be made to ensure that a woman is not pregnant when she enters a trial as determined by a negative pregnancy test detecting the β-subunit of the human chorionic gonadotropin (HCG) molecule. Reliable contraceptive methods include abstinence, homosexuality, barrier methods, hormonal contraception, and willingness to consider interruption of pregnancy.

The IOM believes that participants should be permitted to select voluntarily the contraceptive method of their choice when no relevant, study-dependent, scientific reasons, such as drug interactions, exist for excluding certain contraceptives (9). "The investigator must have knowledge of interactions that might compromise the efficacy of certain contraceptives, such as failure of hormone-based contraception in women on liver cytochrome P_{450}-inducing drugs."

When an unintended pregnancy occurs in an investigational drug trial, the woman and her physician will need to consider whether termination is appropriate (6). The IOM recommends that "pregnancy termination options (should) be discussed as part of the consent process in clinical studies that pose unknown or foreseeable risks to potential offspring" (9). In recent trials of antiepileptic drugs, many women have chosen to terminate their pregnancies.

Investigative Issues

Gender-Specific Analysis

In 1993, the FDA released guidelines for the study and evaluation of gender differences in the clinical evaluation of drugs that called for careful characterization of drug effects by gender (6). This followed a 1988 FDA guideline (Center for Drug Evaluation and Research, 1988) that called for analysis of data to identify variations in efficacy and adverse effects of drugs according to subjects' age group, race, and gender. In 1983 and 1989, the FDA examined the relative numbers of women in the database of New Drug Applications (NDAs). In general, women were represented to the same extent that women were affected by the disease. The General Accounting Office conducted a larger study of drugs approved during 1988–1991, with similar results. However, although women comprised an acceptable percentage of research subjects, gender-specific analyses were not necessarily conducted (6).

In 1993, the FDA stated, "Over the past decade there has been a growing concern that the drug development process does not produce adequate information about the effects of drugs on women. For phase III trials . . . women and minorities and their subpopulations must be included such that valid analysis of differences in intervention effect can be accomplished" (6). To detect efficacy and safety differences related to physiologic gender differences, such as the effects of hormones, substantial representation of both sexes is expected, as is analysis by gender of effectiveness, rates of adverse events, and dose response.

One rationale for gender-specific analysis comes from the increasing recognition of differences in pharmacokinetics in women and men. Gender-related differences in pharmacokinetics are partly caused by variations in body size and composition; women are generally smaller and have a higher percentage of body fat and a lower percentage of body water. Hormones may also affect pharmacokinetics. Changes in pharmacokinetics might be expected at puberty, during the menstrual cycle, and at menopause. Pharmacokinetic variations could also be caused by interactions with steroid hormones taken for contraception or postmenopausal hormone replacement therapy.

The FDA encourages pharmacokinetic screening by gender (6). A small number of steady-state concentration measurements are obtained in most phase II and phase III subjects, which are then analyzed by gender to determine any important differences. If such differences are detected, then formal pharmacokinetic studies are undertaken. The FDA also encourages that an evaluation be conducted of potential interactions between the test drug and contraceptive steroids.

Reproductive Toxicology

Studies of reproductive toxicology must be completed before large-scale exposure of women of childbearing potential to investigational drugs takes place. The FDA guidelines for reproductive toxicology studies (14) call for a three-segment design that evaluates fertility and general reproductive performance, teratology, and perinatal and postnatal status in rodents and other nonprimate mammals.

Reproductive toxicology studies as currently utilized may not be specific predictors of human teratogenic potential. Animals may be more sensitive to the teratogenic effects of new drugs because of differences in metabolism and because dose exposures usually substantially exceed the expected dose range in humans. In vitro techniques might permit a more accurate and specific analysis of mechanisms of teratogenesis. For example, properties of a drug that could promote teratogenesis include the propensity to form arene oxide metabolites or produce antifolate effects. Cell culture techniques could identify drug effects on specific organ formation, such as the palate (15) and the neural tube (16).

POSTMARKETING ISSUES

Defining Appropriate Use in Women of Childbearing Potential

Effects on Contraception

Any pharmaceutical that will be given to women of reproductive age must be evaluated for potential interactions with therapeutic steroid hormones (e.g., contraceptives and hormone replacement therapy). Hormone-dependent contraceptive devices—including oral contraceptive pills, long-acting Depo hormone preparations, and hormone-impregnated intrauterine devices—represent the most effective method of family planning. However, these methods may fail if interactions with other drugs increase steroid metabolism or protein binding, as occurs with drugs that induce the cytochrome P_{450} system of the liver.

Effects on Reproductive Health

Women with epilepsy are at risk for disturbances in reproductive health. As many as one third of women with epilepsy have irregular or abnormal menstrual cycles. Ovulatory function and reproductive hormones released from the hypothalamus, pituitary gland, and gonads may be disrupted. Disorders of sexual desire and arousal are also more frequent in women with epilepsy. Drugs that alter hormonal release and metabolism contribute to this disruption in reproductive function and could partly account for the higher rates of infertility in women with epilepsy. The extent to which a new antiepileptic drug affects reproductive health would influence its use in women of reproductive age (17).

Effects on Bone Mineral Metabolism

Many of the established antiepileptic drugs appear to compromise bone health by placing women at increased risk for osteoporosis, osteopenia, osteomalacia, and fractures—particularly after menopause (18,19,20). Routine examination of the effects of a new antiepileptic drug on bone metabolism and bone density would provide valuable information to determine appropriate use in women.

Use in Pregnant and Lactating Women

Management after Conception

In every evaluation of pregnancy outcome after exposure to the established antiepileptic drugs, preconception antiepileptic drug monotherapy at the lowest effective dose is associated with the lowest risk of adverse outcome (21). This principle of therapy should also be applied to management with the new antiepileptic drugs. To enable selection of the best single agent, the efficacy of each new antiepileptic drug must be clearly defined by seizure or epilepsy type and, ideally, by gender.

The FDA provides risk categories for each approved antiepileptic drug. If a new antiepileptic drug is selected for a woman of childbearing potential, she must be informed of what is understood to be the risk should she become pregnant. As shown in Table 1, the established and new antiepileptic drugs carry the pregnancy risk category C, except for phenytoin and valproate, which carry the risk of category D.

TABLE 1. *FDA use-in-pregnancy drug categories*[a]

The use-in-pregnancy categories of the FDA are based on the degree to which available information has ruled out risk to the fetus, balanced against potential benefits of the drug to the patient.
Category A: Controlled studies show no risk.
Adequate, well-controlled studies in pregnant women have failed to demonstrate risk to fetus.
Category B: No evidence of risk to human fetus.
Either animal findings show risk but human findings do not, or, if no adequate studies have been done, animal findings are negative.
Category C: Risk cannot be ruled out.
Human studies are lacking, and results of animal studies are either positive for fetal risk or lacking. However, potential benefits may justify the potential risk.
Category D: Positive evidence of risk.
Investigational or postmarketing data show risk to the fetus. Nevertheless, potential benefits may outweigh potential risk.
Category X: Contraindicated in pregnancy.
Studies in animals or humans, or investigational or postmarketing reports, have shown fetal risk that clearly outweighs any possible benefits to the patient.

[a]From ref. 24.

These risk categories are not sufficiently specific to be of clinical benefit. Therefore, appropriate risk counseling requires that all information regarding outcome after human pregnancy exposures be available to physician and patient, including pregnancy complications, incidence of fetal malformations and anomalies, and potential problems of cognitive development. A review of the animal reproductive toxicology studies is appropriate. The physician must also know the most effective means to evaluate for abnormal morphogenesis, including appropriate use of level II fetal ultrasonography, measurement of maternal serum α-fetoprotein, and amniocentesis.

Folate supplementation has been conclusively shown to prevent the occurrence (22) and recurrence (23) of neural tube defects and other congenital malformations. All women of childbearing potential should receive folate supplementation of at least 0.4 mg/d, with women at risk for folate deficiency receiving more. The established antiepileptic drugs interfere with folate absorption or folate-mediated biochemical processes. If it is not known whether a new drug has antifolate properties, then folate supplementation >0.4 mg/d should be considered.

For the best management of antiepileptic drug therapy in the pregnant woman with epilepsy, the physician must be able to anticipate pharmacokinetic changes. Changes in drug absorption, protein binding, volume of distribution, metabolism, and clearance must be defined. Pharmacodynamic changes may occur as a result of interaction of the antiepileptic drug with neuroactive hormones of pregnancy.

Surveillance after Conception

Whether women are included or excluded from preclinical trials, it is clear that postmarketing data regarding outcome after pregnancy exposures to a new pharmaceutical must be pursued aggressively.

Observational methods have typically been employed to monitor risks of birth defects associated with marketed medications.[3] Adequate clinical surveillance also requires that the exposed group be identified and that the timing and extent of fetal exposure to the antiepileptic drug be documented. With the present surveillance systems, these goals are not always possible. Also, the sensitivity and specificity of observational databases are limited. It is unlikely that a medication can be determined to be free of risk to the fetus, because extremely large sample sizes are needed to rule out an increased risk for a specific defect.

Surveillance has traditionally been conducted by governmental agencies. The FDA relies on postmarketing surveillance of voluntarily reported adverse events. However, only 10% of these adverse outcomes are likely to be reported. The FDA, Centers for Disease Control (CDC), and industry have also engaged in other surveillance activities. The CDC administers a birth defects program, which includes the National Birth Defects Monitoring Program and the International Clearing House on Birth Defects. These and other large observational databases, such as Medicaid, provide clues regarding adverse outcomes in an epidemiologically diverse population. Industry has recently established registries to evaluate pregnancy and fetal outcomes after exposure to antiepileptic drugs. Other methods that can be utilized to capture pregnancy exposures to an antiepileptic drug include use of automated medication databases and case-control surveillance of birth defects, so that hypotheses can be generated regarding associations between medications and specific birth defects. Ultimately, only mandatory postmarketing epidemiologic safety monitoring can be expected to permit rapid and thorough accumulation of information regarding human exposure to an antiepileptic drug. Postmarketing pregnancy registries that are easily accessible to health care providers will permit medication-related adverse outcomes to be identified in an appropriately short period of time. Information should be obtained regarding time and duration of exposure, maternal dose, exposure to polytherapy, and identification of other variables affecting fetal outcome, including adequacy of prenatal care. At the time of this writing, a prospective antiepileptic drug pregnancy registry is being established.

Counseling after Conception

A discussion of the advisability of breastfeeding is part of postconception counseling for the woman with epilepsy. Pharmaceutical compounds concentrate in breast milk in inverse relation to their degree of protein binding. The greater the protein-bound fraction, the lower the transmission into breast milk. Knowledge of the extent of protein binding of an antiepileptic drug permits an estimate of concentration in breast milk. Other informa-

[3]Andrew EB. Use of observational methods to monitor the safety of marketed medications for risks of birth defects. Presented at the Regulated Products and Pregnant Women Workshop. Food and Drug Administration, Crystal City, Virginia, November 8, 1994.

tion necessary to provide adequate counseling concerns the concentration and effects of the pharmaceutical in the neonate. Neonatal pharmacokinetics are likely to differ from maternal pharmacokinetics, so that the effective concentration in the neonate will vary depending on the its capacity to metabolize and clear the drug. Finally, any acute or chronic effects on development and behavior after neonatal exposure should be defined. This information would enable the mother to make an informed choice regarding breast-feeding.

CONCLUSION

The development of a new drug ideally takes into consideration issues relevant to the women who will use that drug. These are likely to include the effects of female physiology on efficacy, tolerability, and pharmacokinetics; interactions with steroid hormones and the effects of the drug on reproductive health, including fertility and sexuality; and the consequences of exposing a fetus to the new antiepileptic drug.

These valid scientific concerns must be balanced by society's wish to protect individuals from the potential harm of an untested compound. For women of childbearing potential, these concerns have led to decades of restriction from participation in investigational drug trials. Regulatory agencies have recently revised guidelines to correct what is now viewed as excessive past restrictions. For pregnant and lactating women with epilepsy, the proper course of action does not seem clear. Although pregnant and lactating women with epilepsy are likely to take a new antiepileptic drug after release, at present this population is excluded from trials of new antiepileptic drugs. This policy is currently being re-examined, prompted by input from consumers, regulatory agencies, and the courts.

With the release of a new antiepileptic drug, health care providers begin to define the optimal use in special populations. The more the efficacy and tolerability of a drug can be defined in special populations, such as women, the more effectively that drug will be used. This provides the greatest benefit to the pharmaceutical company, the health care provider, and especially the patient.

REFERENCES

1. FDA. General considerations for the clinical evaluation of drugs. Washington, DC: US Government Printing Office; 1977 (Publication No. HEW(FDA)77-3040).
2. Merkatz RB, Temple R, Sobel S, Feiden K, Working Group on Women in Clinical Trials. Women in clinical trials of new drugs: a change in Food and Drug Administration policy. *N Engl J Med* 1993;329:292–296.
3. NIH. NIH/ADAMHA. Policy concerning the inclusion of women in study populations. NIH guide for grants and contracts. 1990.
4. NIH. NIH Revitalization Act. 1993. Public Law (Pub.L.) 103-143.
5. NIH. NIH guidelines on the inclusion of women and minorities as subjects in clinical research. *Federal Register* 1994;59(59):14508–14513.
6. FDA/DHHS. Guidelines for the study of and evaluation of gender differences in the clinical evaluation of drugs. *Federal Register* 1993;58(139):39406–39416.
7. DHHS. Additional DHHS protections pertaining to research, development, and related activities involving fetuses, pregnant women, and human in vitro fertilization. Title 45. Code of Federal Regulations. Part 46, subpart B. March 15, 1994.
8. NIH/Office for Protection from Research Risks (OPRR). Protection for human subjects. 1991;45:CFR 46.
9. Institute of Medicine. Women and health research: ethical and legal issues of including women in clinical studies. Washington, DC: National Academy Press; 1994:1–25.
10. Pregnancy Discrimination Act of 1978.92 Statute 2076, 42 United States Code Section 2000e (k).
11. Civil Rights Act of 1964 (as amended), 42 United States Code Section 2000d et seq.
12. Annas G. Fetal protection and employment discrimination—the Johnson Controls case. *N Engl J Med* 1991; 325:740–743.
13. International Union, United Automobile, Aerospace, and Agricultural Implement Workers, UAW v. Johnson Controls, Inc. 111S. Ct. 1196(1991).
14. FDA/DHHS. International Conference on Harmonization; guideline on detection of toxicity to reproduction for medicinal products; availability. *Federal Register* 1994;59(183):48746–48752.
15. Mino Y, Mizusawa H, Shiota K. Effects of anticonvulsant drugs on fetal mouse palates cultured in vitro. *Reprod Toxicol* 1994;8:225–230.
16. Regan CM, Gorman AMC, Larsson OM, Maguire C, Martin ML, Shousboe A, Williams DC. In vitro screening for anticonvulsant-induced teratogenesis in neural primary cultures and cell lines. *Int J Dev Neurosci* 1990;8:143–150.
17. Morrell MJ. Reproductive health in women with epilepsy. In: *Treatment of Epilepsy*. Ed: W.E. Lew Febiger 1996:179–187. In: Wyllie E. ed. *The Treatment of Epilepsy: Principles and Practice*. 2nd ed. (*in press*).
18. Valimaki M, Tiihonen M, Laitinen K, et al. Bone min-

eral density measured by dual-energy x-ray absorptiometry and novel markers of bone formation and resorption in patients on antiepileptic drugs. *Min Res* 1994;9: 631–637.

19. Sheth R, Wesolowski C, Jacob J, et.al. Effect of carbamazepine and valproate on bone mineral density. *J Pediatr* 1995;127:256–262.
20. Chung S, Ahn C. Effects of antiepileptic drug therapy on bone density in ambulatory epileptic children. *Brain Dev* 1994;16:382–385.
21. Morrell MJ. Pregnancy and epilepsy. In: Porter RJ, Chadwick D, eds. *Epilepsies II*. Boston: Butterworth-Heinemann; 1997:313–332.
22. Czeizel AE, Dudas I. Prevention of the first occurrence of neural tube defects by periconceptional vitamin supplementation. *N Engl J Med* 1992;327:1832–1835.
23. Medical Research Council Vitamin Research Group. Prevention of neural tube defects: results of the Medical Research Council Vitamin Study. *Lancet* 1991; 338:131–137.
24. FDA. Use-in-pregnancy drug categories. 21 CFR§201.57 (f)(6)(i)(a)–(e).

Antiepileptic Drug Development.
Advances in Neurology, Vol. 76,
edited by J. French, I. Leppik, and M. A. Dichter.
Lippincott–Raven Publishers, Philadelphia © 1998.

15

Antiepileptic Drug Trials in Children and Adolescents: Is There a Need?

Jeffrey R. Buchhalter

Division of Child and Adolescent Neurology, Mayo Clinic, Rochester, Minnesota 55905.

AGE-RELATED EPIDEMIOLOGY OF SEIZURES AND EPILEPSIES

It is recognized that seizures and epilepsies are common among children. Although 4% to 10% of children will have one or more seizures, by the age of 20 years approximately 1% will maintain the diagnosis of epilepsy. A striking and important age distribution exists within the pediatric population. The overall incidence of seizures in this population is 50 to 100/100,000. However, the rates are stratified by age: <1 year old, 72 to 250/100,000; <9 years old, 72 to 87/100,000); <14 years old, 45 to 83/100,000 (1). It is only in persons >65 years of age that the disorder becomes as frequent as in children. Thus, the epidemiology of seizures and epilepsy raises several issues. The first is that a large proportion of the people for whom treatment for seizures is considered are children. Therefore, it is prudent that medications used to treat seizures in this age group are demonstrated to be effective and safe. The age distribution is relevant in that pharmacologic properties that influence loading and maintenance dosing of medication (e.g., volume of distribution, plasma half-life, protein binding) vary with age, particularly in the youngest age range, in which seizures are so frequent. Finally, the potential impact of any medication on cognitive and motor development is a special issue that needs to be considered in this population.

The need for additional antiepileptic agents will, in part, be determined by the success of currently available drugs. Whereas measures of efficacy are frequently defined by type of epilepsy syndrome, antiepileptic drugs have traditionally been developed against seizure types. The limitation of the latter approach is illustrated by the example of a generalized tonic-clonic seizure in the context of the syndrome of benign epilepsy with centrotemporal spikes (BECTS) versus a generalized tonic-clonic seizure in the syndrome of symptomatic partial seizures with secondary generalization. Because of the self-limited natural history of BECTS, treatment with any medication is an area of debate, whereas the same seizure type in the latter syndrome can be refractory to anticonvulsant medication and severely limit educational, professional, and social activities.

CURRENTLY AVAILABLE ANTIEPILEPTIC DRUGS

It is useful to summarize briefly the indications for some of the most commonly used antiepileptic drugs available in the United States and note what information is provided by the manufacturer for pediatric dosing. The following information was obtained from Physicians' Desk Reference and more recent product information sheets.

Phenobarbital is indicated for the treatment of generalized and partial seizures. No specific pediatric use is stated. A milligram-per-kilogram dosage is provided. Warning is given regarding possible cognitive effects in children given phenobarbital for febrile seizures.

Phenytoin is indicated for tonic-clonic seizures, psychomotor seizures, and seizures associated with neurosurgery. No pediatric indication is noted. Its use is implied for patients <6 years of age and is explicit for patients >6 years of age in the milligram-per-kilogram dosage guidelines.

Ethosuximide is indicated for the treatment of absence (*petit mal*) seizures. No specific pediatric use is stated, although a milligram-per-kilogram dosing regimen is provided.

Carbamazepine is indicated for partial seizures, generalized tonic-clonic seizures, and "mixed seizure patterns that include the above." Dosage and administration guidelines are provided for children 6 to 12 years old and for adults and adolescents >12 years old. Recently, an indication for the use of carbamazepine in children <6 years of age has been approved, with milligram-per-kilogram dosing guidelines for the suspension and tablet formulations.

Valproic acid is indicated for use in simple and complex absence seizures and adjunctively in patients with multiple seizure types that include absence seizures. Although no pediatric indications are stated, warnings are provided regarding congenital metabolic disorders and severe seizure disorder associated with mental retardation in children <2 years old. A milligram-per-kilogram dosage is provided.

Felbamate has been approved as monotherapy and adjunctive therapy for seizures of partial onset in adults and as adjunctive therapy for seizures associated with the Lennox-Gastaut syndrome in children. As a consequence of the latter indication, pharmacokinetic and dosing information is available for children. Unfortunately, the occurrence of unexplained aplastic anemia and hepatic failure has limited the use of this medication.

Gabapentin is indicated as adjunctive therapy for partial seizures in individuals >12 years old. No pharmacokinetic data are available for individuals <18 years old. Specific milligram-per-kilogram dosage information is not provided.

Lamotrigine has recently been approved as an adjunctive agent for the treatment of partial seizures in adults. A specific caveat is included, which indicates that efficacy and safety have not been established in patients <16 years of age. No pediatric dose range or milligram-per-kilogram dosing is recommended. The most recent product information sheet indicates that the risk for life-threatening rash is significantly higher in children than in adults (see below).

Topiramate is approved as adjunctive therapy for adults with partial-onset seizures. Although the manufacturer is careful to state that efficacy and safety for children have not been established, pharmacokinetic studies in children 4 to 17 years old indicate that clearance is independent of dose and is somewhat higher in children than in adults. Neither an age-related or milligram-per-kilogram dose range is recommended.

Adrenocorticotropic hormone (ACTH), prednisone, and intravenous immunoglobulin have been used to treat epilepsies of childhood, particularly infantile spasms and the Lennox-Gastaut syndrome. Although not specifically approved for the treatment of seizures, a significant literature exists for ACTH and prednisone with regard to dosing protocols.

It should be noted that trials are currently under way for further testing of gabapentin, lamotrigine, vigabatrin, and oxcarbazepine in children.

FREQUENCY OF SEIZURE TYPES

A variety of studies provide information regarding the frequency of different seizure types. In most series in which children are included, partial seizures account for approximately 60% to 75% of all seizure types (1–4). One of the most interesting and relevant of the studies is that derived from a population-based sample in Rochester, Minnesota (1). In this survey, it was found that the incidence of generalized tonic-clonic seizures (10 to

15/100,000) and partial seizures (20/100,000) did not vary significantly with age. However, absence seizures declined markedly from 18 to 1/100,000 at 20 years of age. Similarly, myoclonic seizures peaked in early childhood (50/100,000), then declined to 3/100,000 at 20 years of age. These results indicate that although some seizure types are predominantly confined to childhood, other types also affect the adult population, suggesting that shared seizure types (partial and generalized tonic-clonic) may be treated by the same agents used in adults, with additional studies necessary to define age- and weight-appropriate dosing regimens. Those seizure (and epilepsy) types that preferentially afflict children and adolescents will require specific models and interventions.

FREQUENCY OF EPILEPSY SYNDROMES

As noted above, the seizure type alone may not predict responsiveness to medication or long-term prognosis (both critical factors in determining if additional antiepileptic drug trials are needed for children). The concept and classification of epilepsy syndromes have been most useful in addressing these issues (5). The following are the most common epilepsy syndromes, with the estimated percentage of total childhood epilepsy indicated in parentheses: febrile convulsions (2% to 4%), infantile spasms (2%), Lennox-Gastaut syndrome (1% to 2%), childhood absence (10% to 15%), juvenile myoclonic epilepsy (5%), and idiopathic localization-related epilepsies (20% to 25%). These may be slight overestimates, as data from studies involving the pediatric epilepsy populations (6–8) indicate a frequency of idiopathic localization epilepsies between 0 and 2% and of idiopathic generalized epilepsies between 3% and 26%.

EFFICACY OF ANTIEPILEPTIC DRUGS

One of the most important factors that will determine the need for additional antiepileptic agents is the efficacy of the currently available drugs. These need to be stratified by seizure type and epilepsy syndrome.

When typical absence is considered as a seizure type, studies report a wide range of control, 46% to 70%. However, if typical absence is considered within the childhood absence epilepsy syndromes, as many as 80% of children become seizure-free (9). From the 1950s until the 1980s, ethosuximide was the drug of choice, as long as no other seizure types (e.g., tonic-clonic) were involved. The introduction of valproic acid allowed both nonconvulsive and convulsive seizure types to be treated with a single medication. More recent studies using valproate monotherapy indicate that 95% of children with only absence seizures can be seizure-free (10). It should be noted that this population represented only 18% of the study group and that the seizure-free rate fell to 76% when other seizure types occurred. Juvenile myoclonic epilepsy is another epilepsy that highlights the importance of analyzing outcome by syndrome type. Patients with this syndrome have an 80% to 88% likelihood of becoming seizure-free on valproic acid, occasionally with the addition of a benzodiazepine (10,11). Other idiopathic generalized epilepsy syndromes, such as juvenile absence epilepsy and generalized tonic-clonic seizures on awakening, probably have the same range of seizure control with ethosuximide, valproic acid, and benzodiazepines. The majority of children who are not seizure-free have a relatively small number of seizures, which can, nonetheless, result in some social, educational, and professional limitations.

The most commonly identified idiopathic partial epilepsy syndromes also have a favorable prognosis. In fact, it is currently controversial whether to treat the most common idiopathic localization-related (partial) epilepsy syndrome, BECTS, because of the likelihood (approximately 98%) of patients "outgrowing" the syndrome by the age of 20 years. In addition, the majority of seizures occur near the time of or during sleep, and there appear to be no long-term consequences of either the partial motor-sensory or secondarily generalized tonic-clonic seizures that define this syndrome. Childhood epilepsy with occipital paroxysms is another idiopathic localization-related epilepsy syndrome associated with a >80% likelihood of seizure control based on a limited amount of data. Because the other syndromes included in this group are so uncommon, comment on the likelihood of seizure control is not warranted.

The symptomatic localization-related epilepsies occur commonly and show the least favorable response to antiepileptic drugs. Among children, only approximately 60% of those with symptomatic temporal lobe epilepsy achieve adequate control with an acceptable frequency and severity of drug-induced side effects (12). The likelihood of seizure control in the symptomatic extratemporal lobe epilepsies (frontal, occipital, parietal) is probably even less. Similarly, control of the symptomatic generalized epilepsies of childhood is less than adequate with currently available antiepileptic drugs. Of patients with infantile spasms and Lennox-Gastaut syndrome (among the "catastrophic" pediatric epilepsy syndromes), the rate of seizure control is frequently <50%, and significant cognitive, behavioral, and systemic antiepileptic drug toxicities are frequent.

Febrile convulsions are classified under special syndromes. Although common in children <10 years old (2% to 5%), febrile convulsions are rarely difficult to control. Treatment options include vigorous antipyresis, intermittent use of benzodiazepines, or prophylactic therapy with valproic acid or phenobarbital.

Currently, there is no evidence to suggest that an antiepileptic drug that is effective treatment for a specific seizure type in adults is not effective in children. Specifically, carbamazepine, phenytoin, and valproic acid have been demonstrated to be efficacious for partial and generalized seizures, with no differences noted in the pediatric and adult populations (13). Drugs that are used (but not necessarily approved by the Food and Drug Administration) in the United States for partial seizures in both children and adults include carbamazepine, valproic acid, gabapentin, phenytoin, lamotrigine, felbamate, and phenobarbital. Agents with demonstrated efficacy against seizures with generalized onset include ethosuximide, valproic acid, felbamate, and probably lamotrigine.

ADVERSE EFFECTS OF ANTIEPILEPTIC DRUGS

The adverse effects that occur most commonly in adults using antiepileptic drugs also occur in children, although the absolute frequencies differ depending on the study (14). However, carbamazepine may exacerbate seizures of generalized onset more frequently in children than in adults. Increased sensitivity to valproic acid occurs in children who are <2 years old, developmentally delayed, and taking more than one anticonvulsant (15). In a European trial, vigabatrin appeared to increase the frequency of generalized seizures in children >2 years old (16). Recently, it has been reported that the incidence of a life-threatening rash induced by lamotrigine may be 50 to 100 times more frequent in children than in adults. Although these adverse effects are serious, most side effects of antiepileptic drugs are qualitatively similar in children and adults. The most significant potential difference in toxicity between age-defined populations involves development and cognition. Although the short-term effects of the antiepileptic drugs (especially the barbiturates) have been reported, the long-term consequences of antiepileptic drugs on the developing nervous system are unknown. Known mechanisms of antiepileptic drug action involve interaction with sodium and calcium channels, facilitation of GABAergic inhibitory systems, and suppression of excitatory amino acid systems that are likely to play direct and indirect roles in synaptogenesis.

PHARMACOKINETICS

The effects of age on the kinetics and distribution of antiepileptic drugs is an important topic that is beyond the scope of this chapter but has been described in detail elsewhere (17). A partial list of processes that are age-dependent and affect drug pharmacokinetics include oral and gastric absorption, total protein quantity, protein binding, gastric motility, and volume of distribution. Specifically, newborns in comparison with adults have a longer and more irregular gastric emptying, a reduced absorption surface area, a significantly less acidic gastric pH (>4), and less drug binding owing to lower levels of albumin. Hepatic enzyme systems responsible for the metabolism of antiepileptic drugs are reduced in newborns. In contrast, infants and young children have a faster gastric emptying time and intestinal mobility, decreased plasma protein binding, and a volume of distribution and excretion rates (renal and hepatic) comparable with those of adults.

CONCLUSIONS

On the basis of the considerations presented above, several recommendations can be made regarding the need for antiepileptic drug trials in children.

1. New antiepileptic drugs are needed to control the symptomatic partial and generalized epilepsies.
   a. Antiepileptic drugs effective for partial seizures in adults are effective in children.
   b. Pharmacokinetic and safety data in children are needed.
2. Additional antiepileptic drugs are needed to control the catastrophic epilepsies of early childhood, which differ from adult epilepsies because of developmental aspects. Age-specific pharmacokinetic and safety data are necessary.
3. Additional antiepileptic drugs to treat the generalized idiopathic epilepsies would benefit the considerable number of patients with epilepsy that is refractory to treatment.
4. The long-term benefit of controlling neonatal seizures is currently unknown, but seizures are very common in newborns and therapeutic agents are limited. Thus, trials of new antiepileptic drugs to assess efficacy, safety, and pharmacokinetics are warranted.
5. Syndromes for which new antiepileptic drugs are not required include febrile seizures and the benign epilepsies of childhood (e.g., BECTS).

REFERENCES

1. Hauser WA, Annegers JF, Kurland LT. Incidence of epilepsy and unprovoked seizures in Rochester, Minnesota: 1935–1984. *Epilepsia* 1993;34:453–468.
2. Senanayake N. Classification of epileptic seizures: a hospital-based study of 1,250 patients in a developing country. *Epilepsia* 1993;34:812–818.
3. Cavazzuti GB. Epidemiology of different types of epilepsy in school-age children of Modena, Italy. *Epilepsia* 1980;21:57–62.
4. Cowan LD, Bodensteiner JB, Leviton A, et al. Prevalence of the epilepsies in children and adolescents. *Epilepsia* 1989;30:94–106.
5. Commission on Classification and Terminology of the International League Against Epilepsy. Proposal for revised classification of epilepsies and epileptic syndromes. *Epilepsia* 1989;30:389–399.
6. Shah KN, Rajadhyaksha SB, Shah VS, et al. Experience with the International League Against Epilepsy classifications of epileptic seizures (1981) and epilepsies and epileptic syndromes (1989) in epileptic children in a developing country. *Epilepsia* 1992;33:1072–1077.
7. Oka E, Ishida S, Ohtsuka Y, et al. Neuroepidemiological study of childhood epilepsy by application of the international classification of epilepsies and epileptic syndromes (ILAE, 1989). *Epilepsia* 1995;36:658–661.
8. Ohtsuka Y, Ohno S, Ohtahara S. Classification of epilepsies and epileptic syndromes of childhood according to the 1989 ILAE classification. *J Epilepsy* 1993;6:272–276.
9. Aicardi J. *Epilepsy in Children*. 2nd ed. New York: Raven Press; 1994:94–117.
10. Bourgeois B, Beaumanoir A, Blajev B, et al. Monotherapy with valproate in primary generalized epilepsies. *Epilepsia* 1987;28:S8–S11.
11. Panayiotopoulos CP, Obeid T, Tahan AR. Juvenile myoclonic epilepsy: a 5-year prospective study. *Epilepsia* 1994;35:285–296.
12. Wyllie E, Lüders H. Complex partial seizures in children—clinical manifestations and identification of surgical candidates. *Cleve Clin J Med* 1989;56:S43–S52.
13. Callaghan N, Kenny RA, O'Neill B, et al. A prospective study between carbamazepine, phenytoin, and sodium valproate as monotherapy in previously untreated and recently diagnosed patients with epilepsy. *J Neurol Neurosurg Psychiatry* 1985;48:639–644.
14. Herranz JL, Armigo JA, Arteaga R. Clinical side effects of phenobarbital, primidone, phenytoin, carbamazepine, and valproate during monotherapy in children. *Epilepsia* 1988;29:794–804.
15. Dreifuss FE, Santilli N, Langer DH, et al. Valproic acid hepatic fatalities: a retrospective review. *Neurology* 1987;37:379–385.
16. Lortie A, Chiron C, Mumford J, et al. The potential for increasing seizure frequency, relapse, and appearance of new seizure types with vigabatrin. *Neurology* 1993; 43:S24–S27.
17. Morselli PL, Pippenger CE, Penry JK, eds. *Antiepileptic Drug Therapy in Pediatrics*. New York: Raven Press; 1983.

Antiepileptic Drug Development.
Advances in Neurology, Vol. 76,
edited by J. French, I. Leppik, and M. A. Dichter.
Lippincott–Raven Publishers, Philadelphia © 1998.

16

Pediatric Trials: Practical Issues. Special Populations and Trial Design

John M. Pellock

Division of Child Neurology, Medical College of Virginia, Virginia Commonwealth University, Richmond, Virginia 23213.

OVERVIEW

As new drugs become available for the treatment of epilepsy, issues arise as to when and how to test the safety and efficacy of these medications in children. Historically, antiepileptic drugs have been developed and approved for use in adults with partial seizures. Both clinical development programs and marketing forces encourage this plan. Pharmacokinetic and efficacy studies in children have rarely been performed in preapproval phases of antiepileptic drug development. Smaller pharmacokinetic and perhaps efficacy studies have sometimes been performed to allow dosing guidelines. A review of Physicians' Desk Reference is disappointing in that it quickly reveals that additional steps to ensure that the Food and Drug Administration has approved these drugs for additional indications in pediatric epilepsy are lacking. In 1978, the Committee on Drugs of the American Academy of Pediatrics estimated that three fourths of prescription drugs marketed in the United States lacked full Food and Drug Administration approval for pediatric use. Little has changed. In 1992, 19 new molecular entities with potential use in children were approved by the Food and Drug Administration, but 79% were not labeled for use in children. Most new drugs have been labeled with disclaimers for pediatric use (1). The typical practice has been to extend the use of antiepileptic drugs approved for adult epilepsy to children. Clinicians use these agents to treat partial and secondarily generalized seizures in children and then sometimes attempt similar efficacy studies, in particular of pediatric epilepsy syndromes, based on mechanism of action, animal model data, or pure empiricism.

A more organized approach for antiepileptic drug development has been discussed by both international and national experts, and particular guidelines for antiepileptic drug trials in children were published in 1994 by the Commission on Antiepileptic Drugs of the International League Against Epilepsy. In their recommendations, specific problems related to epilepsy in childhood, including diagnosis and selection of patients, pharmacokinetics, behavior and cognition, and ethical considerations, were delineated. A consensus, despite these difficulties, suggested a need for early studies in children, once phase II and phase III studies had been completed in adults. It was suggested that these studies should at first be open and should determine tolerability, pharmacokinetics, and dose ranges and provide an estimate of efficacy before controlled studies or special syndromes are attempted. It was further recommended that patients in control groups should be treated with well-tolerated, standard antiepileptic drugs, marketed for that indication, when available. It was felt that placebo could be administered only when there was no reference agent or when a study drug appeared to be rapidly effective or could be added to previous medication.

The Committee on Drugs of the American Board of Pediatrics recently has also addressed the issue of "unapproved uses of approved drugs" (2,3) and the difficulties of conducting studies to evaluate medications in children (4). Antiepileptic drugs used to treat seizures in children have been identified as a particular class of agents in which generalization from adult protocols has been modified for pediatric use (3). Knowledge concerning dosage may be inadequate or inexact, and specific advantages or adverse effects that may be seen in children are unidentified.

ISSUES CONCERNING ANTIEPILEPTIC DRUG TRIALS IN CHILDREN

Ethical issues are paramount when children participate in investigative or therapeutic procedures. Legal regulations vary significantly among countries, because children are unable to provide informed consent. Children, however, are particularly vulnerable and should provide assent (active agreement) to the study if they have reached an intellectual age of 7 years or greater (5). In general, most studies cannot be undertaken without proof that there is a direct benefit to the child, that there is no risk (or minimal risk), and that the information gained through the study is beneficial for other children. For this reason, healthy children are almost never included as volunteers in pediatric pharmacokinetic studies, as is the rule in preliminary adult antiepileptic drug studies. Children cannot ethically volunteer, nor can they or their families be rewarded for their participation. The families, however, may receive compensation for expenses and be provided with medical care and "study" medication. This ethical dilemma of not overrewarding makes it sometimes difficult to repay children and their families fully for participating in drug trials.

The performance of single drug versus placebo comparative studies is also difficult. This design has been used to demonstrate the efficacy of gabapentin in the treatment of rolandic epilepsy, because there is no standard of care known and because the epilepsy is thought to be benign whether or not seizures occur (5). When no specific treatment seems superior or when none is known to be efficacious, many patients may consider the option of no therapy. Also, once a drug has been approved for use in adults, parents who select treatment prefer that their child receive it and not possibly be randomized to receive placebo for some extended period. This design of a treatment protocol in a benign epilepsy has led to extremely slow patient recruitment. Double-blind, add-on versus placebo studies are usually acceptable. One must, however, question whether there is any need for trials of antiepileptic drugs in children ages 4 to 12 years with partial seizures, as there is no evidence that their partial seizures differ from those seen in adults. Pharmacokinetic dose ranging and longer safety studies in children at various age levels with otherwise open designs may be sufficient.

Patient selection requires a careful definition of the seizure and epilepsy diagnosis in the populations studied. Because of the size of the population available for study in some relatively rare syndromes, recruitment for studies in a reasonable period of time may be a significant issue. The incidence of epilepsy in children and adolescents ranges from 50 to 100/100,000 (6). Those with truly refractory epilepsy make up a much smaller proportion of the entire group. Those with West syndrome are limited by age and make up only about 2% of cases of childhood epilepsy. Depending on other criteria of inclusion or exclusion for this group, only a small population may be available for study. Similarly, children with the Lennox-Gastaut syndrome account for 1% to 2% of all cases of childhood epilepsy. These children frequently have combined medical and behavioral conditions that require the administration of additional long-term medications. A limit to total seizure number, episodes of status epilepticus, or clusters also may be necessary. The study design will very much define how many of these children can be included. Childhood absence epilepsy may account for up to 10% to 15% of all cases of childhood epilepsy, but if they are to be entered into a trial early in treatment, the numbers quickly decrease. Thus, decisions regarding early treatment versus refractory patients, which concomitant medications will be allowed, the number of seizures that each patient is to have, and inclusion or exclusion of comorbid states definitely affects the available study population. Syndromes are certainly age-related and some study populations must be restricted, whereas others, such as those with the Lennox-Gastaut syndrome, can be extended through a greater age range (7). Diversity of opinion exists as to whether all children with refractory epilepsy should first be studied in open-label pilot studies in less specific syndromes. Those placed in early open studies cannot, however, be later enrolled into blinded studies, and a portion of the otherwise eligible population for pivotal studies is no longer available.

Appropriate dosing during a clinical trial is of paramount importance. Early pharmacokinetic determinations must be accomplished in nearly all studies. Even in open studies, a dose versus level versus efficacy determination should begin to be established, so that it can be compared with available data from animal and adult studies. If the dose-response range is not well determined, a childhood trial design that allows escalation of dose and levels to efficacy or toxicity needs to be considered. An early study of gabapentin in absence seizures used a dose of 20 mg/kg, but blood levels were quite low and insufficient information may have resulted from these trials (8). Whenever possible, dosing of children should depend on blood levels and effect rather than be determined arbitrarily so that maximal information can be obtained. This design modification ensures a therapeutic trial, which may otherwise be complicated by insufficient dosing because of changes in renal and hepatic clearance.

A very practical issue in neonates and young children is the amount of blood that can be sampled. Also, in neonates and in patients with seizures that are difficult to count, investigators must fully establish parameters defining specific events. Limitations exist in both safety and pharmacokinetic studies. The alternative methodology of using discarded or stored blood samples (ex vivo) for simple pharmacokinetic dose determinations such as protein binding should be considered early in drug development in young children. The development of stable isotope techniques and micromethods for drug and metabolite determinations should be a priority for industry and academia when antiepileptic drug studies are contemplated in children <5 years old.

Efficacy parameters should be carefully specified for each trial. Total seizure numbers may not be accurate or sufficient in encephalopathic epilepsy with mixed seizures. Seizure types in children participating in the study might be defined through video-electroencephalographic recording, so that caregivers could be educated and reference could be made to the initial naming or classification throughout the study. The use of total seizure numbers, specific seizures by type per unit time, a specific number of seizure recurrences following treatment, the recording of electroencephalographic seizures for a 24-hour period, or counts per unit time before and after the treatment period should all be considered as efficacy endpoints. Difficulty still exists when children with encephalopathic epilepsy and frequently occurring seizures have clusters or go into status epilepticus. In some studies, rescue with benzodiazepine or other intermittent agents is allowed. In other trials, background medications must be kept stable in regard to to type and dose, and no rescue medications are allowed. The use of time-to-*X*th-seizure or time to a point of failure may allow for shorter studies. Data and times, however, must be determined after adequate dosing has been established.

The use of subjective scales and assessment of cognitive and behavioral affects of new antiepileptic drugs in children is much more difficult than in adults. Scales of quality of life and seizure severity are particularly difficult to apply in young children, and no meaningful neuropsychologic testing can really be performed in children <5 years of age. In children with motor handicaps or mental retardation, even greater difficulties arise. Studies of behavioral and cognitive affects in children in the past have frequently shown that variability between testing dates results from many factors in a child's life other than the effects of medication. These issues, however, are exceedingly important, because children sometimes have exaggerated reactions to anticonvulsants with possible sedative or other behavioral properties. Newer antiepileptic drugs, such as felbamate and lamotrigine, have revealed an alerting property in both children and adults. Seeming overstimulation and insomnia must be documented. Behavior and mood must be specifically tested when possible and observer responses and global assessments recorded over time to allow accurate assessment of the full effect of medication on children's quality of life.

Issues with either open or blinded studies include dosing and the need for special formulations for infants and young children. If only children who can take capsules are allowed in the protocol, certainly the available population is significantly lessened, and medication can be administered by having caregivers empty capsule contents into food or other substances. Tablets are crushed and then mixed. If studies do not allow this technique of administration, one must question what information is really known about drug delivery to young children before release. Do all antiepileptic drugs need to be available as liquids, dispersible tablets, sprinkle preparations, or other palatable formulations before they are approved? Perhaps we should test existing preparations and make recommendations concerning their best use in children who cannot swallow tablets or capsules.

Above and beyond all the above technical considerations, professionals must consider the effect on parents, families, and children with epilepsy of the lack of availability of antiepileptic drugs approved for pediatric use. The recent practice of families importing vigabatrin to treat their children with refractory epilepsy shows their need and dedication. For parents to enroll their children in clinical trials, they must first know about them. Not every family has access to the Internet! Even after learning about the study and the medication involved, parents and children should feel comfortable that they are receiving the best available treatment. If a placebo arm exists, patients (parents) demand that they be allowed to receive active drug in a reasonable time period. They must be assured of excellent, comprehensive medical care. How do study personnel communicate and interact with the child's primary care physician? Many of these families are already overextended in regard to time and monetary commitments; the antiepileptic drug trial must reasonably and adequately reimburse them for both these commitments but not be coercive. And perhaps most importantly, emergency treatment and contact must be built into the trials. Managed health care may not approve a visit not covered by the protocol; other funds must. Those physicians and personnel who perform pediatric antiepileptic drug trials must interact with the entire family. They cannot isolate the epilepsy from other handicaps of the child anymore than they can isolate the child from the family. Thus, the investigator, industry, and government must be aware of the added complexity for patients, families, and caregivers.

CONCLUSIONS

Drug trials should certainly be conducted in children and need to be done early in the development of new antiepileptic drugs. The Epilepsy Branch of the National Institutes of Health held a workshop in 1994 to consider the development of antiepileptic drugs for use in children. The specific aims of this meeting were to (a) determine when pediatric trials are appropriate and necessary; (b) discuss developmental, cognitive, and age-related issues that differentiate studies of drugs in children from those in adults; (c) identify specific characteristics of epileptic syndromes and seizure types in children that need to be addressed in clinical trials; (d) examine features of pediatric pharmacokinetics, including drug interactions, that influence trial design; and (e) explore informed consent and other ethical considerations. New antiepileptic are needed for pediatric epilepsy. The recommendations proposed by the workshop concluded with seven recommendations that were published in 1996 (4).

1. Antiepileptic drugs are needed for pediatric epilepsy; trials for new antiepileptic drugs should include trials for children.
2. If a drug is shown to be effective for partial seizures in adults, this is sufficient to justify approval for use in partial seizures in children, provided that safety and pharmacokinetic considerations are appropriate.
3. As antiepileptic drugs that are approved for use in adults are certain to be used in children, pharmacokinetic data and dosing schedules for children should be provided to the professional community at the time of drug approval.
4. Putative antiepileptic drugs should be tested in immature animals as well as adult animals to identify agents that may be age-specific. New models should be developed for specific age-related syndromes.
5. The development and standardization of new outcome measures of drug effects, especially in the areas of cognition and behavior, are recommended for the evaluation of new antiepileptic drugs in pediatric epilepsy.
6. Postmarketing surveillance for long-term development and cognitive and other safety issues needs to be developed for all new antiepileptic drugs.
7. Governmental agencies, such as the National Institute of Neurological Disorders and Stroke, are strongly urged to identify and support a system or systems to identify and track patients for antiepileptic drug development.

Specific types of epilepsy refractory to existing therapies must receive high priority for testing. Despite the difficulties involved in antiepileptic drug trials in neonates, recent data would suggest that existing medications are less than optimal and that others must be developed.

Many practical issues present significant challenges, and additional trial designs for special populations of children will be necessary. I believe, however, that despite all the challenges, adequate trials of antiepileptic drugs should be well planned and at least begin before the marketing of new antiepileptic drugs. This recommendation is shared by others (2,3) and will allow for the most efficient use of new therapies in children with epilepsy. Until then, lack of approval for use in children should not prevent physicians from prescribing available agents in the best interests of their pediatric patients (2).

REFERENCES

1. Medical Economics Data Production Company. *Physicians' Desk Reference*. Montvale, NJ: Medical Economics Data Production Company; 1994.
2. Committee on Drugs. Unapproved use of approved drugs: the physician, the package insert, and the Food and Drug Administration: subject review. *Pediatrics* 1996;98:143–145.
3. Committee on Drugs. Is the "therapeutic orphan" about to be adopted? Commentaries. *Pediatrics* 1996;98: 118–122.
4. Sheridan PH, Jacobs MP. Conference review: the development of antiepileptic drugs for children. Report from the NIH Workshop, Bethesda, Maryland, February 17–18, 1994. *Epilepsy Res* 1996;23:87–92.
5. Bouma PA, Bovenkerk AC, Westendorp RG, Brouwer OF. The course of benign partial epilepsy of childhood with centrotemporal spikes: a meta-analysis. *Neurology* 1997;48:430–437.
6. Hauser WA, Hesdorffer DC, eds. *Epilepsy: Frequency, Causes and Consequences*. New York: Demos Publications; 1990.
7. The Felbamate Study Group in Lennox-Gastaut syndrome. Efficacy of felbamate in childhood epileptic encephalopathy (Lennox-Gastaut syndrome). *N Engl J Med* 1993;328:29–33.
8. Leiderman D, Garofalo E, LaMoreaux L. Gabapentin in patients with absence seizures: two double-blind, placebo-controlled studies. *Epilepsia* 1993;34(Suppl 6):45(abst).

Antiepileptic Drug Development.
Advances in Neurology, Vol. 76,
edited by J. French, I. Leppik, and M. A. Dichter.
Lippincott–Raven Publishers, Philadelphia © 1998.

17

Clinical Trials for Status Epilepticus

David M. Treiman

Department of Neurology, UCLA School of Medicine, Los Angeles, California 90095.

INTRODUCTION

Status epilepticus (SE) is a medical emergency that requires immediate effective treatment to prevent neuronal damage and even death. Because of the requirement for immediate treatment, clinical trials in the treatment of SE pose a number of special problems not encountered in studies of drugs for the long-term management of epilepsy. This chapter reviews these problems and provides examples of their solutions. Many of the examples are derived from a recently completed large, multicenter comparison of four intravenous regimens in the initial management of generalized convulsive status epilepticus (GCSE), the Veterans Administration Cooperative Studies Program (VACSP) Study No. 265 (1).

STATUS EPILEPTICUS

SE is operationally defined as recurrent epileptic seizures without full recovery of consciousness between seizures, or as more or less continuous clinical and/or electrical seizure activity lasting longer than 30 minutes, whether or not consciousness is impaired. However, recent treatment protocols have suggested that continuous seizure activity persisting beyond 10 minutes should be considered SE, because of documentation that convulsive activity during an isolated, self-limited seizure never lasts more than 2 minutes (2). The implication of this definition is that any epileptic seizure that recurs frequently enough or lasts long enough can be considered a type of SE. Although simplified classification schemes have been proposed (3–5), the International Classification of Epileptic Seizures (6) is the most appropriate classification of SE for use in clinical trial designs. Certain epilepsy syndromes, particularly in childhood, also can be viewed as forms of SE (e.g., electrical SE of slow-wave sleep, Landau-Kleffner syndrome), but these are rare syndromes that are unlikely to be the subject of clinical trials.

GCSE is by far the most common and most dangerous presentation of SE, and is therefore the most appropriate type of status to study in clinical trials. Treiman (4) has characterized GCSE as a condition characterized by paroxysmal or continuous tonic and/or clonic motor movements; these may be overt or quite subtle, but they are associated with profound coma and bilateral, although frequently asymmetric, ictal discharges. Furthermore, he distinguishes between overt GCSE, in which the convulsive movements are unequivocally ictal, and subtle GCSE, in which convulsive movements are so subtle that electroencephalographic confirmation is necessary to make the diagnosis of SE.

SE is far more common that has been previously appreciated. Hauser (7) estimated that there are about 65,000 cases of SE in the United States each year, based on data from Rochester, Minnesota. More recently, DeLorenzo and colleagues (8) suggested that >150,000 cases occur in the United States each year, based on extrapolation of the incidence data from Richmond, Virginia. In any event, better drugs are needed for the treatment of SE. Success rates of 39% to 100% have been reported for the treatment of SE. However, most studies have been based on retrospective chart reviews, and all but two (1,9) were conducted without electroencephalographic confirmation of success. Only four studies (1,9–11) compared treatments assigned in a prospective, randomized fashion. By far the largest was a recently completed VA cooperative study that compared four intravenous drug regimens in the initial management of GCSE: phenytoin alone, diazepam followed by phenytoin, phenobarbital alone, and lorazepam alone (1). In this study, the first drug to which the patient was randomly assigned was successful in overt GCSE only 56% of the time, with a range between 65% success for the best treatment (lorazepam) and 44% success for the least successful drug (phenytoin alone). Among the patients with subtle GCSE, only 15% responded to the first drug, and no statistically significant differences in efficacy of the four treatments were noted.

Mortality associated with SE has been reported in the range of 5% to 50% in previous series (5). In the VA study, outcome was assessed 30 days after the episode of SE. Twenty-seven percent of the patients with overt GCSE and 65% of those with subtle GCSE died within 30 days of their episode of status. It is clear from the outcome data of this most recent and largest study of the treatment of GCSE that more effective drugs are needed to treat SE, including drugs, such as neuroprotective agents, that might improve outcome.

NEED FOR NEW DRUGS

A number of new antiepileptic drugs currently are undergoing evaluation for the long-term management of epilepsy. It is possible that one or more may be an effective agent for the management of GCSE. However, many have been tested in a cobalt/homocysteine model of secondarily generalized convulsive SE (12), and none of the new drugs thus far appears especially promising (13–19). It may be that improvement in the pharmacologic management of GCSE will depend on the development of a new and different approach to therapy, rather than the identification of a highly effective single drug. Experimental data suggest that the most effective treatment of SE may be polytherapy, in which drugs with different mechanisms of action are combined to block excitation and enhance inhibition simultaneously (20). The order in which such drugs are administered appears to be important. We have observed a substantial increase in the efficacy of a combination of low doses of NPC-17742, a competitive NMDA (*N*-methyl-D-aspartate) receptor blocker, and diazepam, which enhances inhibition mediated by GABA (τ-aminobutyric acid), in one rat experiment and of phenytoin and diazepam in another experiment when the excitatory blocker or sodium-channel stabilizer is given 10 minutes before the benzodiazepine (20,21). Of course, these drugs are usually given in the opposite order. The administration of a benzodiazepine before phenytoin is based on pharmacokinetic considerations. Because it is possible to inject a benzodiazepine intravenously far more rapidly than to infuse an effective dose of phenytoin, the benzodiazepines are usually given first. However, our rat data suggest that the traditional order of administration is not the most effective. It appears that when excitation is decreased, the potential for a benzodiazepine to enhance GABA-mediated inhibition is increased. Kapur et al. (22,23) have reported attenuation of GABA-mediated inhibition during SE that can be blocked by administration of an NMDA receptor blocker (24).

CLINICAL TRIALS IN STATUS EPILEPTICUS

If new drugs or new ways to administer old drugs are to be studied in clinical trials of the management SE, several fundamental questions must be considered in the development of such trials. The objective of any clinical

TABLE 1. *Comparative trials of antiepileptic drugs and neuroprotective agents in status epilepticus: potential populations that could be studied*

Specific types of status epilepticus	
	Generalized convulsive status epilepticus
	Nonconvulsive status epilepticus
	Complex partial status epilepticus
	Absence status epilepticus
Specific presentations of status epilepticus	
	Overt versus subtle generalized convulsive status epilepticus
	Treatment-responsive versus refractory status epilepticus
Special populations	
	Children
	Women (eclampsia)
	Encephalopathic patients
	Elderly patients

trial of the management of SE is likely to be to compare the utility of potential treatments for (a) stopping ongoing seizure activity and (b) providing protection against status-induced neuronal damage. However, such treatment comparisons might be conducted in a number of different clinical situations, as outlined in Table 1. Furthermore, comparative clinical trials in SE might also be designed to test specific hypotheses relating to etiology, clinical presentations, clinical features, predictors of response to treatment, and outcome.

Trial Design

As in all clinical trials, rigorous design of a clinical trial for SE management is important to its ultimate success. Essential elements in the design of SE trials include (a) prospective randomization of assignment to treatment groups; (b) double-bind parallel group design, and (c) unambiguous operational definitions of diagnostic criteria and outcome parameters. Because of the potential morbidity associated with delay in successful treatment, a placebo-control group is not ethically acceptable. Unambiguous operational definitions of success are essential. Yet most reports of drug efficacy in SE have failed to provide operational definitions for both diagnosis of SE and ascertainment of success. In the VACSP Study No. 265, the diagnostic criterion for overt GCSE was two or more convulsions without completely recovery of consciousness between the convulsions or continuous convulsive activity for >10 minutes. Subtle GCSE was diagnosed when coma was associated with convulsive activity so subtle that ictal activity on the electroencephalogram was considered necessary by the evaluating physician to make the diagnosis. Treatment was considered successful if seizures stopped within 20 minutes after the start of infusion and no clinical or electrical evidence of seizure activity was observed from 20 to 60 minutes after starting intravenous infusion. Blinding of the evaluating physician to treatment assignment is essential because of the potential for subjective bias during observation of what appears to be clinical seizure activity, especially when ictal activity on the electroencephalogram is assessed. When patients exhibit discrete electroencephalographic seizures, ascertainment of cessation of seizure activity is not difficult. However, during GCSE there is frequently a gradual conversion from ictal to postictal patterns. Determination of the exact time at which all ictal discharges have stopped can be extremely difficult, and it is therefore essential to avoid the possible introduction of subjective bias by utilizing a double-blind design.

Electroencephalographic monitoring to verify successful treatment is also essential in clinical trials of SE. In the VACSP Study No. 265, 26 of 130 patients (20%) with overt GCSE in whom an electroencephalogram had been started within 30 minutes of the onset of treatment continued to exhibit ictal activity on the electroencephalogram, even though all convulsive activity had stopped (25). If only clinical criteria had been used, treatment in these patients would have been considered successful.

Relevant considerations for determination of sample size in status studies, similar to those presented by Pocock (26) for all clinical trials, are listed in Table 2. The most important issue is to determine what difference in

TABLE 2. *Considerations relevant to the determination of sample size in a controlled clinical trial of treatment modalities*

What is the purpose of the trial?
What is the principal outcome measure?
How will the data be analyzed to detect a treatment difference?
What results would be expected with standard treatment?
How small a treatment difference is it important to detect, and with what degree of certainty?

From Leppik et al., ref. 10.

efficacy is clinically relevant. For a life-threatening disorder such as GCSE, most clinicians would agree that a 10% improvement in the success rate would be clinically meaningful. Such trials should be conducted with substantial power, so that the probability of finding such a difference, if it exists, is high.

Informed Consent

The problem of informed consent in emergency treatment research has not yet been fully resolved. A number of issues make informed consent in emergency treatment protocols problematic: (a) The patient's mental status may be impaired, as certainly will be the case in study of GCSE; (b) an acceptable proxy may not be available at the time the emergency treatment must be rendered; (c) truly informed and freely given consent may not be possible under the duress of a serious medical emergency, even if a proxy is available; (d) research is an ongoing process. It involves more than the immediate administration of a therapeutic intervention. In most protocols, the research continues after the acute treatment phase. If a waived consent procedure has been utilized, as was the case in the VACSP Study No. 265, then it is essential to obtain permission to collect research data from the patient or the patient's proxy after emergency care has been rendered. The VA cooperative study was conducted with a waiver of the requirement for consent before randomization. The request for waiver of the consent requirement was accepted by the institutional review board at each of the participating hospitals. The rationale for the waiver was that each of the four treatments being compared was considered by some American physicians to be the best treatment for the initial management of GCSE and no published data demonstrated one of the treatments to be superior to any other. Therefore, the four study treatments were thought to be the best available. The patient was presumed to wish to be treated with one of the best treatments available. Thus, permission to assign the patient randomly to one of these four "best treatments" was waived, but consent was required for the continued collection of research data once the initial treatment had been rendered. In my opinion, this is an appropriate consent mechanism for maintaining patients rights while at the same time facilitating emergency treatment research. However, the waived consent approach is acceptable only if the available data suggest that the treatments being compared are the best available. If a new and still experimental drug for the treatment of SE is to be studied, there is no ethical basis for waiving the requirement for consent. Under such circumstances, consent from a surrogate will be essential before treatment is initiated.

Practical Considerations

A number of practical and logistical issues are likely to influence the success of a clinical trial in SE. These considerations include (a) selection of sites and investigators, (b) patient recruitment, and (c) procedures for drug preparation and blinding of the study. Site selection is crucial. SE does not occur very frequently, even in the busiest emergency rooms and hospitals. There tends to be an inverse relationship between the frequency of status at a specific site and the feasibility of conducting clinical research. Thus, in general, sites with the most cases are the most chaotic. When a site is being considered for inclusion, the frequency of cases of SE should be documented in a prospective manner, and the feasibility of conducting a prospectively randomized, blinded protocol in that clinical environment should be critically assessed. The probability of successfully conducting emergency treatment research also depends on the quality of the site investigators. SE is an emergency that must be treated immediately, and it is not possible to predict when cases of SE will occur. Therefore, the site investigator must be committed to enrolling SE cases when and where they occur. Such a commitment requires a strong and passionate desire to conduct clinical trials research and particularly to recruit for an SE treatment protocol. In general, successful investigators in a status protocol are young, passionate, idealistic, and personally committed to the success of the protocol. To ensure such a commitment, investigators need to be made to feel that they have a personal investment in the success of the clinical trial, that there will be substantial academic credit to be gained, and that participation in the trial is, despite the associated hardships, something of value in which pride can be taken. If investigators have other priorities, they are unlikely to succeed as investigators in clinical trials.

Patient recruitment is best accomplished by organizing an SE treatment team that consists of the site investigator as the physician head of the team, a study coordinator, and an electroencephalographic technician. Such a team can be publicized as being comparable to the cardiopulmonary arrest team that exists in most hospitals. If the status team is perceived as being helpful and offering something of value, the team will be called. If the team is perceived as unhelpful or unduly demanding, the team will not be called and recruitment will suffer. Sometimes, it is effective to offer the contact physician a material award, perhaps in the form of a book credit of cash payment, for every eligible patient for whom this team is called.

A critical element in the design of a blinded clinical trial of SE is drug preparation. In the VACSP Study No. 265 (1), patients were randomly assigned to one of four different drug regimens in a blinded fashion. This was possible because of the development of drug treatment kits that allowed administration of all drugs at the same solution volume and rate of administration. Phenytoin, phenobarbital, and diazepam were packaged in identical vials at appropriate concentrations so that each of the drugs could be administered at 1 mL/min to produce the maximal rates of drug infusion specified in the study. Lorazepam was administered via Tubex injection at a maximal rate of 0.5 mL/min.

Identical-appearing drug treatment kits were prepared for each patient, with each kit containing a first, second, and third treatment box. The first treatment box consisted of one Tubex and five vials, labeled A through E. A nomogram, based on the patient's weight, was used to determine the volume of solution administered from the Tubex and each vial to produce the desired dose without compromising the blind. The Tubex solution and the solution from vial A were injected simultaneously so that treatment always began with active drug. Active drugs in the second and third boxes of a treatment kit were determined by the identity of the active drug(s) in the first box. The treatment team was blinded to the identity of these drugs to maintain the blind for the first treatment.

CONCLUSION

Clinical trials for the management of SE represent a significant challenge because of the necessity of providing emergency treatment that is rapidly effective. Clearly there is a need for better drugs to stop seizure activity during SE and protect neurons from status-induced damage. New antiepileptic drugs need to be evaluated for possible use in the management of SE as they become available. However, it may be that rational polypharmacy, with drugs having different mechanisms of action administered in an optimal order, will be the most effective approach to treatment.

SE protocols require rigorous designs that ensure proper control and blinding of treatment assignment, careful attention to the development of unambiguous operational definitions, and attention to the ethical issues revolving around informed consent. However, a number of practical and logistical considerations also contribute to the success or failure of a specific protocol. A passionate commitment to the protocol on the part of a young and ambitious investigator will do a great deal to ensure the success of the protocol.

REFERENCES

1. Treiman DM, Meyers PD, Walton NY, et al. Treatment of generalized convulsive status epilepticus: a randomized double-blind comparison of four intravenous regimens. *N Engl J Med* (*submitted*).
2. Theodore WH, Porter RJ, Albert P, et al. The secondarily generalized tonic-clonic seizure: a videotape analysis. *Neurology* 1994;44:1403–1407.
3. Celesia GG. Modern concepts of status epilepticus. *JAMA* 1976;235:1571–1574.
4. Treiman DM. Generalized convulsive status epilepticus in the adult. *Epilepsia* 1993;34(Suppl 1):S2–S11.
5. Treiman DM, Delgado-Escueta AV. Status epilepticus. In: Thompson RA, Green JR, eds. *Critical Care of Neurological and Neurosurgical Emergencies*. New York: Raven Press; 1980:53–99.
6. Commission on Classification and Terminology of the International League Against Epilepsy. Proposal for revised clinical and electroencephalographic classification of epileptic seizures. *Epilepsia* 1981;22:489–501.
7. Hauser WA. Status epilepticus: epidemiologic considerations. *Neurology* 1990;40(Suppl 2):9–13.
8. DeLorenzo RJ, Pellock JM, Towne AR, Boggs JG. Epidemiology of status epilepticus. *J Clin Neurophysiol* 1995;12:316–325.
9. Treiman DM, DeGiorgio CM, Ben-Menachem E, et al. Lorazepam vs. phenytoin in the treatment of generalized convulsive status epilepticus. Report of an ongoing study. *Neurology* 1985;35(Suppl 1):284.
10. Leppik IE, Derivan AT, Homan RW, Walker J, Ramsay RE, Patrick B. Double-blind study of lorazepam and diazepam in status epilepticus. *JAMA* 1983;249: 1452–1454.
11. Shaner DM, McCurdy SA, Herring MO, Gabor AJ. Treatment of status epilepticus: a prospective comparison of diazepam and phenytoin versus phenobarbital and optional phenytoin. *Neurology* 1988;38:202–207.
12. Walton NY, Treiman DM. Experimental secondarily generalized convulsive status epilepticus induced by D,L-homocysteine thiolactone. *Epilepsy Res* 1988;2:79–86.
13. Walton NY, Gunawan S, Treiman DM. Treatment of experimental status epilepticus with the GABA uptake inhibitor tiagabine. *Epilepsy Res* 1994;19:237–244.
14. Walton NY, Jaing QB, Hyun B, Treiman DM. Lamotrigine vs. phenytoin for treatment of status epilepticus: comparison in an experimental model. *Epilepsy Res* 1996;24:19–28.
15. Walton NY, Treiman DM. Efficacy of ACC-9653 (a phenytoin prodrug) in experimental status epilepticus in the rat. *Epilepsy Res* 1990;5:165–168.
16. Walton NY, Treiman DM. Motor and electroencephalographic response of refractory experimental status epilepticus in rats to treatment with MK-801, diazepam, or MK-801 plus diazepam. *Brain Res* 1991;553:97–104.
17. Walton NY, Treiman DM. Valproic acid treatment of experimental status epilepticus. *Epilepsy Res* 1992;12: 199–205.
18. Walton NY, Treiman DM. Efficacy of a new NMDA receptor antagonist in treatment of experimental status epilepticus. *Epilepsia* 1993;34(6):52.
19. Walton NY, Treiman DM. Remacemide versus phenytoin for treatment of experimental status epilepticus. *Epilepsia* 1996;37(Suppl 5):212.
20. Walton NY, Treiman DM. Rational polytherapy in the treatment of status epilepticus. *Epilepsy Res Suppl* 1996;11:123–139 (Leppik IE, Homan RW, eds; *Rational Polypharmacy*).
21. Walton NY, Treiman DM. Rational polypharmacy in the treatment of experimental status epilepticus produces increased efficacy with decreased side effects. *Neurology* 1994;44(Suppl 2):A117.
22. Kapur J, Coulter DA. Experimental status epilepticus alters gamma-aminobutyric acid type A receptor function in CA1 pyramidal neurons. *Ann Neurol* 1995;38: 893–900.
23. Kapur J, Lothman EW, DeLorenzo RJ. Loss of $GABA_A$ receptors during partial status epilepticus. *Neurology* 1994;44:2407–2408.
24. Kapur J, Lothman EW. NMDA receptor activation mediates the loss of GABAergic inhibition induced by recurrent seizures. *Epilepsy Res* 1990;5:103–111.
25. Craven W, Faught E, Kuzniecky R, et al. Residual electrographic status epilepticus after control of overt clinical seizures. *Epilepsia* 1995;36(Suppl 4):46.
26. Pocock SJ. *Clinical Trials. A Practical Approach.* Chichester: John Wiley & Sons; 1983. 266 p.

Antiepileptic Drug Development.
Advances in Neurology, Vol. 76,
edited by J. French, I. Leppik, and M. A. Dichter.
Lippincott–Raven Publishers, Philadelphia © 1998.

18

Clinical Trials for Seizure Prevention

Nancy R. Temkin, Sureyya S. Dikmen, and H. Richard Winn

Departments of Neurological Surgery and Biostatistics,
Departments of Neurological Surgery, Rehabilitation Medicine, Psychiatry, and Behavioral Sciences,
and Department of Neurological Surgery, University of Washington, Seattle, Washington 98104.

INTRODUCTION

Epilepsy is a common neurologic condition, and much effort has been devoted to stopping seizures or limiting their impact. One might argue that preventing the seizure disorder from ever occurring is an optimal way to treat or control epilepsy. In contrast to most of the chapters in this book, this chapter deals with trials aimed at that goal—that is, trials for people who do not have epilepsy but are at high risk for acquiring it. We first discuss some of the differences between prevention trials and the more common treatment trials. Second, we provide some background information on posttraumatic seizures, the type of unprovoked seizures most studied in prevention trials, and describe some of the trials that have been performed in an attempt to prevent them. Third, we briefly discuss other conditions in which seizure prophylaxis may be used. Finally, design issues for prophylaxis trials are reviewed.

PROPHYLAXIS TRIALS COMPARED WITH TREATMENT TRIALS

Participants in prophylaxis trials have not had seizures but are at some risk for acquiring them. The probability for seizure development may be quite remote. Of patients considered at high risk for posttraumatic seizures, more than three fourths remain free of epilepsy without any prophylactic treatment. Participants in treatment trials, on the other hand, are having seizures, usually often enough for them to be a problem. This leads to differences in motivation, compliance, and willingness to tolerate side effects.

Prevention trials generally must last much longer than treatment trials—posttraumatic seizure trials frequently continue for 2 years, rather than the several months generally required for outpatient treatment trials, or even the few days for inpatient trials when other treatments for seizures have been withdrawn. Despite the long observation time for prevention trials, the typical endpoint is the time to first seizure; in treatment trials, it is usually the seizure count in some time period or the time to the fourth or later seizure. Furthermore, uncertainty about whether or not a reported event is a seizure is much higher in prevention trials. In a treatment trial, the patient or companion can describe the typical seizures the patient has experienced and video-electroencephalographic monitoring may be performed in some studies. For a prevention trial, any unusual behavior or feeling is a possible seizure manifestation—and the endpoint is typically the time to the first occurrence. To our knowledge, no prevention trial has asked patients to wear electroencephalographic monitors for years to obtain confirmation that a reported event was truly a seizure. All have relied on the judgment of an experienced neurologist, with information coming from patients' or witnesses' reports of the event, and sometimes a short-term electroencephalogram. Blinding is vital in prevention studies, because there is much room for subjectivity.

Differences in the study populations are also relevant. In treatment trials, the investigators often know the eligible patients and can be somewhat selective in whom they encourage to participate. In posttraumatic seizures trials, except for the minimal inclusion/exclusion criteria pertaining to the severity of injury, little is known about potential subjects. Frequently, patients are comatose. As prompt treatment may be necessary to interrupt the process of epileptogenesis, protocols often require treatment within 24 hours of injury. If relatives or friends can be found within that time window, they are usually so distraught that they can give little coherent information about the patient, especially information relevant to a clinical trial, such as the likelihood of compliance.

Given the difficulties associated with prevention trials, an important question is whether they are worth performing. To us, the answer is clearly yes. At least 15% of epilepsy is potentially preventable by pharmacologic prophylaxis (1). This would include epilepsy attributable to cerebrovascular and infectious causes as well as traumatic brain injury. In epidemiologic studies, this remote symptomatic epilepsy tends to be more intractable than idiopathic epilepsy (2). Once seizures develop, they often require lifelong treatment and create emotional, social, and economic burdens for the patient and for society at large. Thus, it is worth much effort to find an effective prevention regimen with few adverse side effects so that this burden can be avoided.

POSTTRAUMATIC SEIZURES

Most of the work done to date concerning the prevention of epileptic seizures has focused on posttraumatic seizures. Posttraumatic seizures are classified according to their time of onset. Early seizures, which are those that occur during the first week, are usually considered provoked seizures, like febrile seizures or alcohol withdrawal seizures. They are often subdivided into immediate seizures and delayed early seizures. Immediate seizures occur within the first hours of injury and generally before a prevention regimen can be instituted. Delayed early seizures take place between 2 and 7 days after injury and are amenable to prevention. Late seizures, occurring after 7 days, are considered unprovoked or epileptic seizures, and a person who has had two or more is usually considered to have epilepsy.

Epidemiology

Late posttraumatic seizures—a more accurate term than posttraumatic epilepsy, as most of the epidemiologic and prevention studies have used the occurrence of at least one late, unprovoked posttraumatic seizure as the endpoint—affect about 2% of patients receiving any medical attention for a head injury (3) and about 5% of people hospitalized with a head injury (4). Annually, this results in about 20,000 new cases of posttraumatic seizures in the United States (4,5). As shown in Table 1, all head injuries are not equally likely to be followed by posttraumatic seizures. Penetrating head injuries received in combat are associated with the highest rate of posttraumatic seizures—about 50% (6). Early seizures are not far behind, and hematoma, contusions, and depressed fractures are all associated with a seizure risk of at least 25% (7). Linear fractures carry much less risk, and those with a mild injury have a still elevated, but much smaller, risk of late posttraumatic seizures (4,8).

The timing of late posttraumatic seizures is not uniform. About a quarter of people in whom late posttraumatic seizures ultimately develop have their first seizure by 3 months after injury, half by 1 year, and three fourths by 3 years (4). Posttraumatic seizures may still make their first appearance up to at least 15 years after war injuries (6). In terms of clinical trials, there clearly are diminishing returns with very long observation periods, but

TABLE 1. *Factors associated with late posttraumatic seizures*[a]

	Incidence of late post-traumatic seizures, %
Penetrating missile wound (6)	53
Early seizure	47
Intracerebral hematoma	40
Subdural hematoma	33
Glasgow Coma Scale score ≤10	32
Depressed skull fracture	31
Cortical contusion	28
Epidural hematoma	26
Linear fracture (8)	5
Mild concussion (4)	<1

Reprinted with permission from from Temkin et al., ref. 7.
[a]Data from the authors' series of 323 cases followed at least 8 days unless indicated otherwise.

trials based on a few weeks or a few months of observation after injury would not capture most of the cases.

Results of Prevention Studies Following Traumatic Brain Injury

At least six observational studies and 11 clinical trials have been performed to assess the effect of antiepileptic drugs on the development of posttraumatic seizures. The most frequently evaluated drugs are phenytoin (Dilantin) and phenobarbital. Results of the observational studies look very favorable (Table 2). Wohns and Wyler (9) and Young et al. (10) used phenytoin and reported an 80% decrease in seizures and a low seizure rate (but no specific control series), respectively. Servit and Musil (11) used phenytoin and phenobarbital and reported a 92% decrease in seizures. Murri et al. (12,13) used phenobarbital in their two studies, and Price (14) used valproate. Seizure rates were very low in all three despite enrollment of high-risk cases. All these observational studies showed substantial reduction in seizures in comparison with nonrandomized controls or historical experience.

Well-controlled studies have demonstrated much less impressive results. As shown in Table 3, three studies in which phenytoin was used reported early seizure findings. The studies of Young et al. (15,16) showed similar low rates on phenytoin and placebo, whereas

TABLE 2. *Summary of observational studies of prophylaxis of posttraumatic seizures*

Investigator (location)	Active treatment	Patients, No.	Length of treatment/ follow-up, mo	Seizure rates: Treated, %	Seizure rates: Untreated, %
Servitt and Musil (Prague, Czechoslovakia)	Low-dose PB/PHT	168	30 mo/8–13 y	2.1[a]	25[a]
Wohns and Wyler (Seattle, WA)	Ther PHT	62	12/6–72	10[a]	50[a]
Young ot al. (Lexington, KY)	Ther PHT	84	12/12	6[a]	2–31[a]
Murri et al. (Pisa, Italy)	Low- and high-dose PB	83	24/24	2	
Murri et al. (Pisa, Italy)	Ther PB	390	12/12	2	7–16
Price (Wakefield, UK)	VPA	143	NA/24	0	15–55

PHT, phenytoin; PB, phenobarbital; VPA, valproate; Ther, therapeutic levels; NA, not available.
[a]Rate for late seizures only.

TABLE 3. *Summary of well-controlled studies of prophylaxis of posttraumatic seizures*

				Seizure rates					
				Early			Late		
Investigator (location)	Active treatment	Patients, No.	Length of treatment/ follow-up, mo	Active, %	Placebo, %	p	Active, %	Placebo, %	p
Hoff and Hoff/Birkmayer (Germany)	Low-dose PHT	100	4 y/>4 y				6[a]	51[a]	τ
Brackett et al. (Kansas City, KS)	Low-dose PB/PHT	125	18/36				23[a]	13[a]	NS
Brackett et al. (Kansas City, KS)	Ther PB/PHT	49	6/18				14[a]	39[a]	0.09
McQueen et al. (Edinburgh, New Castle, UK)	Ther PHT	164	12/24				10	9	NS
Marshall et al. (San Diego, CA)	Ther PB/PHT	154	6/18				24[a]	16[a]	τ
Locke et al. (Los Angeles, CA)	Ther PB, PHT, PB/PHT	303	6/18				4[a]	12[a]	τ
Young et al. (Lexington, KY)	Ther PHT	244	18/18	4	4	NS	12	11	NS
Temkin et al. (Seattle, WA)	Ther PHT	404	12/24	4	14	.001	27	21	NS
Glötzner et al. (Wurzburg, Germany)	Ther CBZ	139	24/24	10	25	.016	27	33	NS
Manaka (Tokyo, Japan)	Ther PB	126	24/60				16	11	NS
Pechadre et al. (Clermont-Ferrand, France)	Ther PHT	86	3–12/24	6	24	.05	6	42	.001

Adapted and reprinted with permission from Temkin et al., refs. 7 and 25.
τ, significance test accounting for loss to follow-up not available; PHT, phenytoin; PB, phenobarbital; CBZ, carbamazepine; Ther, therapeutic levels; NS, not significant.
[a]Rate for early and late seizures combined.

the studies of Temkin et al. (17) and Pechadre et al. (18) showed reductions in early seizures that were both clinically and statistically significant. However, these early seizures were provoked, rather than epileptic, seizures. When late (i.e., epileptic) seizures were considered, three of the six phenytoin studies showed slightly higher seizure rates with phenytoin than with placebo. The results of the other three studies were more favorable, but all had substantial problems. Locke has not, to our knowledge, reported late seizures separately. Thus, the reduction in seizures overall may reflect just a reduction in early seizures. This study also had a low follow-up rate, so any late findings would be based on a small number of cases. The studies of Hoff and Hoff (19), Birkmayer (20), and Pechadre et al. (18) perhaps should have been discussed with the observational studies. They used no treatment control and no blinding. Pechadre et al. used alternate-day assignment, and Hoff and Hoff did not specify the treatment-assignment mechanism. In these cases, the controls were concurrent and from the same population, so the studies are included here. However, with the difficulties alluded to earlier about seizure identification in prevention trials, one should be quite skeptical of results from unblinded studies, such as those of Pechadre et al. (18), Hoff and Hoff (19), and Birkmayer (20).

All these studies had substantial rates of noncompliance and protocol violation. A concern is that the largely negative results for phenytoin in the prevention of epileptic sei-

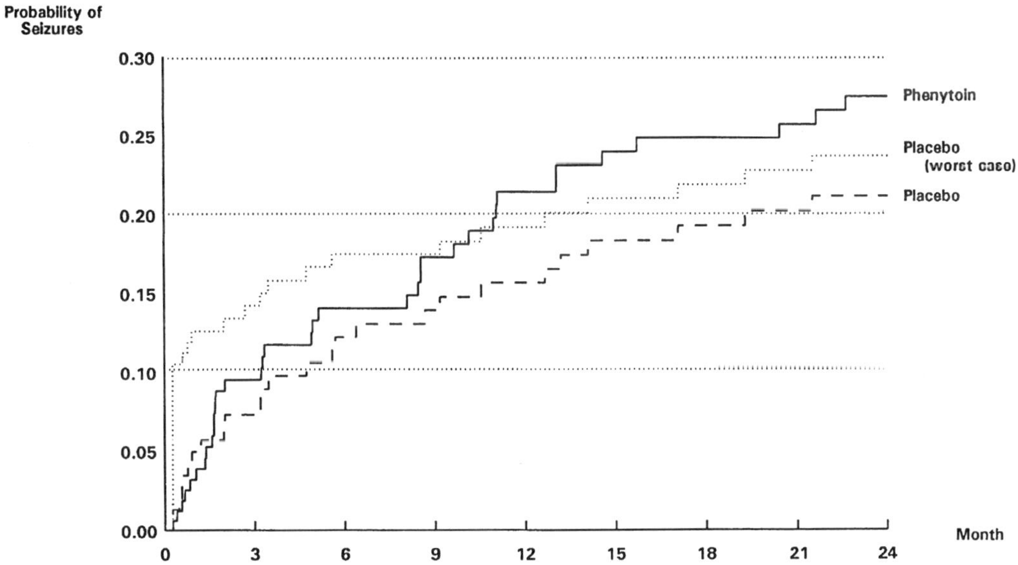

	Subjects At Risk									Total Seizures
Phenytoin	170	123	108	101	95	88	86	85	74	36
Placebo	153	113	106	100	94	90	87	86	77	26
Placebo (worst case)	153	107	101	98	92	88	85	84	74	32

FIG. 1. Cumulative fraction of patients with late seizures (on or after day 8) for patients assigned to phenytoin and placebo, analyzed as intent-to-treat, and for placebo-assigned patients, analyzed as if all patients given phenytoin had had a seizure on day 8. Even compared with this worst-case scenario for the placebo group, the phenytoin-assigned group had a higher cumulative seizure rate by 12 months. (Reprinted with permission from Temkin NR et al., ref. 17. Copyright 1990, Massachusetts Medical Society. All rights reserved. Adapted.)

zures were caused not by an ineffective drug but by studies that were so weakened that they could not detect whether the drug was effective. This is a very valid concern. These studies depend on the patients for compliance and on the patients and nonstudy medical personnel for protocol adherence. Primary analyses for these studies have been on an "intent-to-treat" basis, so noncompliance and protocol violations can seriously weaken the ability of a study to detect an effective drug. In our study, two major problems that might have masked a positive effect of phenytoin are (a) the treatment with phenytoin of patients assigned to placebo who had early seizures and (b) subtherapeutic blood levels of drug, whether caused by noncompliance or by the changes in metabolism that frequently occur following a serious head injury. Despite the protocol specifying that early seizures should be stopped, if necessary, with short-acting drugs such as valium or lorazepam, almost all patients who had early seizures were removed from the treatment protocol by the physicians in charge of their clinical care and were treated clinically with phenytoin. Thus, >10% of the placebo-assigned cases were treated with active drug. To assess the possible effect of this protocol violation, we assumed that each phenytoin-treated, placebo-assigned patient had a late seizure on day 8, the first possible time. As seen in Fig. 1, this causes the seizure rate on placebo in this worst-case scenario to be very high early on. However, by 12 months the cumulative seizure rate on phenytoin was even higher than in this worst-case representation.

Controlling for subtherapeutic levels is more difficult. Levels were measured three times a week for the first week, weekly during the acute hospitalization, and at 1, 3, 6, 9, and 12 months after injury, in addition to being measured after a seizure, a change in drug dosage, or an adverse event. Doses were adjusted after each assessment of phenytoin level, with the goal of keeping the level in the high therapeutic range. Levels were at least therapeutic in >75% of cases on blinded drug at each scheduled assessment time except at 1 week, when changes in metabolism were particularly rapid. Despite this, most patients did not have therapeutic levels at every assessment. To get some idea of the effect of phenytoin in those who seemed to be adequately treated, we performed a supplementary analysis that removed patients from observation as soon as they had a subtherapeutic level (defined as a free level of serum phenytoin of <0.75 mg/L) or if they were known to have stopped taking the drug. As shown in Fig. 2, the cases with continuous therapeutic levels had late seizure experience very similar to the entire group analyzed as intention-to-treat. Thus, in our study at least, it does not appear that protocol violations or subtherapeutic phenytoin levels caused the negative results for late seizures.

Other drugs have not fared much better than phenytoin in randomized trials (Table 3). Most investigators have not presented late seizures separately. The low-dose study of Brackett et al. (21) and the study of Marshall et al. stopped with a higher seizure rate on the combined phenobarbital/phenytoin arm. This is especially disappointing because the rates include early as well as late seizures, and the studies using phenytoin alone have shown that phenytoin is effective against early seizures. Early results from the study of Brackett et al. using therapeutic doses of phenobarbital and phenytoin looked promising, but the study was stopped because of a low accession rate. Early results from the phenobarbital and phenobarbital/phenytoin study arms of Locke et al. were favorable, but they were affected by the same problems as the phenytoin arm of the study—a low follow-up rate and no separation of results on early and late seizures. The studies of Locke and Marshall and the therapeutic dose study of Brackett were stopped prematurely for administrative reasons—either low accession or insufficient follow-up. The study of Glötzner et al. (22) using carbamazepine found a significant reduction in early seizures but no effect on late, epileptic seizures. These results with carbamazepine are very similar to our results with phenytoin.

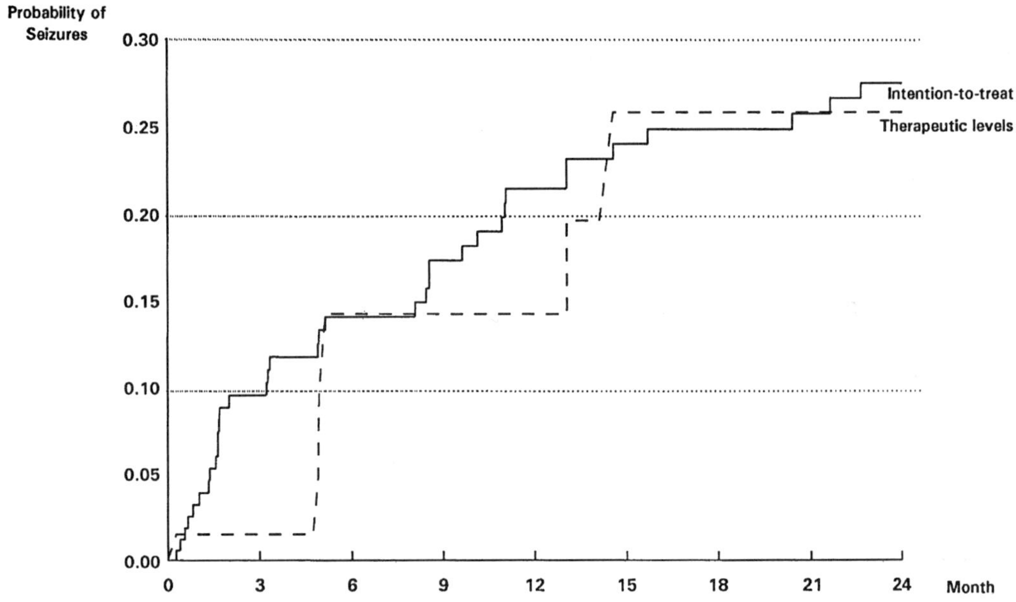

Subjects At Risk										Total Seizures
Phenytoin Intention-to-treat	170	123	108	101	95	88	86	85	74	36
Phenytoin Therapeutic levels	71	23	18	17	16	12	12	12	9	6

FIG. 2. Cumulative fraction of patients with late seizures (on or after day 8) for patients assigned to phenytoin, analyzed as intent-to-treat, and for patients excluded when they had a subtherapeutic phenytoin level or when they stopped taking drug before the end of the 1-year treatment period. The seizure rates are very similar for all phenytoin-assigned patients and for those with therapeutic levels of phenytoin. (Reprinted with permission from Temkin NR et al., ref. 17. Copyright 1990, Massachusetts Medical Society. All rights reserved. Adapted.)

POSTCRANIOTOMY SEIZURES

The two randomized antiepileptic drug trials for prevention of unprovoked seizures that involve other populations were both performed in patients having a craniotomy (23,24). Results of both studies reinforce those of the posttraumatic seizure trials. Although North et al. (23) reported that prophylaxis with phenytoin was effective until about 70 days, a careful look at the results indicates that all the benefit was in the first week, and it took until 70 days for the late seizures on phenytoin to overcome the early advantage. The results of Foy et al. (24) with carbamazepine and phenytoin also show no significant effect. An interesting aspect of the Foy study is that drug administration began 24 hours prior to the surgery, so the drug levels should have been therapeutic by the time of the craniotomy.

CURRENT STATUS OF PROPHYLAXIS

Based on the evidence from well-controlled trials, we do not have any drugs that have been shown to prevent epileptogenesis, that is, the process whereby a normal brain turns into one that generates unprovoked seizures. Most of the newer drugs have not been tried for prophylaxis in humans. Several studies are planned or under way. Our group at the University of Washington has an ongoing study evaluating valproate for preventing posttraumatic seizures. Parke-Davis has a study evaluating phosphenytoin to prevent early seizures after stroke and may extend it to evaluate late seizures as well (E. Garofolo, *personal communication*). A study to evaluate vitamin E in the prevention of posttraumatic seizures is in the planning stage (A. Salazar, *personal communication*). Until these or other trials demonstrate some regimen to be effective, the use of long-term prophylaxis against late seizures is not justified by scientifically rigorous evidence. For such evidence to be obtained, additional trials are likely to be needed.

CONSIDERATION OF DESIGN FOR PROPHYLAXIS TRIALS

When prevention trials are being planned, some design issues to consider include the condition and patient population, outcome measures, when to start treatment, duration of treatment, duration of follow-up, and sample size. All these may have an impact on the power of the trial, and many possible combinations can yield the desired power.

Patient Population

The condition most often studied has been traumatic brain injury. Strokes and aneurysm repairs also are sometimes followed by epilepsy, and it may be appropriate to consider some patients with these conditions for seizure prophylaxis. Patients with brain tumors may be another population to consider. Craniotomy for a variety of reasons has also been studied. Combining seizure types in treatment studies is discussed by Drs. French (Chapter 10) and Pellock (Chapter 16). Many of the points they make apply to combining conditions for prevention trials. Within these general conditions, there are subgroups with different seizure risks. A high-risk group is usually preferred for prophylaxis trials for two reasons: It allows a smaller sample size (as discussed later), and if the seizure risk is too low, one has to question whether prophylaxis is worthwhile. For example, in our studies, we have tried to include only head injuries associated with at least a 20% chance of seizures. In our first trial, we included the first eight factors shown in Table 1 as inclusion criteria (17). Because in the phenytoin trial the seizure rate was <5% for those with a low Glasgow Coma Scale score but no other inclusion criteria, we have removed a low Glasgow Coma Scale score as a basis for entry into the valproate study. Even though a low Glasgow Coma Scale score or linear fracture is accompanied by a seizure rate much higher than that expected in the general population, maybe even 100 times the expected rate, we do not feel it is worth treating >19 people in whom seizures would not develop anyway based on the possibility of preventing them from occurring in one person. Antiepileptic drugs are not free of medical and neurobehavioral side effects and financial costs. In choosing a population for a trial, as in deciding on a clinical treatment for a patient, careful consideration of whether benefits are likely to outweigh costs is necessary.

Outcome Measures

Conceptually, the outcome of interest in prevention trials is whether the treatment prevents the epileptogenic process from evolving to a point where spontaneous seizures occur. Operationally, whether a late posttraumatic seizure occurs during the follow-up period and time to the first unprovoked seizure are the endpoints that have been used. The latter allows investigators to account for patients who have been lost to follow-up more reasonably by using survival analysis methods. Because a drug that suppresses seizures but does not influence the epileptogenic process will produce a low seizure rate during the period of active treatment but not influence the rate after treatment has been stopped, analyses need to account for this possibility. Comparison of the estimated cumulative seizure rates at fixed times provides some insight. A difference at the end of active treatment that narrows considerably or disappears after a period of no treatment (when suppressed seizures can become overt) suggests a treatment that suppresses seizures without altering the process; a difference that remains despite a substantial period of no treatment suggests that the epileptogenic process has been affected. It should be noted that methods such as the Cox proportional hazard model, which assumes a constant treatment effect over time, might give misleading results for a treatment that suppresses seizures without altering the underlying process.

Timing and Duration of Treatment and Follow-up

In studies, treatment has begun anywhere from within 24 hours (most commonly) to 1 month after injury. Duration of prophylactic treatment has ranged from a month to 4 years, with follow-up from 18 months to >5 years. Very little seems to be known about the process of epileptogenesis, including when it starts and how long it is amenable to interruption. The trend has been toward starting treatment more quickly. In some situations, such as planned aneurysm repair or craniotomy, prophylaxis can begin before the surgery. With conditions such as head trauma or stroke, it is not possible to have the drug on board before the insult occurs.

With respect to treatment duration, extending the length of treatment increases the cost, the chance of side effects, the rate of loss to follow-up, and the likelihood of noncompliance, but it may also increase the chance of successful prophylaxis. Most of the decisions here have been more in the realm of art than science. More recently, shorter treatment periods have come into fashion. Hoff and Hoff, in a study first reported in 1947, treated for 4 years (19). Our phenytoin study treated for 1 year (17). Based on the recommendations from a workshop on prophylaxis of posttraumatic seizures sponsored by the National Institutes of Health in 1990, our current study with valproate evaluates 1 and 6 months of treatment.

Duration of follow-up needs to extend beyond the period of treatment if one hopes to determine whether the treatment has influenced the epileptogenic process rather than merely prevented seizures while being taken. The true indication of success for prophylaxis is that the patients have no seizures despite having stopped taking the drug. A fairly prolonged period off treatment may be needed to differentiate suppression from interruption of the epileptogenic process, as seizures may be relatively rare. Annegers et al. (2) found 56% of people had a second seizure within a year of their first remote symptomatic seizure and 77% had another within 5 years. Duration of follow-up also needs to be considered in designing prevention trials because it influences the observed seizure rate. As just over half of people in whom late seizures develop following traumatic brain injury have their first seizure during the year after injury (4), a study with a 12-month follow-up will see a seizure rate only about half that seen in a study with a 10-year follow-up.

Sample Size

The observed seizure rate is a major determinant of the needed sample size. If the seizure rate is 25% on the control regimen and decreases by half in the treatment group, a sample size of 384 will give 80% power to detect such a difference. If the control rate is only 10%, the power is only 43% with that sample size. A sample size of 1094 would be needed to detect a halving of the seizure rate from 10% to 5%.

All the design elements discussed need to be considered together when a trial for prevention is planned. For example, if the population chosen for study has a very high risk for development of seizures, adequate detection of an effective treatment may be possible with a shorter follow-up time or smaller sample size. On the other hand, a large sample size may compensate for lower-risk patients, a shorter follow-up period, or lower drug effectiveness resulting from a short treatment period.

CONCLUSION

Although clinical trials for seizure prevention differ in many respects from trials that develop treatments to control epilepsy, they share a common goal—reducing the number of people whose lives are made more difficult by seizures. As no treatments have yet been shown to be effective in preventing the development of epileptic seizures, additional trials are likely to be necessary.

ACKNOWLEDGMENT

This work was supported in part by grant R01-NS19643 from the National Institutes of Health, National Institute of Neurologic Disorders and Stroke.

REFERENCES

1. Hauser WA, Annegers JF, Kurland LT. Incidence of epilepsy and unprovoked seizures in Rochester, Minnesota: 1935–1984. *Epilepsia* 1993;34:453–468.
2. Annegers JF, Shirts SB, Hauser WA, Kurland LT. Risk of recurrence after an initial unprovoked seizure. *Epilepsia* 1986;27:43–50.
3. Annegers JF, Grabow JD, Groover RV, Laws ER Jr, Elveback LR, Kurland LT. Seizures after head trauma: a population study. *Neurology* 1980;30:683–689.
4. Jennett B. *Epilepsy After Nonmissile Head Injuries*. Chicago: Year Book Medical Publishers; 1975.
5. Kraus JF. Epidemiology of head injury. In: Cooper PR, ed. *Head Injury*. Baltimore: Williams & Wilkins; 1987:1–19.
6. Salazar AM, Jabbari B, Vance SC, Grafman J, Amin D, Dillon JD. Epilepsy after penetrating head injury. I. Clinical correlates: a report of the Vietnam Head Injury Study. *Neurology* 1985;35:1406–1414.
7. Temkin NR, Haglund MM, Winn HR. Posttraumatic seizures. In: Youmans JR, ed. *Neurological Surgery*. 4th ed. Philadelphia: WB Saunders; 1996:1834–1839.
8. Jennett WB. *Epilepsy After Blunt Head Injuries*. London: William Heinemann Medical Books; 1962.
9. Wohns R, Wyler A. Prophylactic phenytoin in severe head injuries. *J Neurosurg* 1979;51:507–509.
10. Young B, Rapp R, Brooks W, Madauss W, Norton J. Posttraumatic epilepsy prophylaxis. *Epilepsia* 1979;20: 671–681.
11. Servit Z, Musil F. Prophylactic treatment of posttraumatic epilepsy: results of a long-term follow-up in Czechoslovakia. *Epilepsia* 1981;22:315–320.
12. Murri L, Parenti G, Bonuccelli U, Lenzi B, DelTacca M. Phenobarbital prophylaxis of posttraumatic epilepsy. *Ital J Neurol Sci* 1980;4:225–230.
13. Murri L, Arrigo A, Bonuccelli U, Rossi G, Parenti G. Phenobarbital in the prophylaxis of late posttraumatic seizures. *Ital J Neurol Sci* 1992;13:755–760.
14. Price D. The effiency of sodium valproate as the only anticonvulsant administered to neurosurgical patients. In: Parsonage M, Caldwell A, eds. *The Place of Sodium Valproate in the Treatment of Epilepsy*. London: The Royal Society of Medicine International Congress and Symposium Series; 1980:23–34.
15. Young B, Rapp RP, Norton JA, Haack D, Tibbs PA, Bean JR. Failure of prophylactically administered phenytoin to prevent early posttraumatic seizures. *J Neurosurg* 1983; 58:231–235.
16. Young B, Rapp RP, Norton JA, Haack D, Tibbs PA, Bean JR. Failure of prophylactically administered phenytoin to prevent late posttraumatic seizures. *J Neurosurg* 1983;58:236–241.
17. Temkin NR, Dikmen SS, Wilensky AJ, Keihm J, Chabal S, Winn HR. A randomized double-blind study of phenytoin for the prevention of posttraumatic seizures. *N Engl J Med* 1990;323:497–502.
18. Pechadre JC, Lauxerois M, Colnet G, et al. Prévention de l'épilepsie posttraumatique tardive par phénytoine dans les traumatismes craniens graves: suivi durant 2 ans. *Presse Med* 1991;20:841–845.
19. Hoff H, Hoff H. Fortschritte in der Behandlung der Epilepsie. *Monatsschr Psychiatr Neurol* 1947;114: 105–118.
20. Birkmayer W. Die Behandlung der tramatischen Epilepsie. *Wein Klin Wochenschr* 1951;63:603–609.
21. Penry JK, White BG, Brackett CE. A controlled prospective study of the pharmacologic prophylaxis of posttraumatic epilepsy. *Neurology* 1979;29:600–601.
22. Glötzner FL, Haubitz I, Miltner F, Kapp G, Pflughaupt KW. Anfallsprophylaxe mit Carbamazepin nach schweren Schadelhirnverletzungen. *Neurochirurgia (Stuttg)* 1983;26:66–79.
23. North JB, Penhall RK, Hanieh A, Frewin DB, Taylor WB. Phenytoin and postoperative epilepsy: a double-blind study. *J Neurosurg* 1983;58:672–677.
24. Foy P, Chadwick D, Rajgopalan N, Johnson A, Shaw M. Do prophylactic anticonvulsant drugs alter the pattern of seizures after craniotomy? *J Neurol Neurosurg Psychiatry* 1992;55:753–757.
25. Temkin NR, Dikmen SS, Winn HR. Posttraumatic seizures. In: Eisenberg HM, Aldrich F, eds. *Changes in Management of Head Injury*. Philadelphia: WB Saunders; 1991:425–435.

Antiepileptic Drug Development.
Advances in Neurology, Vol. 76,
edited by J. French, I. Leppik, and M. A. Dichter.
Lippincott–Raven Publishers, Philadelphia © 1998.

19

Alternate Endpoints for Seizure Measurement

Joyce A. Cramer

Departments of Neurology and Psychiatry, Yale University School of Medicine, New Haven, Connecticut 06516.

INTRODUCTION

The measurement of seizures traditionally is the primary outcome in epilepsy clinical trials. With few exceptions, the approach to seizure measurement has been a parochial dedication to quantification of the frequency of complex partial seizures. In primary generalized epilepsy, another single seizure type is selected for studies. One of the reasons that most protocols are written with a simple endpoint for seizures is the wish to provide the Food and Drug Administration with the type of data they have seen in previous trials. Innovative protocol designs can result in delays during Food and Drug Administration review of a New Drug Application (NDA). Nonetheless, with so many new antiepileptic drugs past the need for a phase III clinical trial as part of their NDA submission, it is timely to consider alternate endpoints for seizure measurement in clinical trials. It might also be appropriate for investigators to reanalyze data from completed studies using different criteria to enhance our understanding of the clinical efficacy and effectiveness of individual drugs.

The differences between phase III clinical trials and studies performed in later stages of drug development suggest the need to move beyond tests of efficacy toward assessment of effectiveness. Efficacy trials are designed to test a drug in a sample of well-defined patients so as to maximize differences in comparison with a control treatment (often a placebo). Effectiveness trials are designed to assess the overall effect of a drug in a general population, relative to actual use. Another aspect of effectiveness studies is an assessment of costs and benefits from a health service perspective, often called pharmacoeconomics. Of course, protocol design must take into consideration the issues pertinent to the type of study planned. Thus, the questions to be asked will become more sophisticated as a drug moves through development. If the developer has not initiated effectiveness studies before the drug is approved for marketing, physicians might not appreciate the usefulness of the new medication. Clinicians cannot make much use of the data reported from phase III studies, because protocol design bears little relationship to the type of problems (and patients) they see in practice. When a physician suggests a new medication to a patient, it is not feasible to present the outcome of a phase III study by stating:

"This drug was better than placebo for 12 weeks in patients with four or more complex partial seizures a month."

The patient wants to know:

"Will the new medication work for me, in my situation, with my type of seizures?"

The similarities in efficacy among most of the new antiepileptic drugs in a typical phase III trial suggest that we are missing something. Is it not likely that drugs with various mechanisms of action should have different effects on seizure propagation? Why are there no clinical trials comparing efficacy in frontal-onset versus temporal-onset complex partial seizures? How well do the new drugs work for simple partial seizures? We will not know more about the clinical effect of drugs unless more careful measurements are made of changes in seizures during treatment.

TRADITIONAL MEASURES OF SEIZURE FREQUENCY

The basic elements of recording seizure frequency include the proper classification of events and the quantification of each type of seizure (seizure counts by type) (Table 1). Inclusion of a time interval allows derivation of a "seizure rate." Another calculation presents the data as percentage of patients whose seizure count or rate decreased by 50% or 75% for an interval. This simple, dichotomous expression of change in seizure frequency is relatively insensitive and may miss important differences between treatments. The mean percentage reduction in seizures can be influenced by outliers, whereas analyses of actual seizure counts can be enhanced by transformation (e.g., log or formula). Recent studies of gabapentin were analyzed for reduction in seizure frequency from baseline as a response ratio, based on the number of seizures in 28 days of baseline (B) and treatment (T). The formula $(T - B)/(T + B)$ provided a ratio ranging from -1 to $+1$, with negative scores indicating improvement. The definition of a responder as a patient having a 50% reduction in seizures was equivalent to a response ratio of -0.33 (1).

Although becoming seizure-free is of great interest to patients, whether this happens is rarely reported after clinical trials. Some studies report the number of seizure-free days or the longest seizure-free interval during a clinical trial. Unfortunately, the sporadic recurrence of seizures minimizes the value of this information. The variability of seizure occurrence among large populations, and the fact that patients participating in phase III trials usually have frequent seizures, make it unlikely that analyses of seizure-free intervals will provide useful information. Most types of data presentation require a lengthy baseline observation period to ascertain a seizure history before the treatment is changed. This step creates two problems. First, patients are not observed untreated. Second, the observation is made at the onset of participation in a clinical trial, when many patients have fewer seizures; this phenomenon can be attributed to the Hawthorne effect, wherein any change in status (e.g., close observation and special attention) often results in improvement.

NONTRADITIONAL MEASURES OF SEIZURES AND EPILEPSY

Approaches that differ from the traditional quantification of seizures might be consid-

TABLE 1. *Traditional measures of seizure activity*[a]

	Drug A	Drug B
Seizure counts by type	100 CPS 20 GTCS	150 CPS 5 GTCS
Seizure rate by interval	4.2 CPS/mo	3.5 CPS/mo
Percentage seizure-free for interval	40% CPS 70% GTCS at 12 mo	30% CPS 55% GTCS at 12 mo
Percentage change from baseline	↓30% CPS ↓50% GTCS	↓22% CPS ↓70% GTCS
Percentage patients with *X*% seizure reduction	65% of patients >50% ↓Sz	55% of patients >50% ↓Sz
No. seizure-free days	12 d in 3 mo	18 d in 3 mo
Longest seizure-free interval	15 d in 3 mo	12 d in 3 mo

CPS, complex partial seizures; GTCS, generalized tonic-clonic seizures; Sz, seizure.

[a]Examples of a variety of traditional endpoints for comparison of two drugs in a clinical trial. Each type of measure is listed with representative scores, points, time interval, or other endpoint for two different treatments (drugs A and B).

ered surrogate endpoints, because they either do not include an account of every seizure or combine several aspects of outcome (Table 2). During planning for the Veterans Administration (VA) Epilepsy Cooperative studies, we tried to conceptualize the impact of epilepsy as an overall composite score based on seizure frequency and severity, coupled with adverse effects (2,3). The composite score differs from the global assessment typically formulated by the investigator during a clinical trial, which compares current with baseline status. The composite score was intended to serve as a representation of treatment effectiveness, not just efficacy, and a 10-point change in this score was considered clinically important (4,5).

Another way to consider overall outcome is to note how long patients continue to take the randomized treatment. Discontinuation could occur because of uncontrolled seizures, intolerable adverse effects, or both, resulting in a high risk-to-benefit ratio. Display of these data could be made as a life table of the time to discontinuation. The results of the VA Epilepsy Cooperative studies can be explained using life tables that describe the proportion of patients who were able to continue on their first medication. The figures have been widely used to demonstrate the likelihood that newly treated patients will stay on the initial medication for several years. Time on initial treatment represents patient satisfaction. The "sensibility" of composite scores or life tables is valuable to clinicians in understanding the overall impact of treatment selection for patients. Remission rates also can be determined during long-term follow-up, providing a valuable view of overall treatment outcome.

Measurement of Seizure Severity

The impact on patient well-being of the severity of seizures and their clinical manifestations (e.g., automatisms) may be equal to or greater than the total number of seizures. Although it is well-known that seizure severity can be diminished with antiepileptic drug treatment, those data are rarely reported. Examples are the reduction in severity from secondarily generalized tonic-clonic seizures to complex partial seizures, and from complex partial seizures, with altered consciousness, to simple partial seizures, with consciousness

TABLE 2. *Nontraditional measures of seizure activity*[a]

	Drug A	Drug B
Duration of treatment	No. weeks on drug (life table)	No. weeks on drug (life table)
Seizure score by type and frequency	25 points CPS 5 points GTCS Frequency score	40 points CPS 10 points GTCS Frequency score
Seizure severity scale with modulators	15 points CPS 3 points GTCS Severity score	25 points CPS 5 points GTCS Severity score
Composite score (Sz and AE)	15 points Sz 10 points AE 25 composite	25 points Sz 15 points AE 40 composite
Remission rates (percentage patients Sz-free for a period)	20% Sz-free for 12 mo	30% Sz-free for 12 mo
Seizure impact scale (patient perception)	5 points Overall score	10 points Overall score
Quality of life, patient satisfaction scale	85 points Overall score	120 points Overall score
Remission rates (percentage patients Sz-free)	20% at 12 mo	30% at 12 mo

[a]Examples of a variety of nontraditional endpoints for comparison of two drugs in a clinical trial. Each type of measure is listed with representative scores, points, time interval, or other endpoint for two different treatments (drugs A and B).

AE, adverse effects.

maintained. If the postictal period is shortened, patients can resume activities rapidly. If automatisms do not occur, the seizure may not be noticed by other people. These examples represent instances in which a patient might consider the treatment successful, even though seizures are not altogether stopped.

Several scales have been developed to assess seizure severity, both objectively (by assigning weights to various states) and subjectively (from the patient's perspective). The VA Seizure Frequency and Severity Rating (2,3) combines quantitation of the total number of each type of seizure experienced in the interval since the previous assessment, categorization of seizure frequency into a graded point system (e.g., 50 points for two generalized tonic-clonic seizures), and modification of the point score based on severity factors (e.g., 60% reduction if all seizures occurred nocturnally, allowing the patient to go to work or school during the day). The scores for simple partial, complex partial, and secondarily generalized tonic-clonic seizures can be used individually or can be combined into a summary score. The Chalfont Seizure Severity Scale (6), like the VA Rating, assigns a score to seizures based on interference with patient function (e.g., more points for a more conspicuous automatism during a complex partial seizure). This scale has been revised and is now called the National Hospital Seizure Severity Scale (NHS-3) (7). Both the VA Rating and the NHS-3 Scale utilize information gathered from the patient and witnesses, if available, during a structured interview. The Liverpool Seizure Severity Scale (8) differs from the others in that it does not include an actual accounting of the number of seizures; rather, it is based on the patient's perception of how seizures occur and an overview of the the frequency of ictal and postictal phenomena (e.g., falling, incontinence). The Liverpool Scale is completed by the patient as a self-rating. Scale scores can be used to further understanding of the action of a medication in modulating seizures in regard to factors other than frequency. It has been used in studies of lamotrigine (9).

Quality of life (QOL) assessment is another surrogate measure of treatment effectiveness. If significant improvement in QOL occurs during a new treatment, superiority over another treatment can be demonstrated, even if the total number of seizures is not changed. QOL scales can provide important information relevant to drug assessment, particularly because so few differences are seen among the new antiepileptic drugs based on seizure counts. Although QOL is usually offered as a secondary endpoint in clinical trials, it will probably attain primary status as we learn more about how to estimate sample sizes for trials and how to estimate clinically important differences.

Other Measures

During the early clinical development of a new medication, researchers often want to make a rapid assessment of the likely efficacy of the drug. Treatment with an investigational drug can be initiated during an inpatient evaluation for epilepsy surgery, when all standard medications are withdrawn to elicit seizures during monitoring (10). The new drug is started in place of the previous, standard medications as soon as the monitoring is completed. The endpoint for the trial is time (days) to the next or *N*th seizure, as defined by patient safety considerations. Although the data derived from this type of study are limited, it can be used as a screen for efficacy for partial seizures (11).

Recent studies of gabapentin used two seizure endpoints to differentiate between a "pseudo"-dose of placebo (300 mg daily) and a standard dose (3600 mg daily) as monotherapy while patients were hospitalized during a presurgical evaluation. The time-to-exit was measured as days from initiation of the study treatment to the occurrence of a specific number of seizures, presented as a life table. The percentage of patients who completed 8 days of study treatment also was presented as a life table. Both measures demonstrated the efficacy of the standard dose. In another trial (945-082), a seizure endpoint was the occurrence of twice the base rate of seizures. Both the time-to-exit and twice-base-rate endpoints represent "escape clauses" that protect patients by stopping the study according to a predefined formula that prevents undue exposure to seizures without adequate pharmacologic protection.

PITFALLS IN SEIZURE MEASUREMENT

Compliance

Partial medication compliance confounds seizure measurement in a clinical trial. Did the drug fail, or did the patient fail to take the drug (12)? Expectations of seizure control are based on the assumption that patients are taking the treatment and dose as randomized. The lower the compliance rate, the more difficult it is to find a difference between treatments (13). Reporting of medication dosing is an area rarely discussed in epilepsy studies. Total reliance is placed on patient reports, for both quantity of dosing and type and number of seizure events.

Outliers

Inclusion criteria that allow patients with a high seizure frequency to enroll can be damaging to analyses. Criteria should be established both for a minimal and maximal number of seizures. Patients whose seizures occur in clusters often have a high seizure count but long intervals between clusters. The protocol should include a plan defining a maximal length of time between seizures and a maximal number of seizures per episode in the inclusion criteria. In some instances, patients who typically have clusters of several seizures might be included with the definition that each cluster would count as a single episode (e.g., Lennox-Gastaut syndrome).

Frequent Seizures

Video-electroencephalography is useful for counting frequent episodes (too numerous to count, or TNTC). The early studies of valproic acid for absence and myoclonic seizures included a 6-hour electroencephalographic recording for quantification of spike-and-wave complexes and duration of episodes (14). In studies of Lennox-Gastaut syndrome, specific periods of each day have been established during which episodes are counted under close observation, rather than being estimated for a whole day or week (15).

Noncompleters

Patients who leave a clinical trial for non-drug-related reasons (e.g., moving to another location, lack of transportation, other medical problems) leave holes in the data. Analyses should include patients for as long as they participated, but extrapolation beyond actual data is hazardous. Effectiveness studies often follow patients for the full duration of the protocol period (e.g., 1 year) even if they discontinue treatment. Data are collected for alternate treatments and study endpoints, including seizure frequency, seizure severity, and QOL (16).

SUMMARY

The type of seizure measurement selected should be tailored to the needs of the clinical trial. These needs change as the development of the investigational agent moves along. Protocol designers who look toward nontraditional outcome measures might acquire valuable data that could be used to differentiate their drug from other new treatments. Most importantly, as clinical trials evolve into effectiveness studies, clinicians are provided with useful data on which to base selection of a drug of first choice to treat each type of seizure disorder.

REFERENCES

1. Chadwick DM. Gabapentin: clinical use. In: Levy RH, Mattson RH, Meldrum B. *Antiepileptic Drugs*. 4th ed. New York: Raven Press; 1995:851–856.
2. Cramer JA, Smith DB, Mattson RH, Delgado-Escueta AV, Collins JF, the VA Epilepsy Cooperative Study Group. A method of quantification for the evaluation of antiepileptic drug therapy. *Neurology* 1983;33(Suppl 1): 26–37.
3. Cramer JA, Mattson RH. Quantitative approaches to

seizure severity, In: Meinardi H, Cramer JA, Baker GA, Martins da Silva A. *Quantitative Assessment of Epilepsy Care: Clinimetric Applications.* eds. New York: Pergamon; 1993:55–72.

4. Mattson RH, Cramer JA, Collins JF, Smith DB, Delgado-Escueta AV, et al. Comparison of carbamazepine, phenobarbital, phenytoin, and primidone in partial and secondarily generalized tonic-clonic seizures. *N Engl J Med* 1985;313:145–151.
5. Mattson RH, Cramer JA, Collins JF, the Department of Veterans Affairs Epilepsy Cooperative Study No. 264 Group. A comparison of valproate with carbamazepine for the treatment of partial seizures and secondarily generalized tonic-clonic seizures in adults. *N Engl J Med* 1992;327:765–771.
6. Duncan JS, Sander JWAS. The Chalfont Seizure Severity Scale. *J Neurol Neurosurg Psychiatry* 1991;54:873–876.
7. O'Donoghue MF, Duncan JS, Sander JW. The National Hospital Seizure Severity Scale: a further development of the Chalfont Seizure Severity Scale. *Epilepsia* 1996; 37:563–571.
8. Baker GA, Smith DF, Dewey M, Morrow J, Crawford PM, Chadwick DW. The development of a seizure severity scale as an outcome measure in epilepsy. *Epilepsy Res* 1991;8:245–251.
9. Smith D, Baker GB, Davies G, Dewey M, Chadwick DW. Outcomes of add-on treatment with lamotrigine in partial epilepsy. *Epilepsia* 1993;34:312–322.
10. Bourgeois B, Leppik IE, Sackellares JC, et al. Felbamate: a double-blind controlled trial in patients undergoing presurgical evaluation of partial seizures. *Neurology* 1993;43:693–696.
11. Pledger GW, Kramer LD. Clinical trials of investigational antiepileptic drugs: monotherapy designs. *Epilepsia* 1991;32:716–721.
12. Cramer JA, Mattson RH. Monitoring compliance with antiepileptic drug therapy. In: Cramer JA, Spilker B, eds. *Patient Compliance in Medical Practice and Clinical Trials.* New York: Raven Press; 1991:123–138.
13. Hasford J. Biometric issues in measuring and analyzing partial compliance in clinical trials. In: Cramer JA, Spilker B, eds. *Patient Compliance in Medical Practice and Clinical Trials.* New York: Raven Press: 1991: 265–282.
14. Sato S, White BG, Penry JK, Dreifuss FE, Sackellares JC, Kupferberg HJ. Valproic acid versus ethosuximide in the treatment of absence seizures. *Neurology* 1982; 32:157–163.
15. Felbamate Study Group in the Lennox-Gastaut syndrome. Efficacy of felbamate in childhood epileptic encephalopathy (Lennox-Gastaut syndrome). *N Engl J Med* 1993;328:29–33.
16. Rosenheck R, Cramer JA, Xu W, et al. A comparison of dozapine and haloperedol in hospitalized patients with refractory schizophrenia. *N Engl J Med* 1997;337 (Sept 18).

Antiepileptic Drug Development.
Advances in Neurology, Vol. 76,
edited by J. French, I. Leppik, and M. A. Dichter.
Lippincott–Raven Publishers, Philadelphia © 1998.

20

Alternate Endpoints: Studies in Quality of Life and Health Economics of Epilepsy

Azmi A. Nabulsi and Karrar H. Ali

Abbott Laboratories, Abbott Park, IL 60064.

INTRODUCTION

Epilepsy is a relatively common condition, with an estimated prevalence of 0.5% in the United States (1). In two cross-sectional studies, trends have shown increases in the prevalence of all types of seizures for both sexes (2). The difficulty in studying and managing epilepsy is its silent disease process. Because seizures may occur infrequently, people may go several years before either realizing or accepting the disorder. In a study of 106 hospital cases, 24 months elapsed before a diagnosis was made in 35% of the cases. Many patients have the condition for years before they can be given a correct diagnosis (3).

As a result, health outcomes of epilepsy have not been well studied. During the past two decades, however, some progress has been made in measuring the quality of life of individuals with epilepsy and the cost effectiveness of both drug therapy and surgical procedures. In this chapter, we review the literature of quality of life and economic studies of epilepsy and its treatment. We summarize study results and discuss methodologies for both quality of life and health economics studies of epilepsy.

QUALITY OF LIFE

Recently, an increasing amount of research has been directed toward the assessment of the effects of disease and treatment on health-related quality of life (HRQOL). QOL studies and instruments (questionnaires) have been used to measure physical, social, and psychologic domains. Depending on the disease and course of treatment, HRQOL instruments have been structured to reflect general health using disease-specific and treatment-specific measures. Even though most questionnaires rely on the patient's perspective and opinion of the particular disease or treatment (some, however, use third-party ratings), these instruments are fairly accurate in determining the patient's health status. Psychometric tests of reliability and validity are used to confirm statistical significance and the proper use of the instrument in several populations. Yet, because of the multifaceted domains of any disease or treatment, it becomes a monumental task to develop an instrument that thoroughly captures all areas of QOL.

In epilepsy, marked progress has been seen in the development of QOL studies and instruments during the last 15 years. Although the effect of epilepsy on patients, family members, and health care providers varies with seizure type, HRQOL assessment is crucial in relating seizure severity and frequency with disease and/or treatment. Those who experience few seizures may not show a significant change in HRQOL, whereas those with refractory epilepsy may be devastated across all domains of HRQOL (4). By using disease-specific HRQOL questions, investigators may be able to assess the extent to which the disease affects the patient; by using treatment-related questions, they may be able to form conclusions regarding the effectiveness of treatment on the patient's health status as well. In addition, generic or non-disease-specific instruments can provide comparative data across different disease states.

Studies of Quality of Life in Epilepsy

Before 1980, there were no instruments or studies that looked directly at QOL in epilepsy patients. The most commonly used instrument was the Minnesota Multiphasic Personality Inventory (MMPI), which was not an HRQOL instrument *per se*; rather, it was developed within a psychiatric context and contained a few items on epilepsy (5). In a 1980 report, Dodrill et al. (6) developed the Washington Psychosocial Seizure Inventory (WPSI) to study psychosocial problems among 127 epilepsy patients. The 132-item questionnaire included scales in the following areas: family background; emotional, interpersonal, and vocational adjustment; financial status; adjustment to seizures, medicine, and medical management; and an evaluation of overall psychosocial functioning. In addition, three scales to test validity were incorporated to account for items left blank, detect attempts to present oneself in an overly favorable state, and identify those questions endorsed by no more than 15% of the patients. To measure reliability, the questionnaire was administered to professional raters and to patients' friends.

The professionals demonstrated a higher internal consistency among themselves than the patients' friends. With each administration, the internal consistency of each scale was evaluated by a split-half method in which the results of odd and even numbered items were correlated. All correlations were statistically significant at the .01 level or better. Although results from this study showed the WPSI to be accurate in assessing problems among patients with epilepsy, there was some concern about overlaps between scales. For example, those with emotional problems tended also to have interpersonal and vocational problems. Interrelated domains such as these are expected to overlap in HRQOL instruments.

The WPSI has been used in other studies to examine the effects of antiepileptic drugs on seizure disorders, diagnose pseudoseizures, evaluate therapy, and screen intellectual and neuropsychologic functioning. An extension of WPSI, the Adolescent Psychosocial Seizure Inventory (APSI), is also available (7). This instrument measures essentially the same domains as the WPSI, but questions are geared to the specific psychologic concerns of adolescents as determined by psychologists or social workers.

Chaplin et al. (8) used a quantitative approach to measure the social effects of epilepsy. Their study population included not only clinic-based patients but also those with well-controlled epilepsy and with recently diagnosed epilepsy in the U.K. This postal questionnaire was based on a total of 21 areas of concern examined through interviews with patients. Overall, statements tended to be similar to those in other questionnaires, especially concerning individual adjustments to seizures. Differences were in the nature of the statements—that is, they were more practical and objective than those in U.S. instruments, which place greater emphasis on the emotional and psychologic aspects of adjustment (9).

Initially, questions were formulated to require yes-or-no answers; however, after further reflection and feedback from patients, shades of agreement or disagreement were used. Statements were also given weight based on the relative significance of the statement by the individual. Validity testing is particularly difficult when an attitude scale is used, such as the one in this study, because there are no objective measures of an individual's attitudes, and correlation between attitude and behavior is often small (10). Results showed that the questionnaire was within the range of acceptance. Reliability was measured using a test-retest procedure. The full questionnaire was administered twice to 20 patients at an epilepsy center with an intervening period of 1 month. Pearson's correlational analysis to determine consistency showed that overall correlations were significant and satisfactorily high. Although this questionnaire is an excellent means to assess social effects and adjustments in patients with epilepsy, it has not been possible to validate all 21 areas. However, the authors feel that the 21 areas are important to capture all social aspects, and that adding more questions to a postal questionnaire would not be feasible.

Jacoby et al. developed a QOL model for epilepsy that incorporates both generic and epilepsy-specific items to describe the way in which an individual's life is affected (11). It is a brief and simple instrument that measures the impact of a condition and its treatment, as perceived by patients. Items were selected on the basis of previous research, discussion with experts, and interviews with patients. In total, eight items considered to encompass the most important areas of everyday life were included in the impact scale: relationship with spouse or partner, relationship with other close family members, social life and social activities, work, health, relationship with friends, feelings about self, and plans and ambitions for the future. In addition to the impact scales, patients also completed the following scales: Hospital Anxiety and Depression (12), Self-esteem (13), Affect Balance (14), Mastery (15), Life Fulfillment (11), and Perceived Quality of Life (16).

Seventy-five patients from a large epilepsy clinic in the U.K. completed the scale. Patients were asked to respond to each item by stating how much a particular aspect of their life was affected by epilepsy and its treatment. Rather than yes-or-no answers, responses ranged from not at all (a score of 1 on the Likert scoring system) to a lot (a score of 4). The higher the score, the greater the perceived impact of epilepsy on the patient.

Statistical analysis showed acceptable reliability of all domains except the work item. Because the patients had intractable epilepsy and were not in paid employment, this item was often omitted. A revised version of the scale is currently being tested in a new population of people with varying degrees of seizure severity, and the work item has been modified to accommodate both employed and unemployed people. Significant correlations showed acceptable validity and supported the hypothesis that the less the perceived impact of epilepsy and its treatment, the better an individual's psychologic profile.

The Quality of Life in Epilepsy Inventory (QOLIE-89) was developed by Devinsky et al. (17) to measure HRQOL for patients with epilepsy whose seizures are controlled or whose seizure frequency is low to moderate. The 36-item RAND Health Survey 1.0 (SF-36) (18) was used as a generic core, which was expanded with additional general items [pictorial chart developed for the Dartmouth COOP (19) and an overall QOL item from the Faces Scale (16)]. Epilepsy-specific items were supplemented to reflect issues commonly reported by epilepsy patients with moderately well-controlled epilepsy. These questions were derived from the experience of health professionals specializing in epilepsy, individual outpatient interviews, and a thorough literature review of studies examining seizure severity and psychosocial aspects of epilepsy (Table 1).

The final measure contained 86 items grouped into 17 multi-item scales and three single items. Factor analysis of the 17 scales yielded four HRQOL dimensions: (a) epilepsy-specific, (b) cognitive, (c) mental health-related, and (4) physical health-related. Patients also completed a battery of neuropsychologic tests (20) and were evaluated for systemic and neurologic effects of medications (21).

Three hundred four patients and patient-designated proxies completed the inventory and were retested 1 to 91 days later. Construct validity was supported by significant patient-proxy correlations for all scales and by correlations between neuropsychologic tests and self-reported emotional and cognitive function. Patients with few or no seizures

TABLE 1. *Measures in the Quality of Life Epilepsy Inventory (QOLIE-89)*

Generic core: RAND Health Survey 1.0 (36 items)
- Includes eight multi-item scales that assess physical functioning and role limitations resulting from physical problems
  - Measures general health perceptions (five items), energy/fatigue (four items), social function (two items), emotional well-being (five items), role limitations resulting from emotional problems (three items), physical function (10 items), and role limitations resulting from physical health problems (four items)
  - Includes two-item scale measuring bodily pain, with one item that examines change in health state

Expansion of the generic core (nine items)
  - Two SF-36 role limitations scales expanded by three items to make scales analogous to one another
  - Two items on general health perceptions added to supplement the general health perceptions scale

From Devinsky et al., ref. 17.

in the preceding year showed a consistent pattern of reporting better HRQOL than patients having more frequent seizures. The epilepsy-specific scale and three of four other scales (Seizure Worry, Work/Driving/Social Function, and Health Discouragement) had the highest relative validities of all scales in relation to seizure severity and HRQOL.

The QOLIE-89 is the latest development to measure health-related QOL for epilepsy (22). Two shorter versions have also been developed, containing subsets of the QOLIE-89. The QOLIE-31 has 31 items grouped into seven multi-item scales, and the QOLIE-10 contains 10 single items (23). The reliability and validity data have been discussed in recent reports (24,25). The methodology used in developing the QOLIE-89 was similar to that used in developing an HRQOL instrument for patients who have had epilepsy surgery (Epilepsy Surgery Inventory, discussed below). Because this instrument also includes questions on antiepileptic therapy, it may be suitable for use in clinical trials to assess the impact of antiepileptic drug therapy. This aspect of the instrument is currently under investigation.

Studies of Quality of Life in Epilepsy Treatment

Studies performed to assess the effects of epilepsy treatment on HRQOL are summarized in Table 2. In the United States, surgical treatment has been on the increase, tripling between 1985 and 1991 (26). A large number of patients still require treatment yet do not receive it because of the failure of primary care physicians to identify surgical candidates or the reluctance of third-party payers to provide coverage (27,28). Although the risk for significant morbidity or death from brain surgery is relatively low, the thought of this procedure evokes fear in patients' minds (29).

Forrow et al. (30) point out four issues to consider in any discussion of surgery-related studies: (a) Altering a disease process or risk factor (like seizures) favorably does not imply that overall health or risk is altered favorably. (b) Measured morbidity or mortality is not reduced in many patients who are treated. (c) Emphasis on population-wide benefits can distort decision making related to individual benefits. (c) Diagnosis and treatment affect many endpoints other the ones that are usually measured and reported.

At the Reed Neurological Research Center, Rausch and Crandall (31) evaluated patients before, 1 month after, and 1 year after temporal lobe surgery. Patients who were not operated on but were given a diagnosis of epilepsy based on stereo-electroencephalography (SEEG) served as controls. Four social ratings were chosen from a comprehensive battery to measure psychosocial QOL (32,33). All four scales were found to be highly reliable, with 10 of the patients rated by two independent raters. Cognitive measures included the Full-Scale IQ and four verbal and nonverbal summary scores derived from the Wechsler Adult Intelligence Scale (WAIS) (34). Three memory tests, two verbal and one nonverbal, were selected to rep-

TABLE 2. *Summary of quality-of-life studies for epilepsy treatment*

Study (ref.)	Methods	Instruments	Results
Rausch and Crandall, 1982 (31)	Prospective psychosocial and cognitive evaluation (preoperative, one month and one year after surgery)	• Four scales for psychosocial measurement • Five scales for cognitive measurement	• Improvement in psychosocial status 1 year post surgery • Improvement in degree of dependency, work/ performance history, non-family relationships • Seizure-free patients showed increase in IQ scores
Vickrey et al., 1992 (36)	Retrospective study of patients who underwent surgical treatment from 1974-1990	Epilepsy Surgery Inventory (ESI-55)	• Completely seizure-free patients scored significantly higher than patients with complex partial or grand mal seizures • Pain scale not different between groups
Smith et al., 1993	Randomized, placebo-controlled, clinical trial of lamotrigine	• Liverpool HRQOL battery • Social Problems Questionnaire • Hospital Anxiety and Depression Scale • Affect Balance Scale • Nottingham Health Profile	• No difference in physical domains for lamotrigine and placebo group • No change in social parameters • Balance (mood) and mastery scales had significant difference between groups
Wagner et al., 1995	Questionnaire administered during regular clinic visit and 14 days after to patients on AED therapy in multicenter trial	• 171 items from 31 scales, measuring general health, AED therapy, and occurrence and impact of symptoms	• Patients seizure-free for at least 6 months from AED therapy had higher HRQOL

resent memory functioning in the patients (35).

The results of this study indicated that seizure relief subsequent to surgical treatment was accompanied by improvement in psychosocial status after 1 year. Patients who became essentially free of seizures following surgery showed a corresponding postoperative increase in intelligence score. However, little evidence was found of improvement in social functioning.

In addition, Vickrey et al. (36) developed the Epilepsy Surgery Inventory (ESI-55) to assess the HRQOL outcomes of patients who had undergone surgical treatment of intractable epilepsy. The 55-item instrument was developed by combining a generic core measure, the 36-item RAND Health Survey 1.0 (SF-36) with a 19-item supplement including areas of cognitive function, role limitations caused by memory problems, epilepsy-specific health perceptions, and overall QOL (Table 3). The ESI-55 was mailed to 224 adults who had been evaluated for resective brain surgery to treat intractable epilepsy between 1974 and 1990. This retrospective evaluation was carried out by mailing the questionnaires to patients who had had surgery at

TABLE 3. *Construct of the Epilepsy Surgery Inventory (ESI-55)*

1. RAND Health Survey (SF-36)
   - Generic core instrument that taps into eight health concepts relevant to people with epilepsy (see Table 1 for full description)
2. Cognitive function
   - Three items used in the RAND Medical Outcomes Study that address attention and cognitive problems
   - Two items that assess verbal and nonverbal memory problems
3. Role limitations

various times in the past. All questionnaires were self-administered, completed at home, and returned by mail to the principal investigator. Determination of construct and content validities showed high correlations between all scales. Reliability coefficients for internal consistency exceeded the standard for group comparisons.

As hypothesized, results showed that completely seizure-free patients scored significantly higher on all scales than did patients with some type of partial seizures. Only the Pain Scale scores did not differ significantly. However, because the questionnaire was administered postoperatively, no comparisons could be made between preoperative and postoperative QOL. Further studies using the ESI-55 in surgical patients in a prospective manner would strengthen conclusions of the impact of surgery on epilepsy patients.

Although surgery has been used for decades to treat epilepsy, drug therapy has also increased since the introduction of carbamazepine in 1974 and valproic acid in 1978. Now, a number of drugs have become available to treat generalized and partial seizures. The recent introduction of felbamate and gabapentin in 1993 and lamotrigine in 1994 has renewed interest in QOL and outcomes studies (37).

However, only a handful of studies examine QOL changes with the administration of antiepileptic drugs. Wagner et al. (38) compiled 31 previously validated and newly developed generic and epilepsy-specific scales to evaluate the impact of antiepileptic drugs. New items and scales were created to test domains for which no previously developed measures could be found. The final questionnaire contained 171 items and were divided into four modules: (a) a general health core measure, (b) additional generic measures of health, (c) measures specific for epilepsy and antiepileptic drug therapy, and (d) items to measure the occurrence and impact of symptoms.

The SF-36 was used to measure general health. This includes eight health domains and a comparison of general health status with health status 1 year previously. Additional questions were attached to the SF-36 to evaluate the effects of epilepsy and its treatment, particularly in regard to psychologic distress, and to test cognitive functioning (39,40,41). An epilepsy-specific module was attached to measure feelings of personal control, the impact of epilepsy and its treatment on daily life, distress and behavioral problems related to epilepsy, and patient-perceived seizure severity (42). Also, 16 items were added to measure the frequency and impact of symptoms often associated with currently available antiepileptic drug therapy. These included questions to detect blurred vision, slurred speech, involuntary movement, slowed reactions, and nausea and vomiting. The validity of all scales was assessed in relation to both disease severity (defined as time since last seizure) and frequency of symptoms possibly associated with antiepileptic drug treatment.

One hundred thirty-six ambulatory patients from three clinics in the U.K. participated in the study. Patients who had been seizure-free for at least 6 months tended to have a higher HRQOL score than patients with recent seizures. Those who were seizure-free also fared better in HRQOL in all SF-36 scales than those who had had a seizure in the last week.

Nearly all scales did well in terms of validity and reliability. The epilepsy-specific scales were among the best in discriminating between patients who differed in respect to time since last seizure. The scales with the highest correlations for validity were the epilepsy-specific Impact Experience and Agitation Scales. As expected, symptoms had a significant negative impact on HRQOL. The only symptom that did not show at least a moderate association was weight loss. Overall, the questionnaire proved to be useful in detecting differences between patients with epilepsy.

Smith et al. (43) are the only investigators who have incorporated an HRQOL questionnaire in a clinical trial. A randomized, double-blinded, crossover study of lamotrigine was conducted in 81 patients with refractory partial seizures. Three areas of efficacy were measured: seizure frequency, seizure severity, and HRQOL. The HRQOL instrument was administered at the end of baseline and each treatment phase; it contained physical, social, and psychological domains to address some common consequences of intractable epilepsy. The physical domain included seizure frequency and a specifically designed scale for seizure severity (44). The Social Problems Questionnaire was used to determine the patient's satisfaction with a range of social issues (45). Several scales were compiled to measure the psychological domain, which includes disturbance of mood, depression, self-esteem, and ability to cope with stress (11–14).

Among the study patients, no significant differences in mean scores for the physical domain were found between lamotrigine and placebo in all six subscales (Energy, Pain, Emotional Reaction, Sleep, Social Isolation, and Physical Mobility). Few patients reported severe dissatisfaction with any of the social parameters tested. There were no significant differences in the mean scores for lamotrigine and placebo except in the scales for Affect Balance (happiness) and Mastery. Although an improvement in mood might be a direct effect, it is unclear that it will change results of the Mastery Scale. Although no association between seizure severity and Mastery was noticed, the Mastery Scale may not have been sensitive enough to detect changes in severity. Nevertheless, from the multiple-regression analysis the authors conclude that seizure severity, Affect Balance, and Mastery are probably independent of each other.

Because the scales used were from previously validated studies, the authors trust in their accuracy to determine QOL. However, as per the protocol, patients who discontinued prematurely did not complete the HRQOL Questionnaire. This could have introduced bias in favor of lamotrigine. Also, changes in psychologic measures could be caused by an improvement in seizure control, whereas changes in seizure severity or frequency could be caused by coincidental improvements in mood attributable to extraneous factors. Although the multiple regression analyses do not support these arguments, more HRQOL studies in clinical trials in epilepsy are needed to assess the potential limitations of this type of study.

Despite the number of instruments to measure QOL in epilepsy, more research needs to be geared to HRQOL in both surgery and drug therapy. To date, there are only a handful of clinical trials with HRQOL measures despite the great strides to develop instruments. Using the ESI-55 as a basis for expansion, the QOLIE-89 seems to be an instrument that may improve HRQOL assessment in clinical trails. Improvement in assessment method will help investigators learn more about the domains most affected by epilepsy and those most sensitive to intervention.

ECONOMIC IMPACT OF EPILEPSY

In a discussion of health economics, several key concepts must be understood. The total cost of illness is the sum of direct and indirect costs. Direct costs are expenditures for the prevention, detection, and treatment of a disease. They include hospital payments, professional fees, personnel, and all applicable drug costs. Hospice care, transportation, and rehabilitation can also add significantly to direct costs (46). Indirect costs include production loss resulting from illness, disability, reduced skill and/or capacity to work, and premature death. Depending on the disease and time of onset, indirect costs can make up a substantial portion of the total cost of an illness (47).

The cost of epilepsy on society and its health system is quite burdensome. To develop better programs to treat the disease, governments have taken an active part in establishing estimates regarding the cost of epilepsy. A 1975 study performed for the Commission for the Control of Epilepsy and its Consequences provided a comprehensive estimate of the annual cost of epilepsy in the United States. Direct cost was estimated at $560 million (or $1.8 billion adjusted in 1991 dollars); indirect cost was estimated at $3.0

billion (or $8.5 billion in 1991 dollars). These figures suggest that the cost of epilepsy exceeds that of many other neurologic disorders and represents >3% of the total cost of all neurologic brain diseases (48).

A more recent study, by the National Foundation for Brain Research (*unpublished report*), examined national cost estimates for hospital care and physician services in 1991. For patients with epilepsy, total hospital costs were estimated at $532.4 million, and costs for physician services at $76.7 million. In contrast, this study found the cost of epilepsy to be <1% of the total cost of all neurologic disorders.

The indirect cost of epilepsy has been studied to determine its burden on individuals and society. Unemployment and reduced income usually contribute most to indirect cost. One study suggested that persons with epilepsy had about twice the unemployment rate of the general population, and if employed, they were less likely to be in professional or managerial occupations and more likely to be in service or skilled occupations (49). For those with severe or frequent seizures, unemployment as high as 50% has been reported, with a high rate of discouragement from participation in the labor force (50). Although the unemployment figures are of great concern, no studies have been able to quantify loss of employment for affected individuals or society.

In a comprehensive study to determine the cost of epilepsy, the total lifetime cost in 1990 dollars for all persons with a diagnosis of epilepsy at the time was $90 billion. The average cost per patient was about $20,000, with indirect cost accounting for 63% of the total economic cost. Indirect cost was mainly attributed to lost work, housekeeping days lost, and excess unemployment. These cost estimates did not adequately account for other indirect costs, such as lost employment of caretakers of patients and reduced QOL, nor did it account for other direct costs, such as dental treatment and side effects associated with antiepileptic drugs, factors that can increase the cost substantially (51).

With only a handful of studies available, it is difficult to assess accurately the economic impact on patients, caretakers, or providers. Unfortunately, the bulk of the cost lies with indirect costs, a domain that is not easily measurable. At least two thirds of the cost of epilepsy is associated with unemployment and reduced productivity, yet there is no firm method to determine these costs. Furthermore, the present studies in the literature fail to provide a comprehensive review of total cost for patients, health care providers, and society. Firm conclusions cannot be based on results from different studies using different methodologies.

Economic Impact of Therapies

The economic impact of the available therapies for epilepsy has not been well studied, although the methodology for conducting economic studies has been fairly well established. As health providers become increasingly concerned with health outcomes and cost effectiveness of interventions, economic evaluation becomes more important.

Currently, a handful of studies have assessed the economic impact of epilepsy treatments. A detailed study estimating the cost of epilepsy and its treatment was carried out by Begley et al. (51). A model incorporating survival, use and cost of medical care, and time lost from work and housekeeping was developed using six prognostic groups with varying degrees of epileptic seizures (Fig. 1). The model specified the sequence of treatment stages that the average person in each group would experience and the major medical services that would be used in each stage. Patterns of services used took into account initial evaluation, follow-up treatment (visits and hospitalizations), changes over time in the type and quantity of antiepileptic drugs, treatment for adverse reactions to antiepileptic drugs, diagnostic testing performed at the time and subsequent to initiation of antiepileptic drugs, and the incidence and effects of surgery. In this hypothetical model, patients in group 1 were postulated to receive

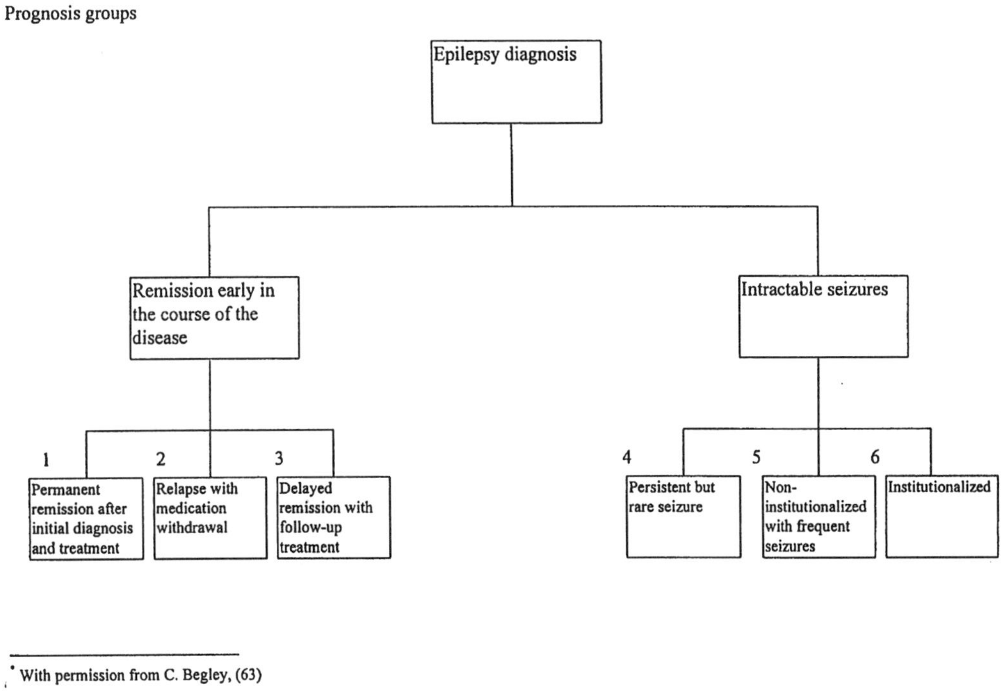

FIG. 1. Prognosis groups. (Reproduced with permission from Begley et al., ref. 51.)

follow-up monitoring after initial evaluation and antiepileptic drug treatment for 1 to 5 years, and after discontinuation of antiepileptic drugs they were expected to remain seizure-free. Patients in group 2 were postulated to respond to initial and follow-up treatments; however, because of relapse they were expected to continue antiepileptic drug treatment to maintain seizure control. Patients in group 3 were postulated to continue to have seizures with their initial therapy but expected to become seizure-free once an appropriate combination of medications had been prescribed. After initial evaluation, patients in groups 4 to 6 were expected to receive more intense follow-up treatment using different antiepileptic drug regimens. All potential surgical candidates were from group 5, and those in group 6 had intractable seizures but were not expected to be considered as surgical candidates.

The authors postulated that antiepileptic drug treatment varied across prognostic groups in terms of the proportion of the group receiving monotherapy and/or polytherapy and the type of antiepileptic drug prescribed. Drug therapy options included carbamazepine, phenytoin, phenobarbital, primidone, and valproate (see article for exact dose composition). The average lifetime cost for epilepsy treatment per patient was estimated to range from \$4272 (in group 1) to \$138,602 (in group 5); indirect costs accounted for 63% of the total cost. Drug treatment accounted for the highest portion of direct cost, followed by physician visits and inpatient hospital care. The only exceptions were in group 6, in which institutionalized patients had greater cost for electroencephalography, and in group 5, in which surgery candidates had greater surgical follow-up cost; both of these exceptions were as expected. Group 5 also had the highest indirect cost, with approximately 70% of total indirect cost attributed to morbidity (lost work, housekeeping days lost, and excess unemployment). In a sensitivity analysis, the high estimate of drug cost added 74% (\$844 million) to direct cost and 28% to the total cost estimate; the low drug cost estimate decreased direct cost and total cost estimates by 35% and 13% ($403 million), respectively.

Despite the comprehensiveness of this study, there were limitations to the model. Known costs, such as for treatment of dental problems related to side effects of antiepileptic drugs, treatment of injuries acquired during seizures, long-term hospital care of persons with status epilepticus, medical equipment, and counseling for patients and family members, were not incorporated in the analysis. Neither the high indirect cost of underemployment of persons whose productivity was reduced by epilepsy nor the cost of pain and suffering or reduction in overall HRQOL of epileptic patients and their caretakers was assessed. One may never be able to capture all costs in an economic model. And, as in all modeling studies, one must consider the reliance on expert judgment and inferences from current literature when determining the accuracy of model assumptions, which is not true in studies in which costs are accrued prospectively.

O'Neill et al. (52) studied the economic consequences of adjunctive anticonvulsant therapies. A decision-analytic model was developed to represent the consequences of treatment with three drugs during 1 year. Cost of treatment was then estimated per patient and for the overall proportion of successfully treated patients during 1 year with alternative therapeutics (clobazam, vigabatrin, or lamotrigine). Patients initially on clobazam were assumed to switch to vigabatrin in the event of failure, and subsequently to lamotrigine if a second failure occurred. For patients initially treated with vigabatrin, lamotrigine was assumed to be given if treatment failed, followed by clobazam; for those treated initially with lamotrigine, vigabatrin was given, then clobazam. If the third therapy failed in any case, gabapentin was administered.

Cost data used included the cost of treatment given, both initially and if treatment was switched, and the cost of extra clinic visits should a patient not be controlled on current therapy. These costs were then incorporated with clinical data from the three drugs. Efficacy rates for clobazam, vigabatrin, and lamotrigine were obtained from published clinical trials (53–55). Sensitivity analyses were performed to test the robustness of the models. Variables tested included efficacy rates, dosage regimens, and number of extra clinic visits incurred for those who failed therapy.

Results show that drug costs for vigabatrin and lamotrigine were approximately seven times higher than those for clobazam, and lamotrigine was slightly more expensive than vigabatrin. The cost of lamotrigine was greatly reduced if used with valproate but was still more than four times as expensive as clobazam. Clinical data were incorporated to obtain cost-effective ratios. The expected cost effectivess per patient for treatment during the 1-year period was 40% higher for patients who started on vigabatrin or lamotrigine rather than on clobazam. Sensitivity analysis revealed no change in outcome when key variables were changed in the model.

Although the study shows sound methodology, there are several assumptions that must be considered. First, comparisons were based on outcomes from previously published clinical trial data, which do not reflect actual clinical practice. Second, once seizures were controlled on either vigabatrin or lamotrigine, the authors assumed patients retained control for the remainder of the treatment period, with no long-term dropout. This could have favored the drugs' long-term effectiveness (there is some evidence of long-term dropouts with clobazam because of tolerance) (56). Third, this study omitted the costs of blood monitoring and treating side effects from the model because they were assumed to be equal for all three drugs. There is evidence that more blood monitoring is required with the newer drugs because the risk for drug interactions is greater (57,58) and side effects can be more severe (43,59). Finally, because this model was based on a British population, the issue of its relevance to the United States may be questioned. Variations in practice undoubtedly affect variables in the model, and one must be cautious when applying international results to the United States.

Navarro and Ashraf (60) conducted a cost-minimization analysis using retrospective data from earlier Veterans Administration efficacy studies (61,62). The cost of medication, pharmacy fees, and initiation and maintenance costs were examined for four drugs: phenytoin sodium (Dilantin), generic carbamazepine, carbamazepine USP (Tegretol), and divalproex sodium (valproate) delayed-release tablets (Depakote). A panel of neurologists was consulted to determine the pattern of therapy, number of clinical visits, laboratory tests required, clinical management, and treatment of adverse effects for an average case. Direct costs were then estimated for patients over 5 years and discounted to the net present value.

In this study, the cost of follow-up laboratory tests and physician visits for all three drugs were approximately the same, ranging from $240 to $248. Determination of the net cost of therapy (discounting 15%) by the usual dosage range, with the annual dispensing fee and cost of adverse effects added, showed that phenytoin was lowest and valproate was highest in cost. Sensitivity analysis was carried out on the cost to treat adverse drug reactions and the annual cost of medication because these variables have the greatest impact on final costs. Results showed that phenytoin continued to remain the least costly in terms of treating adverse drug reactions associated with its use. Unfortunately, the authors did not include phenobarbital, an inexpensive drug that was also evaluated in the Veterans Administration study.

This study was strictly a cost-minimization analysis of three drugs. Although conclusions point to the cost of medication and therapy, one must consider the cost effectiveness of the three drugs. One drug may be more expensive, but this analysis does not incorporate effectiveness of the drug, which affects the cost-to-effectiveness ratio and alters the economic advantage of a particular drug over another.

CONCLUSION

The current literature in epilepsy research is disparate, in regard to both QOL and economic outcomes. The diagnosis of epilepsy signifies a chronic disorder that requires lifelong treatment. The disease not only affects the patient but also the patient's family, friends, and health care providers. It is imperative we evaluate all aspects of epilepsy and its burden on society.

QOL research has seen some progress during the last 15 years. We now have adequate instruments that measure psychosocial parameters for both the disease itself and its associated treatment. With the upcoming trials using the QOLIE-89 and related versions, more information will become available on the impact of intervention on epilepsy. Future research should provide fine tuning of the existing instruments. In addition, we need to study on those domains that affect the patient's QOL the most and compare treatments from the patient's perspective.

In epilepsy, economic research is still lagging. Despite the established methodologies to collect and analyze economic data, little attention has been given to epilepsy. What exists currently in the literature is either outdated or has too many limitations to assess the economic burden accurately. There are few cost-effective studies on either antiepileptic drug therapy or surgery. There is still no firm conclusion that one therapy is better than another. Furthermore, there are no cost-utility studies in epilepsy. These types of studies not only account for cost of therapy, but also incorporate QOL and patient preferences regarding a specific therapy and outcome. If more such studies become available, then we may be able to determine the impact of epilepsy on individuals, their families, and society more accurately, and we may be able to assess the impact of interventions on the treatment of epilepsy.

ACKNOWLEDGMENT

The authors would like to thank Dr. Kenneth Summerville, Jr., Dennis Revicki, Joyce Cramer and Jan Lips for their valuable comments.

REFERENCES

1. Hauser WA, Kurland LT. The epidemiology of epilepsy in Rochester, Minnesota, 1935–1968. *Epilepsia* 1975; 16:1–66.
2. Cockerell OC, et al. Epilepsy in a population of 6000 re-examined: secular trends in first attendance rates, prevalence, and prognosis. *J Neurol Neurosurg Psychiatry* 1995;58:570–576.
3. Shorvon SD. *The drug treatment of epilepsy: towards more effective anticonvulsant assessment and therapeutics* (Thesis). Chicago, IL: University of Chicago, 1982.
4. Santilli N, Kessler BL, Schmidt WT. Quality of life in epilepsy: perspective of patients. In: Trimble MR, Dodson WE, eds. *Epilepsy and Quality of Life.* New York: Raven Press; 1994.
5. Dahlstrom WG, Welsh GS, Dahlstrom LE. *An MMPI Handbook.* Minneapolis: University of Minnesota Press; 1972 (vol 1).
6. Dodrill CB, Batzel LW, Queisser HR, Temkin NR. An objective method for the assessment of psychological and social problems among epileptics. *Epilepsia* 1980; 21:123–135.
7. Batzel LW, Dodrill CB, Dubinsky BL, et al. An objective method for the assessment of psychosocial problems in adolescents with epilepsy. *Epilepsia* 1991;32: 202–211.
8. Chaplin JE, Yepez R, Shorvon S, Floyd M. A quantitative approach to measuring the social effects of epilepsy. *Neuroepidemiology* 1990;9:151–158.
9. Hunt SM, McEwen J, McKenna SP. Measuring health status: a new tool for clinicians and epidemiologists. *J R Coll Gen Pract* 1985;35:185–188.
10. Wicker AW. Attitudes versus actions: the relationship of verbal and overt behavioural responses to attitude objects. *J Soc Issues* 1969;25:41–78.
11. Baker GA, Jacoby A, Smith DF, Dewey ME, Chadwick DW. Development of a novel scale to assess life fulfillment as part of the further refinement of a quality of life model for epilepsy. *Epilepsia* 1994;35:591–596.
12. Zigmond AS, Snaith RP. The hospital anxiety and depression scale. *Acta Psychiatr* 1983;67:361–370.
13. Rosenberg M. *Society and the Adolescent Self-image.* Princeton: Princeton University Press; 1965.
14. Bradburn NM. *The Structure of Psychological Well-being.* Chicago: Aldine; 1969.
15. Pearlin LI, Schooler C. The structure of coping. *J Health Soc Behav* 1978;19:2–21.
16. Andrews FM, Withey SB. *Social Indicators of Well-being. Americans' Perception of Life Quality.* New York: Plenum Press; 1976.
17. Devisnky O, Vickrey BG, Cramer JA, et al. Development of the quality of life in epilepsy inventory. *Epilepsia* 1995;36:1089–1104.
18. Hays RD, Sherbourne C, Mazel E. The RAND 36-item health survey 1.0. *Health Econ* 1993;2:217–227.
19. Nelson EC, et al. The functional status of patients: how can it be measured in physicians' offices? *Med Care* 1990;28:1111–1126.
20. Perrine KR. A new quality-of-life inventory for epilepsy patients: interim results. *Epilepsia* 1993;34(Suppl 4): S28–S33.
21. Cramer JA, Smith DB, Mattson RH, Delgado-Escueta AV, Collins JF. A method of quantification for the evaluation of antiepileptic drug therapy. *Neurology* 1983;33(Suppl 1):26–37.
22. Devinsky O. Clinical uses of the quality of life in epilepsy inventory. *Epilepsia* 1993;34(Suppl 4):S39– S44.
23. Cramer JA. Quality of life assessment for people with epilepsy. In: Spilker B, ed. *Quality of Life and Pharmacoeconomics in Clinical Trials.* 2nd ed. Philadelphia: Lippincott-Raven; 1996.
24. Cramer JA, Perrine K, Devinsky O, Meador K. A brief questionnaire to screen for quality of life in epilepsy: the QOLIE-10. *Epilepsia* 1996;37:577–583.
25. Vickrey BG, Perrine KR, Hays RD, Hermann BP, Cramer JA, Meador KJ, Devinsky O. *Scoring Manual for the QOLIE-31, Version 1.0.* RAND; 1993.
26. Engel J, Shewmon DA. Overview: who should be considered a surgical candidate? In: Engel J Jr, ed. *Surgical Treatment of the Epilepsies.* 2nd ed. New York: Raven Press; 1993.
27. Hauser WA. The natural history of drug-resistant epilepsy: epidemiologic considerations. *Epilepsy Res Suppl* 1992;5:25–28.
28. Engle J. Update on surgical treatment of the epilepsies. *Neurology* 1993;43:1612–1617.
29. The Commission on Neurosurgery of Epilepsy of the International League Against Epilepsy. *A Global Survey on Epilepsy Surgery, 1980–1990. Epilepsia* 1992;38(2): 249–255.
30. Forrow L, Wartman SA, Brock DW. Science, ethics, and making clinical decisions. Implications for risk factor intervention. *JAMA* 1988;259:3161–3167.
31. Rausch R, Crandall PH. Psychological status related to surgical control of temporal lobe seizures. *Epilepsia* 1982;23:191–202.
32. Horowitz MJ, Cohen FM. Temporal lobe epilepsy: effects of lobectomy on psychosocial functioning. *Epilepsia* 1968;9:23–41.
33. Taylor DC, Falconer MA. Clinical, socioeconomic, and psychological changes after temporal lobectomy for epilepsy. *Br J Psychiatry* 1968;114:1247–1261.
34. Wechsler D. *Wechsler Adult Intelligence Scale.* New York: Psychological Corporation; 1955.
35. Wechsler D, Stone CP. *Wechsler Memory Scale.* New York: Psychological Corporation; 1945.
36. Vickrey BG, Hays RD, Graber J, Rausch R, Engel J Jr, Brook RH. A health-related quality of life scale instrument for patients evaluated for epilepsy surgery. *Med Care* 1992;30:299–311.
37. Wilder BJ. The treatment of epilepsy: an overview of clinical practices. *Neurology* 1995;45(Suppl 2):S7–S11.
38. Wagner AK, Keller SD, Kosinski M, et al. Advances in methods for assessing the impact of epilepsy and antiepileptic drug therapy on patients' health-related quality of life. *Qual Life Res* 1995;4:115–134.
39. Stewart AL, et al. Psychological distress/well-being and cognitive functioning measures. In: Stewart AL, Ware JE, eds. *Measuring Functioning and Well-Being: the Medical Outcomes Study Approach*, Durham, NC: Duke University Press; 1992.
40. Russell D, Peplau LA, Ferguson ML. Developing a measure for loneliness. *J Pers Assess* 1978;42:290–294.
41. Bergner M, Bobbitt RA, Carter WB, et al. The Sickness Impact Profile: development and final revision of a health status measure. *Med Care* 1981;19:787–805.
42. Jacoby A. Epilepsy and the quality of everyday life:

findings from a study of people with well-controlled epilepsy. *Soc Sci Med* 1992;34:657–666.
43. Smith D, Baker G, Davies G, Dewey M, Chadwick DW. Outcomes of add-on treatment with lamotrigine in partial epilepsy. *Epilepsia* 1993;34:312–322.
44. Hunt SM, et al. A quantitative approach to perceived health status: a validation study. *J Epidemiol Community Health* 1980;34:281–286.
45. Corney RH, Clare AW. The construction, development, and testing of a self-report questionnaire to identify social problems. *Psychol Med* 1985;15:637–649.
46. Lindgren B. *The Cost of Illness in Sweden, 1964– 1975.* Lund: Institutet for Hälso-och sjukvärdsekonomi; 1981. 163 p.
47. Bootman JL, Townsend RJ, McGhan WF, eds. *Principles of Pharmacoeconomics.* Cinncinnati: Harvey Whitney Books; 1990.
48. Commission for the Control of Epilepsy and Its Consequences. Economic cost of epilepsy. In: *Plan for Nationwide Action on Epilepsy.* Washington, DC: National Institutes of Health; 1978; DHEW publication No. 78-279:177–178 (vol 4).
49. Trostle JA. *Managing epilepsy: a community study of chronic illness in Rochester, Minnesota* (Thesis). San Francisco, CA: University of California, 1987.
50. Fraser RT, Clemmons D, Trejo W, Temkin NR. Program evaluation in epilepsy rehabilitation. *Epilepsia* 1983; 24:734–736.
51. Begley CE, Annegers JF, Lairson DR, Reynolds TF, Hauser WA. Cost of epilepsy in the United States: a model based on incidence and prognosis. *Epilepsia* 1994;35:1230–1243.
52. O'Neill BA, Trimble MR, Bloom DS. Adjunctive therapy in epilepsy: a cost-effectiveness comparison of alternative treatment options. *Seizure* 1995;4:37–44.
53. National Association of Health Authorities and Trusts. *Healthcare Economic Review* 1990;22.
54. Richens A, Yuens AWC. Overview of the clinical efficacy of lamotrigine. *Epilepsia* 1991;32(Suppl 2): S12–S16.
55. Canadian Clobazam Cooperative Group. Clobazam in the treatment of refractory epilepsy. *Epilepsia* 1995; 32: 407–416.
56. Faulkner-Connelly J. Vigabatrin. *Ann Pharmacother* 1993;27:197–203.
57. Robertson MM. Current status of the 1,4- and 1,5-benzodiazepines in the treatment of epilepsy. *Epilepsia* 1986;27(Suppl 1):S527–S541.
58. Trimble MR. Clobazam. In: Trimble MR, ed. *New Anticonvulsant Drugs.* New York: John Wiley; 1994.
59. Brodie MJ. Drug profiles. Lamotrigine. *Lancet* 1992; 339:1397–1400.
60. Navarro RP, Ashraf T. Cost analysis of carbamazepine, phenytoin, and valproate for use in complex partial seizures. *Med Interface* 1993;6:113–118.
61. Mattson RH, Cramer JA, Collins JF, et al. Comparison of carbamazepine, phenobarbital, Dilantin, and primidone in partial and secondarily generalized tonic-clonic seizures. *N Engl J Med* 1985;313:145–151.
62. Mattson RH, Cramer JA, Collins JF, the Department of Veterans Affairs Epilepsy Cooperative Study No. 264 Group. A comparison of Depakote with carbamazepine for the treatment of complex partial seizures and secondarily generalized tonic-clonic seizures in adults. *N Engl J Med* 1992;327:765–771.

Antiepileptic Drug Development.
Advances in Neurology, Vol. 76,
edited by J. French, I. Leppik, and M. A. Dichter.
Lippincott–Raven Publishers, Philadelphia © 1998.

21

Alternate Endpoint: EEG Assessment of Antiepileptic Drug Efficacy and Toxicity

Eli M. Mizrahi

Section of Neurophysiology, Department of Pediatrics, Baylor College of Medicine, Houston, Texas 77030.

INTRODUCTION

Quantitative alternatives to the clinical assessment of the efficacy and toxicity of antiepileptic drugs (AEDs) are needed because of the relatively imprecise nature of the clinical evaluation. Traditionally, clinical evaluation is based on reports of seizure occurrence by observers or the patient and on the report or observation of signs of clinical toxicity by the patient, observers, or physicians. Doses of AEDs are adjusted to obtain an optimal balance between seizure occurrence and signs or symptoms of toxicity.

This traditional "trial-and-error" method is the cornerstone of clinical management of patients with epilepsy, but it has its limitations. Titration to seizure occurrence or to toxicity may be time-consuming—particularly if seizure frequency is low and the increase in doses of AEDs is conducted in small and infrequent increments. Seizure detection, either by the patient or observers, may be imprecise; patients may be unaware or not remember that seizures have occurred, and observers may not be sufficiently trained to recognize specific seizure types or may not be present when seizures occur. In addition, signs of toxicity can be difficult to identify; their onset may be insidious, specific neuropsychologic testing may be required, or they can be confused with an underlying neurologic disorder.

Efforts to develop alternatives to the clinical assessment of effectiveness and toxicity of AEDs have been based on the application of electroencephalography (EEG), since specific features of the EEG can be quantified and may provide an objective basis for AED assessment. A basic strategy of application is based on a comparison of the EEG findings before and soon after initiation of treatment. If this technique is to be useful, the EEG should be recorded before the onset of therapy and then immediately after AED steady state is achieved. The occurrence and morphology of interictal epileptiform discharges or changes in EEG background activity can be determined and compared. Comparison of the two recordings may provide a basis for the clinician to determine the likelihood of future seizure control or toxicity.

Unfortunately, when this strategy is based solely on visual analysis of EEG, its utility has been limited for a number of reasons. The duration or timing of recording may limit the acquisition of critical data. The degree of changes in EEG waveform morphology or background frequencies may not be sufficient to be detected by visual inspection. In addition, specific types of epilepsy may require different types of EEG assessment.

Efforts to improve upon visual analysis of EEG have been a focus of research activities for several years at the Epilepsy Research

Center, Baylor College of Medicine and The Methodist Hospital, Houston, Texas. This report presents the results of these efforts. The relevant investigations of others are discussed, but the focus of this report is on the results of clinical investigations at this institution. The discussion is divided into two parts: determination of AED efficacy and determination of AED toxicity.

DETERMINATION OF ANTIEPILEPTIC DRUG EFFICACY

Clinical Problems in Assessment of Antiepileptic Drug Efficacy

The assessment of AED efficacy has been traditionally based on clinical observation and the reports of the patient, family, or caregivers. However, as noted above, this can be unreliable. The sources of limitations of clinical assessment include the following: observer or reporter bias or degree of expertise, duration of the observation period ("sampling error"), time period of observation (e.g., daytime versus nocturnal sleep), and the variable intervals between assessments. In some instances, clinical seizures may appear to be controlled by clinical assessment, but EEG recording may prove otherwise. In addition, there may be varying degrees of reported control in a given time period because of variations in AED serum levels.

Principles of Application of Electroencephalographic Quantification

Ideally, if EEG is to be a more effective tool in the assessment of AED efficacy than clinical assessment alone, it should be able to detect seizure occurrence consistently, characterize seizure type accurately, quantify seizure frequency, and most importantly predict the probability of future seizures. All these goals cannot yet be attained for all types of epilepsy in all age groups. However, significant progress has been made in achieving some of these goals. The critical factor in application is the tailoring of specific methods of quantitative EEG analysis to the specific characteristics of various seizure types.

The application of EEG in AED assessment depends on seizure type, age of the patient, the epileptic syndrome, and the epileptiform features that characterize the interictal and ictal EEG. These determine whether analysis should be directed toward ictal or interictal EEG events. Thus, the EEG can be analyzed by occurrence of electrographic seizure activity, morphology of interictal focal spike discharges, or occurrence of interictal generalized spike-and-wave activity in relation to the sleep-wakefulness cycle. Not all applications are suitable for all clinical circumstances.

In this report, the use of EEG in the determination of the efficacy of AED therapy is discussed for four specific seizure types: neonatal seizures, infantile spasms, partial seizures (either simple or complex), and generalized seizures.

Neonatal Seizures

The clinical and electrical seizure activity of the newborn are relatively unique. The clinical events have been classified as focal clonic, focal tonic, myoclonic, generalized tonic posturing, or motor automatisms (i.e., oral-buccal-lingual, ocular, or progression movements) (1). Although some clinical events are closely associated with electrical seizure activity and are considered to be of epileptic origin, others occur in the absence of EEG seizure activity and have clinical features suggesting they are not of epileptic origin but rather are exaggerative reflex behaviors—so-called "brain stem release phenomena" (1,2). In addition, it is not uncommon for electrical seizures to occur in the absence of any clinical seizure activity.

The diagnosis of neonatal seizures and the decision to treat neonatal seizures with AEDs are based on clinical observation and EEG findings. Seizure types thought to be consistently of epileptic origin include focal clonic, focal tonic, and some myoclonic events. These cannot be provoked or enhanced by stimulation of the patient and cannot be suppressed by restraining the infant. Electrical seizure activity consistently appears with each clinical seizure, and typically the motor activity is time-locked to electrical discharges. These electroclinical seizures are typically treated with AEDs. Seizure types thought to be of nonepileptic origin include generalized tonic posturing, some myoclonic events, and motor automatisms (also referred to as "subtle" seizures). These can be provoked or enhanced by stimulation of the infant and can be suppressed or arrested by restraint. Electrical seizure activity is not associated with these clinical seizure types. These are not treated with AEDs. In addition, electrical seizure activity unassociated with clinical signs is typically treated with AEDs.

There are no reliable EEG markers of potential epileptogenesis in neonates, as there are in older children and adults. In older children and adults, the findings of interictal focal spikes or sharp waves or of generalized spike-and-slow waves can be interpreted, within appropriate clinical circumstances, to identify patients who may have had a seizure or have the potential to experience a seizure in the future. However, there are no such reliable interictal markers in neonates—sharp-wave transients may be normal variants, of uncertain diagnostic significance, or abnormal (but not specifically epileptiform) (3). Thus, whereas interictal epileptiform EEG activity in older children and adults may be the basis for EEG assessment of AED efficacy, in neonates only the actual recording of electrical seizure activity can serve this purpose.

This poses a number of limitations in the application of EEG to determine efficacy. First, one of the goals of EEG analysis as an endpoint of AED therapy is to predict whether an individual patient may have further seizures after AED treatment. Because in the neonate electrical seizure activity itself is the only finding indicating epileptogenesis, this goal cannot be achieved. Another goal of EEG analysis as an endpoint of therapy is to determine whether a patient may be experiencing seizures. Although EEG can document electrical seizure activity, its effectiveness may be directly related to the length of recording—the longer the recording, the more likely the possibility of recording an electrical seizure. If none are recorded, it may simply be a consequence of the duration of the study (sampling error).

Despite these limitations, there is a clear role for the utilization of EEG in the assessment of AED therapy during *acute administration.* In neonates with electroclinical seizures, the initial response to effective acute AED administration may be cessation of the clinical seizure with persistence of electrical seizure activity (Fig. 1). This is followed in many instances by the eventual cessation of electrical seizure activity also. This phenomenon of initial control of clinical seizures with persistence of electrical seizure activity is referred to as "decoupling" (1,4). Consequently, if EEG is not utilized during the acute administration of AEDs in neonates with electroclinical seizures and clinical observation alone is relied on, AEDs may be considered effective even though electrical seizures may persist.

In addition to EEG recording during acute AED administration, longer-term EEG surveillance can be helpful in circumstances in which electrical seizure activity may occur in the absence of clinical seizures, as in neonates with diffuse encephalopathies and EEG findings of the paroxysmal alpha pattern ("alpha seizure pattern") or electrical seizures of the depressed brain (5), in neonates paralyzed pharmacologically, and in neonates after acute administration of AEDs ("decoupled" seizures). Again, in these instances the length of recording is critical. Sampling error in detecting seizures can be reduced by increasing the duration of recording, but this strategy involves limitations in the availability of trained personnel to provide real-time interpretation of the EEG at the bedside.

Although computer-based, automated electrical seizure detection systems have been reliably utilized in the care of older children and adults, experience in neonates has been limited. Recently, a computerized neonatal seizure detection system has been developed and tested in several centers (6–8). These preliminary studies indicate that most electrical seizures can be automatically detected in

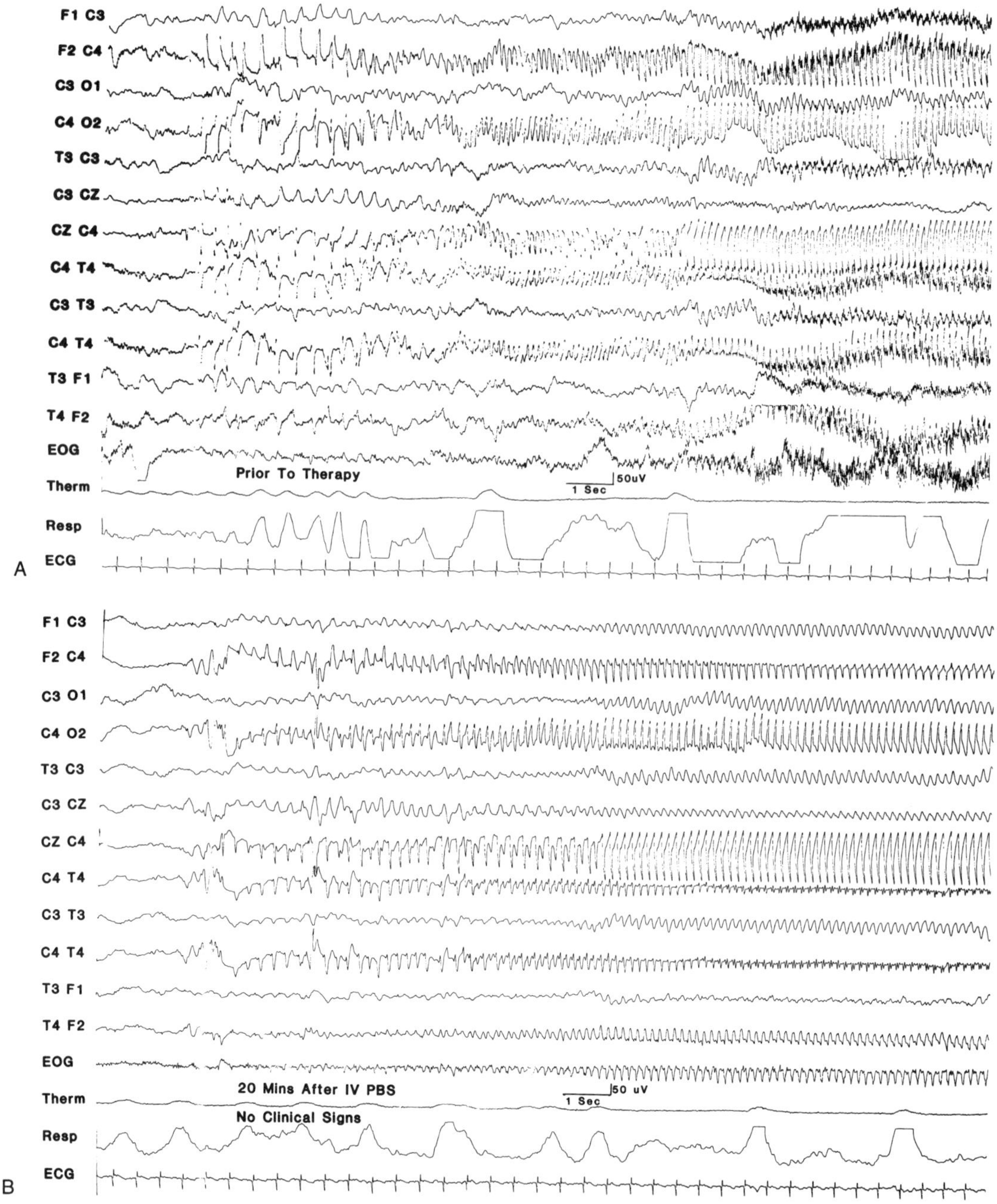

FIG. 1. Decoupling response of neonatal electroclinical seizures to acute AED therapy. **A:** Before administration of phenobarbital electrical seizure activity is present in the right centrotemporal region in association with clinical clonic seizure activity of the left arm and leg. **B:** Following administration of a loading dose of phenobarbital (20 mg/kg IV), the infant has no clinical seizures (e.g., by observation, seizures are controlled), but electrical seizure activity persists ("decoupled" from clinical seizure activity). (Reproduced with permission from Kellaway and Mizrahi, ref. 28.)

neonates; however, false-positive and false-negative detections do occur. The number of false-negative detections is smaller when the technical quality of the EEGs is optimal. Thus, this technique can reduce the need for continuous bedside interpretation of the EEG by a clinical neurophysiologist, but visual analysis for confirmation of some detections is still required. However, computer-based automatic seizure detection is promising overall and may eventually have an important role in the assessment of AED efficacy in neonates treated for seizures.

Infantile Spasms

The disorder characterized by infantile spasms is unique to infants and young children. The presence of infantile spasms in association with the clinical findings of developmental delay and the EEG findings of hypsarrhythmia is often referred to as West syndrome. In addition to its clinical and EEG features, the disorder is also unique for its response to hormonal therapy (9–11). This treatment cannot be technically referred to as AED therapy. However, because prednisone or adrenocorticotropic hormone (ACTH) is given to eliminate infantile spasms, a seizure type with distinctive clinical and EEG features, the determination of the efficacy of this therapy utilizing EEG as an endpoint is discussed here. Furthermore, the same techniques should be used in any future prospective evaluation of new AEDs used to treat this disorder.

Clinically, a spasm consists of contractions of muscles of the neck, trunk, or extremities and is usually bilateral and symmetric. Spasms are of flexor, extensor, or mixed flexor-extensor types (12). In an individual infant, the same number of spasms may occur during the day as at night, but they rarely occur when the infant is asleep. Spasms can be sporadic but most often occur in clusters.

A number of EEG findings have been associated with infantile spasms. The most common interictal pattern is hypsarrhythmia (Fig. 2), either the prototypic or a modified pattern (13). However, other interictal patterns can be associated with infantile spasms, including normal background activity. A number of ictal patterns have been associated with spasm occurrence. The most common is a generalized slow-wave transient followed by a sudden, generalized voltage attenuation of background activity (12) (Fig. 2).

Traditional therapy of infantile spasms has been with ACTH or prednisone, either in low-dose, short-duration (14) or high-dose, long-duration (15,16) regimens. Other medical treatments include administration of traditional AEDs such as valproate and nitrazepam. Other, new AEDs are also being used, such as vigabatrin and felbamate. In addition, some advocate surgical excision of a "zone of cortical abnormality" to treat infantile spasms (17). However, the treatment of infantile spasms is not without controversy. This in part relates both to the selection of therapy (regimens of hormonal therapy, standard AED therapy, or surgery) and to the methods of assessment of outcome of treatment. Outcome may be determined by cessation of spasms or improved interictal EEG or long-term developmental status. In the acute period of treatment, cessation of spasms and EEG are assessed, and cessation of spasms is considered the only true determinant of short-term therapeutic efficacy.

Determination of acute outcome of therapy by either clinical assessment of spasm occurrence or analysis of interictal EEG has been shown to be unreliable. Clinical assessment is limited by a number of factors. In some infants, spasms spontaneously resolve. The cumulative spontaneous remission rate of spasms in the first 12 months after onset of infantile spasms in untreated patients is 25% (18). Thus, in some infants it may be difficult to ascertain whether improvement is based on specific treatment or on the natural history of the disorder. Most significantly, the sporadic mode of occurrence of spasms makes parental reporting of the presence or absence and the frequency of infantile spasms in a given infant unreliable (14,19) (Fig. 3).

Determination of outcome by assessment of interictal EEG is also limited. Traditionally, one measure of outcome has been improve-

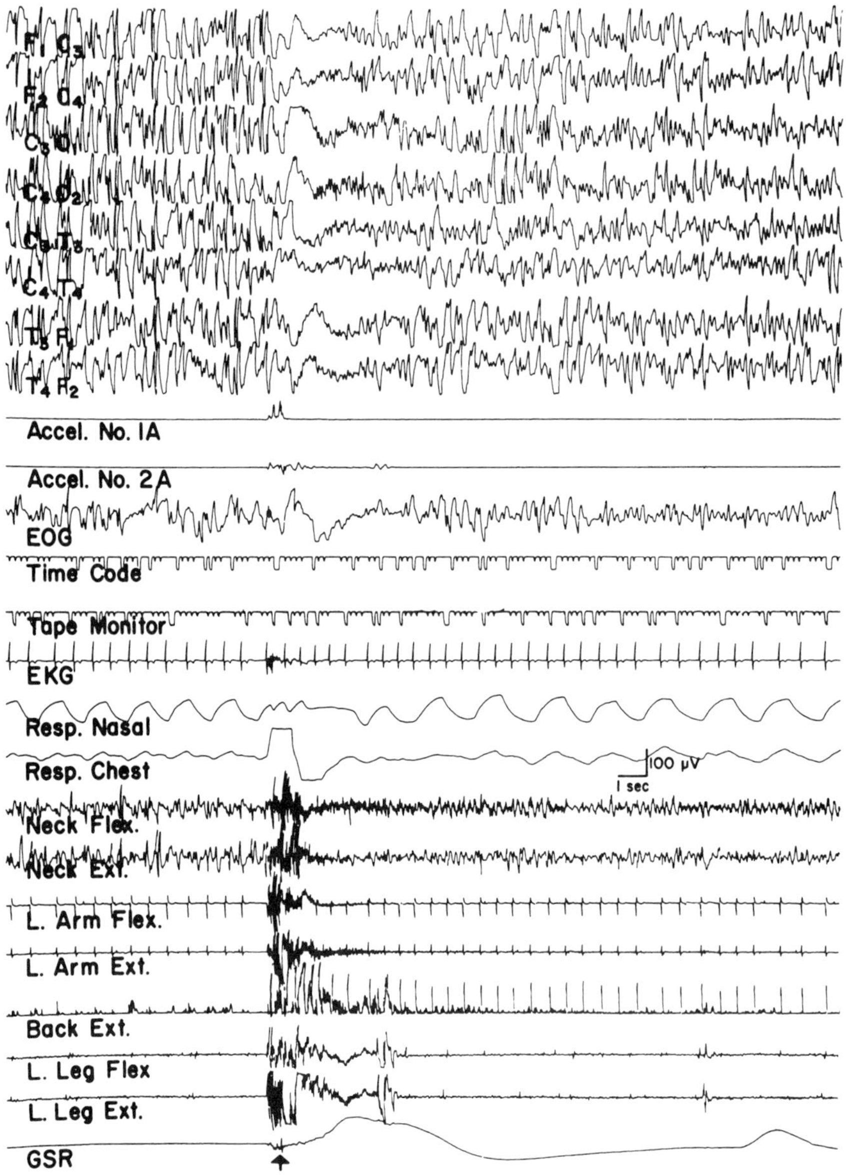

FIG. 2. EEG-polygraphic recording in a child with infantile spasms obtained simultaneously with video. A clinical spasm (*arrow*) is recorded. On EEG, it is associated with a high-voltage, sharp-and-slow wave followed by a brief period of generalized voltage attenuation. The background EEG preceding the spasm is hypsarrhythmic but normalizes transiently following the ictal event. Movement, recorded by triaxial accelerometers, is shown by an upward deflection (*Accel. channels*). Electromyographic electrodes placed over various muscle groups indicate that the clinical spasms involved both flexors and extensors. (Reproduced with permission from Kellaway, ref. 24.)

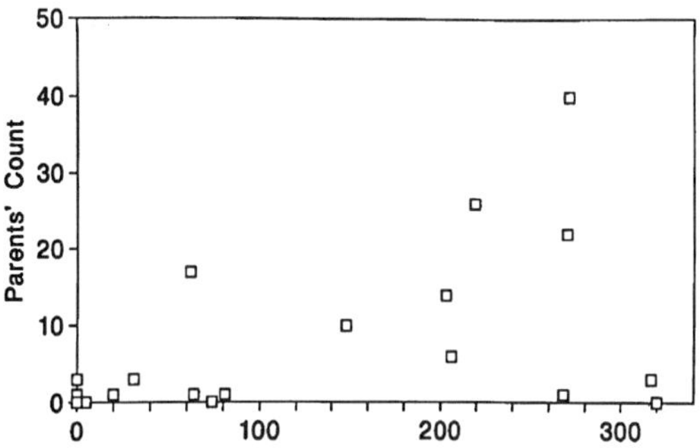

FIG. 3. Comparison of parents' estimation of spasm frequency with results of 24-hour EEG-polygraphic-video monitoring 2 to 4 weeks after institution of ACTH or prednisone therapy. The coefficient of determination (r^2) between the parents' count and the count obtained by video monitoring was .26. (Reproduced with permission from Hrachovy et al., ref. 29.)

ment of the interictal EEG from hypsarrhythmia to normal background activity. However, not all infants with infantile spasms demonstrate hypsarrhythmia on the initial EEG, and spasms can persist after therapy even when the background activity has improved (9,13).

The acute response to therapy—the cessation of spasms—has been characterized in investigations utilizing prolonged EEG-polygraphic-video monitoring studies (12,19,20). A response was defined as cessation of the clinical spasms and their ictal EEG accompaniment and has been determined to be an "all-or-nothing" phenomena. Thus, detection of any events, rather than determination of their frequency of occurrence in a given time period, is the critical factor in assessment. In clinical practice, physicians typically rely on parental observations to determine efficacy. However, parental observations are unreliable as a method of determining that spasms have stopped (Fig. 3). On the other hand, the witnessing of a spasm indicates that spasms persist. In addition, because of the episodic and inconsistent distribution of spasms over time, the reliability of assessment during relatively brief periods of observation is limited by sampling error; although the observation (or EEG recording) of spasms is significant, failure to detect spasms during a given time period is inconclusive.

Thus, it has been concluded that the only reliable method to document the cessation of infantile spasms as a result of therapy is prolonged EEG-polygraphic-video monitoring. Relatively brief routine EEGs can be adequate if spasms are present, because frequency of spasms is not an appropriate measure of treatment efficacy. However, a 12-hour monitoring study, recording both clinical and EEG features during wakefulness and sleep, is the single best method to document the absence of spasms and therapeutic efficacy (9,12,20).

Partial Seizures

The clinical assessment of AED efficacy in the treatment of partial seizures is limited by the features of the seizures themselves. The clinical character of either simple or complex partial seizures may prevent accurate seizure identification by observers or limit recognition by the patient that a seizure had occurred. Some seizures may occur primarily during nocturnal sleep and thus escape detection or determination of frequency. Most importantly, partial seizures may be infrequent, making it difficult to determine whether an absence of seizures for a long period of time can be attributed to AED efficacy.

Traditionally, the finding of focal spikes or sharp waves on the interictal EEG has been interpreted as a sign of potential epileptogenesis. However, spikes found in an untreated patient may persist following treatment with AEDs regardless of whether seizures are controlled or not. Change in the number of spikes in an individual patient following the initiation of AED therapy has also proved to be of limited value (21).

Quantitative studies focusing on the predictive value of the changes in the morphology of the spike induced by AED therapy have resulted in more promising findings. Frost and colleagues (22) devised a computer-assisted method of analyzing spike morphology that utilizes measurements of amplitude, duration, and sharpness (Fig. 4). The combined mea-

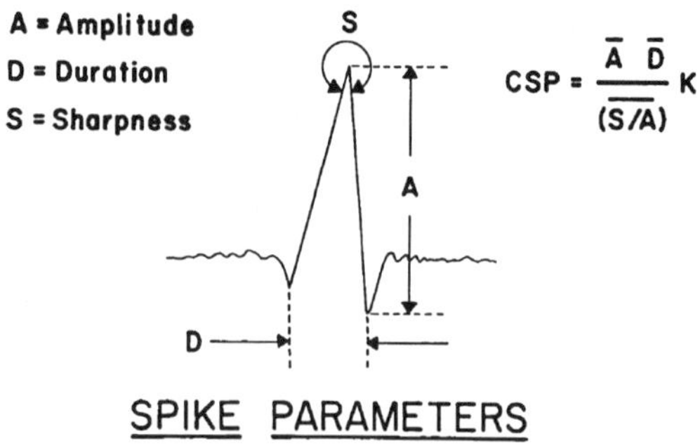

FIG. 4. Scheme used for determining spike parameters. *A*, amplitude; *D*, duration; *S*, sharpness; *A̅*, average amplitude; *D̅*, average duration; *S/A*, average normalized second derivative value at the peak (sharpness); *K*, constant scaling factor; *CSP*, composite spike parameter. (Reproduced with permission from Frost et al., ref. 22.)

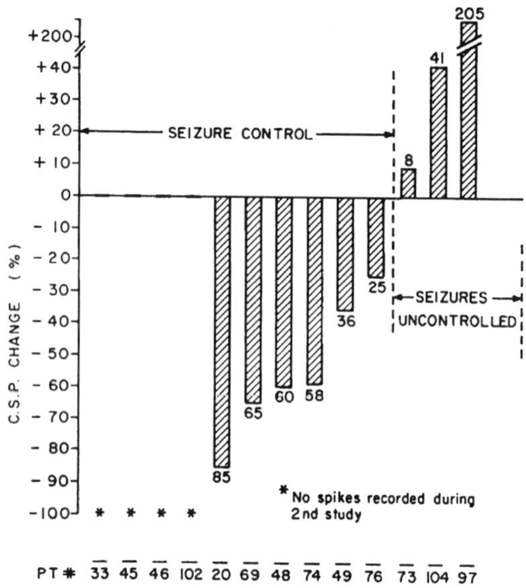

FIG. 5. Relationship between change in CSP after institution of therapy and seizure control outcome. Patient numbers are indicated on the horizontal axis. (Reproduced with permission from Frost et al., ref. 22.)

surements and a mathematical constant are calculated to provide a single score, referred to as the composite spike parameter (CSP). In their experimental design, a fixed number of spikes recorded during non-rapid-eye-movement (NREM) sleep were detected and analyzed by computer before initiation of AED treatment in patients with partial seizures. A single CSP score was determined for each patient before treatment began. The process was repeated after initiation of therapy with AEDs appropriate for the treatment of partial seizures once it had been determined that pharmacologic steady state had been achieved. A steady-state CSP score was then calculated for each patient. Each patient was followed clinically for a predefined time period extending well beyond the time of assignment of the steady-state CSP, so as to determine the occurrence and frequency of clinical seizures.

Changes in the pretreatment CSP in relation to the steady-state CSP were correlated with the long-term clinical outcome of each patient. A reduction in the CSP at steady state consistently predicted whether individual patients would experience seizure control (Fig. 5). Thus, application of CSP as an *acute* measure can be utilized to predict long-term AED efficacy and can serve as an objective method of assessment of AED therapy in patients with partial seizures.

Generalized Epilepsy with 3-Hz Spike-and-Wave Activity

Generalized epilepsy associated with 3-Hz spike-and-wave activity is characterized by absence, myoclonic, atonic, or tonic-clonic seizures, or combinations of these types. Absence seizures may be brief, frequent, and at times difficult for observers to detect or patients to recognize. When absence seizures occur in association with other types of generalized seizure, they may be infrequent and thus difficult to quantify. Similarly, when the other generalized seizure types are present alone, their relatively low frequency and sporadic occurrence make their assessment prone to sampling error by observers or the patient.

Determination of the occurrence of interictal generalized spike-and-wave activity during EEG-video monitoring studies for 24 to 36 hours in untreated patients with generalized epilepsy and 3-Hz spike-and-wave activity revealed a characteristic distribution of activity over time (23). Generalized spike-and-wave activity is typically most abundant during NREM sleep in comparison with REM sleep or the awake state (Fig. 6). Although the amount of spike-and-wave activity in a 24-hour period can vary widely between patients, the amount recorded in an individual patient on successive days is relatively constant.

Studies were made comparing the findings of sequential, continuous, 12- to 36-hour EEG-video recordings conducted before AED therapy with those obtained following incremental increases in AED serum levels (12,23–25) (Fig. 7). The absolute and relative changes in the abundance of spike-and-wave activity were determined for the entire period of each study for each patient, and the absolute reduction of spike-and-wave activity was determined for each stage of the sleep-wakefulness cycle in each patient. Seizure

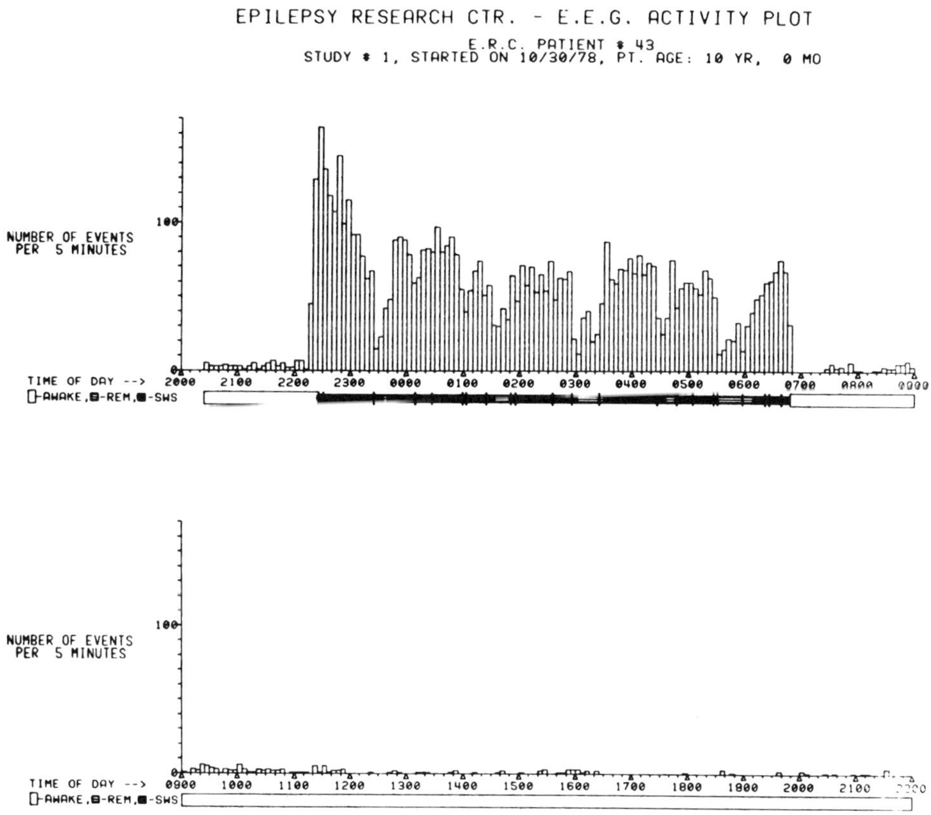

FIG. 6. Time modulation of generalized spike-and-wave in an untreated patient with absence epilepsy. The plot is made in 5-minute intervals to demonstrate details of the modulatory process. The onset of sleep is associated with an abrupt, steplike increase in spike activity that reaches its peak in about 15 minutes. Thereafter, there is a progressive decline throughout the remainder of the first slow-wave sleep cycle, which is independent of REM sleep. The first REM episode is very brief and appears to have little further effect, but as soon as the REM episode is over and the second slow-wave sleep cycle occurs, the spike activity again progressively increases, and the cycle is repeated five times throughout the night. With the onset of arousal, the spike activity is greatly attenuated and remains at zero level for the first 17 minutes of the awake state. The level of spike activity remains very low throughout the day, and there is a period between 16:20 and 20:00 hours when only six spikes occur. (Reproduced with permission from Kellaway, ref. 25).

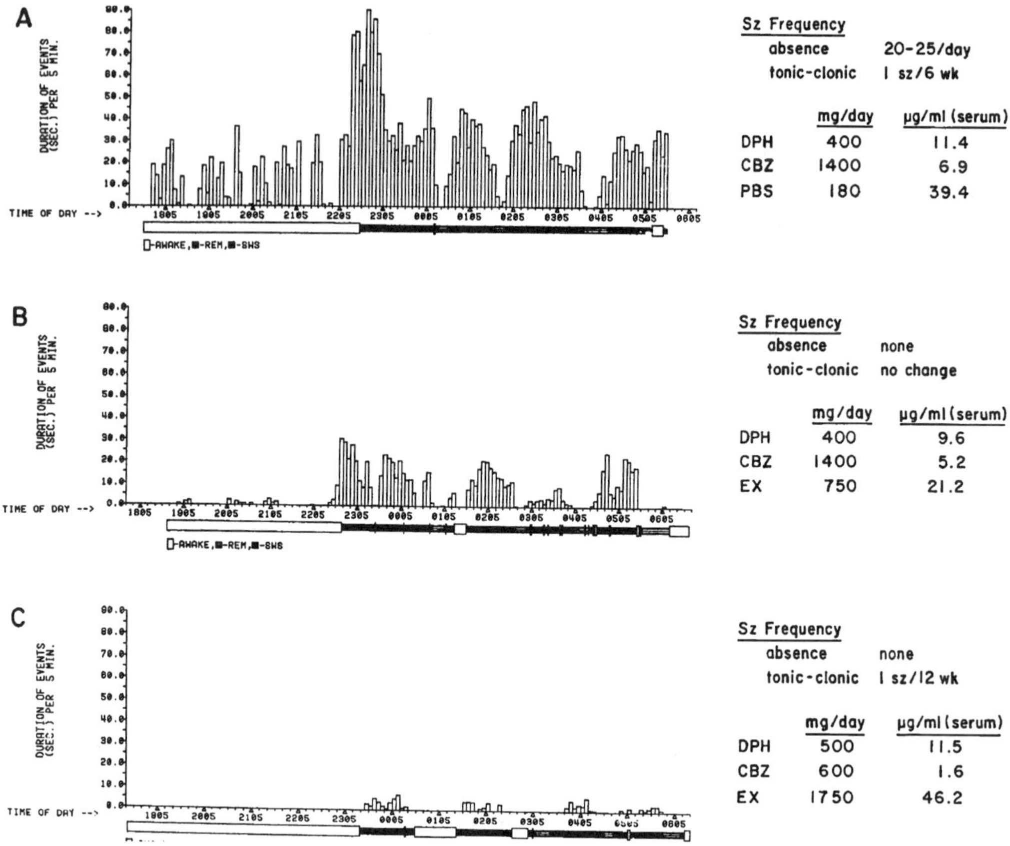

FIG. 7. Time plots of serial 12-hour monitoring sessions, showing amount of spike-and-wave activity in relation to wakefulness, REM sleep, and slow-wave sleep in patient with absence and generalized tonic-clonic seizures. **A:** Characteristic time-modulated distribution of spike-and-wave activity shows greatest activity in early slow-wave sleep, less activity in later slow-wave sleep, marked attenuation in REM sleep, and variable activity while the patient is awake. **B:** Treatment with ethosuximide (*EX*) reduces the amount of activity throughout the sleep-wake cycle. Activity is significantly reduced during wakefulness and REM sleep but persists in slow-wave sleep. **C:** Increased ethosuximide dose abolishes spike-and-wave activity in REM sleep and in the awake state and markedly reduces this activity in slow-wave sleep. Abolition of spike-and-wave activity in the awake state is consistent with the abolition of absence seizures. However, in patients with generalized tonic-clonic seizures as well as absences, persistence of spike-and-wave activity in any state is compatible with persistence of generalized tonic-clonic seizures. Further medical management in this patient included withdrawal of carbamazepine (*CBZ*), which did not alter her clinical course when used in maximal tolerated doses, and a gradual increase in ethosuximide to abolish remaining spike-and-wave activity in slow-wave sleep. *DPH*, phenytoin; *PBS*, phenobarbital. (Reproduced with permission from Mizrahi, ref. 30.)

occurrence was documented acutely by EEG-video monitoring and long-term by historical reporting of observers and patients.

These studies demonstrated the following: (a) There is a direct quantitative relationship between the incidence of seizures of absence, atonic, and/or myoclonic type and the overall measure of interictal spike-and-wave activity. (b) AEDs such as ethosuximide and valproate reduce and may eventually abolish spike-and-wave activity in EEG recordings of sufficient duration to include nocturnal sleep. (c) The rate of reduction of spike-and-wave activity in relation to increasing drug levels is a measure

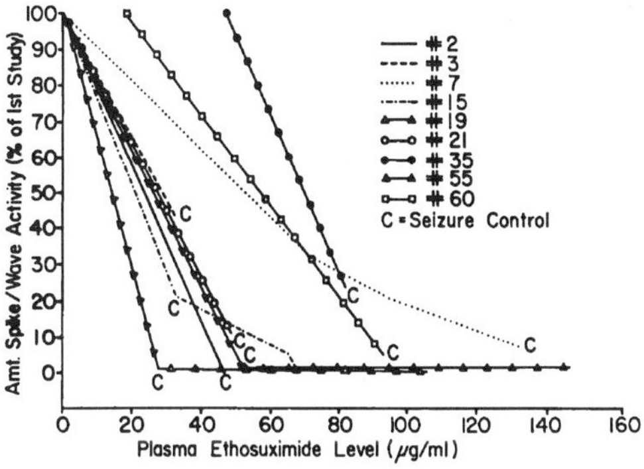

FIG. 8. Relationship between serum levels of ethosuximide, abundance of generalized spike-and-wave activity, and control of absence seizures. (Reproduced with permission from Kellaway, ref. 24.)

of drug effectiveness (Fig. 8). (d) With treatment, spike-and-wave activity disappears first in REM sleep, then in wakefulness, and last in nocturnal NREM sleep (Fig. 7). (e) At a serum AED level at which spike-and-wave activity is no longer present in wakefulness or REM sleep, absence, myoclonic, and atonic seizures no longer occur. (f) If any spike-and-wave activity occurs within the prolonged recording period, generalized tonic-clonic seizures can persist. (g) The relationship between reduced spike-and-wave activity and increasing serum levels of ethosuximide is initially linear, but it may become asymptotic at higher AED levels, with marked increases in levels producing only small further reductions in spike-and-wave activity (Fig. 8).

These findings indicate that for some types of generalized epilepsy, EEG can be used to predict the likelihood of further seizures in individual patients and provide an objective measure of AED effectiveness. Some applications may require overnight EEG studies with nocturnal recordings of slow-wave sleep. However, some findings of the studies of prolonged EEG records can be applied to the interpretation of shorter, routine EEGs recorded during the day. For example, the presence of spike-and-wave activity during the awake state on even a routine EEG is evidence that serum AED levels are not adequate to prevent absence seizures. However, a lack of spike-and-wave activity in a brief recording may reflect a sampling error (24,25).

In addition, the findings of a relatively brief, routine, daytime recording may suggest a degree of seizure control that under optimal clinical circumstances is characterized by absence of seizures but that under circumstances that stress the patient (e.g., sleep deprivation) is marked by breakthrough seizures despite stable AED serum levels. This has been referred to as a state of "fragile" seizure control (24) and is indicated by EEG findings of no spike-and-slow activity during wakefulness but an abundance of such activity during sleep (even daytime sleep). Further reduction of spike-and-wave activity in sleep can limit the potential for breakthrough seizures in such patients.

DETERMINATION OF ANTIEPILEPTIC DRUG TOXICITY

Analysis of the EEG in the determination of toxicity of AEDs is not as helpful as in assessment of efficacy for a number of reasons. Some AED-induced changes of the EEG background activity have no clinical significance, such as the induction of low- to moderate-voltage symmetric beta activity. Other AED-induced changes, such as generalized slowing of the background activity, usually are associated with signs of clinical toxicity (21,26). For the EEG to provide useful information concerning AED safety, any AED-induced finding should precede and predict the eventual onset of toxicity or should detect toxicity that may be too subtle to be noticed during standard neurologic examination such as the presence of cognitive dysfunction.

Recently, Frost and colleagues (27) conducted a prospective study of children treated with carbamazepine for partial seizures to identify associated EEG alterations. Their goal was to identify EEG changes immediately following institution of therapy that were predictive of subsequent decline in specific cognitive parameters for each patient. A complete neuropsychologic assessment and an EEG were performed before the initiation of AED therapy. The neuropsychologic tests included a standard Wechsler Intelligence Scale for Children, Revised (WISC-R) and age-appropriate instruments to evaluate language, motor, perceptual, and performance skills and academic achievement. A 30-second segment of EEG, with the child awake and with eyes closed, was selected for computer analysis. A quantitative summary of average frequency and amplitude characteristics was obtained from the electrodes derived from the occipital regions; thus, the alpha rhythm of each patient was objectively characterized.

Children were restudied 2 weeks after attainment of a therapeutic AED level with EEG only (initial treatment study) and 1 year after initiation of therapy with both neuropsychologic testing and EEG. The alpha frequency decreased slightly in the initial treatment study in most patients. However, a decline of >0.5 Hz in the initial treatment EEG was observed in a subset of children who subsequently demonstrated a decline in neuropsychologic performance 1 year after onset of AED therapy (Fig. 9). These findings suggest that quantitative analysis of the alpha rhythm frequency can be useful to identify individuals early in the course of AED treatment who are at increased risk for the subsequent development of cognitive changes related to their medical therapy.

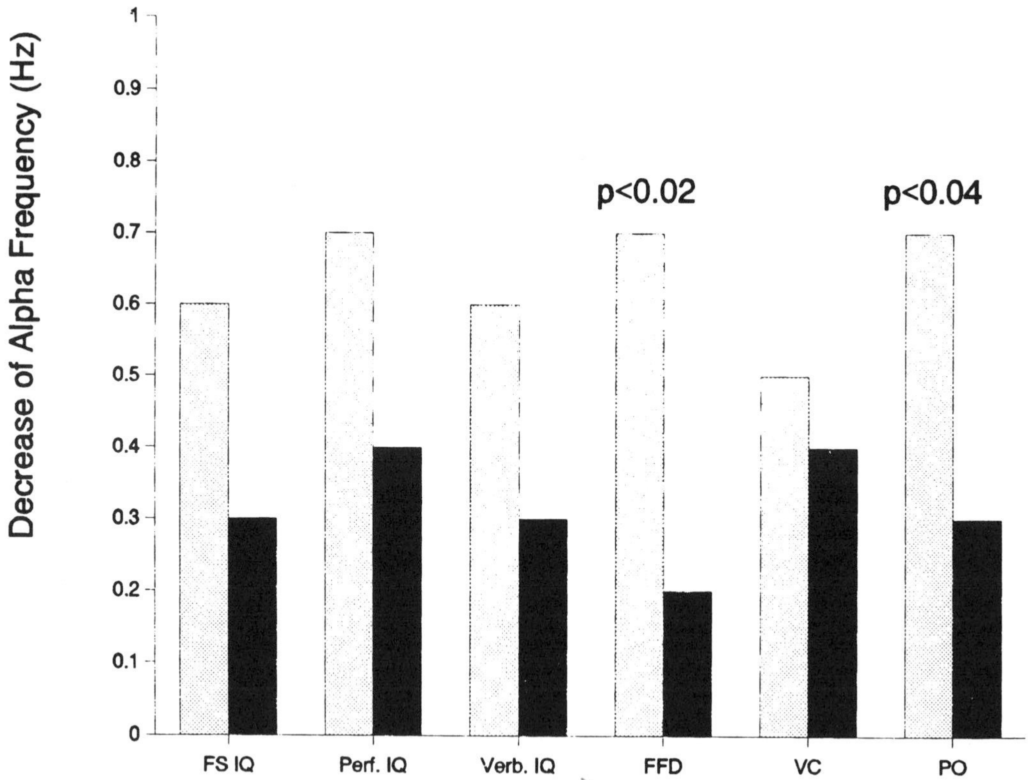

FIG. 9. Average decrease in alpha frequency observed following initiation of carbamazepine therapy in children exhibiting decreased performance on the WISC-R (–) (*gray bars*) compared with the change in alpha frequency documented in patients whose neurologic status improved or showed no change (+ or 0) (*black bars*) for each of the categories. *FS IQ*, Full-Scale IQ; *Perf. IQ*, Performance IQ; *Verb. IQ*, Verbal IQ; *FFD*, Freedom From Distractibility factor; *VC*, Verbal Comprehension factor: *PO*, Perceptual Organization factor. (Reproduced with permission from Frost et al., ref. 27.)

ACKNOWLEDGMENT

Investigations cited here and conducted at the Epilepsy Research Center were supported by Grant No. NS11535, National Institute of Neurological Disorders and Stroke, NIH.

REFERENCES

1. Mizrahi EM, Kellaway P. Characterization and classification of neonatal seizures. *Neurology* 1987;37: 1837–1844.
2. Kellaway P, Hrachovy RA. Status epilepticus in newborns: a perspective on neonatal seizures. *Adv Neurol* 1983;34:93–99 (Delgado-Escueta AV, Wasterlain CG, Treiman DM, Porter RJ, eds. *Status Epilepticus*).
3. Hrachovy RA, Mizrahi EM, Kellaway P. Electroencephalography of the newborn. In: Daly D, Pedley TA, eds. *Current Practice of Clinical Electroencephalography*. 2nd ed. New York: Raven Press; 1990:201–242.
4. Mizrahi EM, Kellaway P. The response of electroclinical neonatal seizures to antiepileptic drug therapy. *Epilepsia* 1992;33(Suppl 3):S144.
5. Kellaway P, Hrachovy R. Electroencephalography. In: Swaiman KF, Wright FS, eds. *The Practice of Pediatric Neurology*. 2nd ed. St. Louis: CV Mosby; 1982;96–114 (vol 1).
6. Gotman J, Flanagan D, Rosenblatt B, Bye A, Mizrahi EM. Automatic seizure detection in newborns: validation with multicenter data. *Epilepsia* 1996;7(Suppl 5):62.
7. Flanagan D, Gotman J, Rosenblatt B, Bye A, Mizrahi EM. Multicenter validation of automated seizure detection in the newborn. *J Clin Neurophysiol* 1997;14(2):162.
8. Gotman J, Flanagan D, Rosenblatt B, Bye A, Mizrahi EM. Multicenter validation of automated seizure detection for the newborn EEG. *Electroencephalogr Clin Neurophysiol* 1997, *in press*.
9. Hrachovy RA, Frost JD Jr. Severe encephalopathic epilepsy in infants: infantile spasms. In: Dodson WE, Pellock, eds. *Pediatric Epilepsy: Diagnosis and Therapy*. New York: Demos; 1993:135–145.
10. Lacy JR, Penry JK. *Infantile Spasms*. New York: Raven Press; 1976.
11. Lombroso CT. Prognosis in neonatal seizures. *Adv Neurol* 1983;34:101–113.
12. Kellaway P, Hrachovy RA, Frost JD Jr, Zion T. Precise characterization and quantification of infantile spasms. *Ann Neurol* 1979;6:214–218.
13. Hrachovy RA, Frost JD Jr, Kellaway P. Hypsarrhythmia: variations on the theme. *Epilepsia* 1984;25:317–325.
14. Hrachovy RA, Frost JD Jr, Kellaway P, Zion TE. Double-blind study of ACTH vs. prednisone therapy in infnatile spasms. *J Pediatr* 1983;103:641–645.
15. Singer WD, Rabe EF, Haller JS. The effect of ACTH therapy upon infantile spasms. *J Pediatr* 1980;96:485–489.
16. Snead OC III, Benton JW, Myers CJ. ACTH and prednisone in childhood seizure disorders. *Neurology* 1983; 33:966–970.
17. Chugani HT, Shields WD, Shewman DA, Olson DM, Phelps ME, Peacock WJ. Infantile spasms: I. PET identifies focal cortical dysgenesis in cryptogenic cases for surgical treatment. *Ann Neurol* 1990;27:406–413.
18. Glaze DG, Hrachovy RA, Frost JD Jr, Kellaway P, Zion TE. Prospective study of outcome of infants with infantile spasms during controlled studies of ACTH and prednisone. *J Pediatr* 1988;112:389–396.
19. Hrachovy RA, Frost JD Jr. Intensive monitoring of infantile spasms. In: Schmidt D, Morselli PL, eds. *Intractable Epilepsy: Experimental and Clinical Aspects*. New York: Raven Press; 1986:87–97.
20. Frost JD Jr, Hrachovy RA, Kellaway P, Zion T. Quantitative analysis and characterization of infantile spasms. *Epilepsia* 1978;19:273–282.
21. Bazil CW, Pedley TA. General principles. Neurophysiological effects of antiepileptic drugs. In: Levy RH, Mattson RH, Meldrum BS, eds. *Antiepileptic Drugs*. 4th ed. New York: Raven Press; 1975:79–89.
22. Frost JD Jr, Kellaway P, Hrachovy RA, Glaze DG, Mizrahi EM. Changes in epileptic spike configuration associated with attainment of seizure control. *Ann Neurol* 1986;20:723–726.
23. Kellaway P. The incidence, significance and natural history of spike foci in children. In: CE Henry (Ed.), *Current Clinical Neurophysiology: Update on EEG and Evoked Potentials*. Elsevier/North-Holland, New York, 1981:151–175.
24. Kellaway P. Childhood seizures. In: Gotman J, Ives JR, Gloor P, eds. *Long-term Monitoring in Epilepsy*. New York: Elsevier; 1985;267–283 (EEG Suppl No. 37).
25. Kellaway P. Intensive monitoring in infants and children. *Adv Neurol* 1986;46:127–137 (Gumnit RJ, ed. *Intensive Neurodiagnostic Monitoring*).
26. Glaze DG. Drug effects. In: Daly DD, Pedley TA, eds. *Current Practice of Clinical Electroencephalography*. 2nd ed. New York; Raven Press; 1990:489–512.
27. Frost JD Jr, Hrachovy RA, Glaze DG, Rettig GM. Alpha rhythm slowing during initiation of carbamazepine therapy: implications for future cognitive performance. *J Clin Neurophysiol* 1995;12:57–63.
28. Kellaway P, Mizrahi EM. Clinical, electroencephalographic, therapeutic, and pathophysiologic studies of neonatal seizures. In: Wasterlain CG, Vert P, eds. *Neonatal Seizures*. New York: Raven Press; 1990: 1–13.
29. Hrachovy RA, Frost JD Jr, Glaze DG. Single-blind study of high-dose vs. low-dose ACTH therapy in infantile spasms. *Epilepsia* 1992;33:113.
30. Mizrahi EM. Electroencephalographic/polygraphic/video monitoring in childhood epilepsy. *J Pediatr* 1984; 105:1–9.
31. Kellaway P. Maturational and biorhythmic changes in the electroencephalogram. In: Anderson VE, Hauser WA, Penry JK, Sing CF, eds. *Genetic Basis of the Epilepsies*. New York: Raven Press; 1982;21–33.
32. Kellaway P, Frost JD Jr. Biorhythmic modulation of epileptic events. In: Pedley TA, Meldrum BS, eds. *Recent Advances in Epilepsy*. New York: Churchill Livingstone; 1983:139–154 (vol 1).

Antiepileptic Drug Development.
Advances in Neurology, Vol. 76,
edited by J. French, I. Leppik, and M. A. Dichter.
Lippincott–Raven Publishers, Philadelphia © 1998.

22

Routine Measurement of New Antiepileptic Drug Concentrations: A Critique and a Prediction

Martin J. Brodie

Epilepsy Unit, Department of Medicine and Therapeutics, Western Infirmary, Glasgow G11 6NT, Scotland.

INTRODUCTION

With the advent of simple, robust, reliable, and convenient assay techniques, therapeutic drug monitoring of antiepileptic drugs has become widely accepted into clinical practice (1). Nevertheless, indiscriminate and unthinking measurement of anticonvulsant levels has attracted criticism (2–4). Accordingly, guidelines for their correct use have been produced by the International League Against Epilepsy (5). What is the situation regarding the likely usefulness of routine monitoring with the newer agents? This chapter concentrates on vigabatrin, lamotrigine, and gabapentin. Felbamate is unlikely now to be used in sufficient numbers of patients for its concentration-effect-toxicity profile to be explored adequately, and there are too few clinical data with oxcarbazepine, topiramate, tiagabine, or zonisamide to allow any useful conclusions to be reached at present.

DEFINITION

Therapeutic drug monitoring can be defined as the pragmatic manipulation of the dose of an antiepileptic drug, using the plasma concentration as a guide, to optimize its efficacy, avoid or identify toxicity, and detect or confirm poor compliance.

CLINICAL FACTORS

For therapeutic monitoring of an antiepileptic drug to be useful in patient care, clinical questions other than "What is the drug level?" must be answered. Such questions would include the following: "Is the current dose likely to provide complete seizure control?" "How much leeway do I have to increase the dose?" "Are the patients' symptoms likely to be caused by drug toxicity?" "Is the patient taking the medication according to instructions?" Monitoring with the established antiepileptic drugs has been found helpful in a number of clinical settings (6), some of which are listed below:

1. A patient has recently started taking an antiepileptic drug.
2. A patient has poor control despite an apparently adequate dose.
3. A patient has symptoms that may be caused by drug toxicity.
4. A patient is suspected of poor compliance with the dosage schedule.
5. A patient is taking more than one antiepileptic drug and is still having seizures.
6. A patient on combination therapy is experiencing side effects.
7. A patient has severe hepatic or renal disease.

8. A drug is being given to a prepubertal child, a pregnant woman, or an elderly patient.

PHARMACOLOGIC CONSIDERATIONS

Comprehensive data now exist on the kinetics of all new antiepileptic drugs (7). For monitoring to be of clinical value, it is axiomatic that the circulating concentration of the drug correlates better with the anticonvulsant effect and/or symptoms and signs of toxicity than does the dose. The minimal effective and maximal safe concentrations of a few drugs can be combined to provide a "target" or "therapeutic" range around which the dose can be adjusted (3). For these criteria to be applicable, a number of pharmacologic requirements must be met; these are listed in Table 1.

With all new antiepileptic drugs, good pharmacokinetic data are always available from volunteers and from epileptic patients who have been given single doses at an early stage in the development program. Attempts are also made to identify pharmacokinetic interactions with other antiepileptic drugs. However, as few patients will have received the drug in clinical trials at a fixed dosage, data to support therapeutic monitoring as an adjunct to clinical practice at the launch of a new moiety are invariably lacking. Such studies, in particular those exploring the relation between concentration and efficacy and/or toxicity, are undertaken only after the drug has been used to treat many patients worldwide.

Chromatography is not a suitable method for routine therapeutic monitoring of an antiepileptic drug, as it is expensive and cumbersome and requires substantial laboratory expertise. The development of a simple enzyme immunoassay method for measuring the compound usually comes along only when this is perceived to be attractive commercially—that is, when the drug has attained an established place in the therapeutic armamentarium and when measurement of the circulating concentration appears to be clinically useful.

TABLE 1. *Pharmacologic requirements determining the suitability of an antiepileptic drug for routine therapeutic monitoring*

1. Accurate kinetic information in epileptic patients taking the drug as monotherapy and in combination with other antiepileptic drugs
2. Poor correlation between the dose and the circulating concentration of the drug—that is, substantial pharmacokinetic variability
3. Good correlation between the concentration of the drug and its antiepileptic effect and/or the emergence of side effects—that is, minimal pharmacodynamic variability
4. Narrow target range between effective and toxic levels of the drug appropriate to the majority of treated epileptic patients
5. Simple, accurate, reliable, widely available, and cheap assay for the drug

NEW ANTIEPILEPTIC DRUGS

In the following sections, the criteria set forth above are considered in relation to the three best-established new antiepileptic drugs. Chromatographic assays are available for all three agents: vigabatrin (8,9), lamotrigine (10,11), and gabapentin (12,13). An immunofluorometric method has also been published for lamotrigine (14). More than 200,000 patients have been treated to date with lamotrigine and more than 100,000 with vigabatrin and gabapentin.

Vigabatrin

Vigabatrin was the first new antiepileptic drug to be licensed in the U.K. in 1989. Since then, it has become available for general prescription as add-on therapy throughout Europe, Africa, and Asia, although it has not yet been approved in the United States. It is a racemate, with the (*S*)-enantiomer responsible for the drug's pharmacologic activity (15). The major mode of action of vigabatrin is unique; the drug acts as a "suicide" inhibitor of γ-aminobutyric acid transaminase (GABA-T), the enzyme responsible for the catabolism of the important inhibitory neurotransmitter GABA. It is excreted unchanged by the kidney and has a short elimination half-life of 5 to 7 hours (16). Correlation between the dose and concentration is poor because of marked interindividual variation in vigabatrin levels during a dosage interval (17). Vigabatrin destroys its target enzyme by binding to it irreversibly, and so *de novo* synthesis is necessary for recovery, a process that takes some days (15). Accordingly, the duration of effect of vigabatrin exceeds 24 hours, and the drug is usually administered once or twice daily (18). Monitoring vigabatrin concentrations, therefore, is not helpful in predicting clinical response (9) or the emergence of side effects (19).

Lamotrigine

Lamotrigine was launched in 1991 as a treatment for refractory epilepsy in the U.K. and Ireland, its first markets. It is now available for general prescription as adjunctive therapy in more than 70 countries. More recently, it has been licensed for use in children as monotherapy in some of these. It exerts its effect, in part at least, by selectively blocking the slow, inactivated state of the sodium channel (20). Its elimination half-life exceeds 24 hours in drug-naïve patients, in whom kinetics are linear at therapeutic dosage (21). Enzyme-inducing antiepileptic drugs reduce the half-life to around 15 hours, whereas sodium valproate inhibits lamotrigine metabolism, lengthening its half-life to 60 hours or more (22). A combination of valproate and an inducer returns the half-life to around 24 hours.

A notional target range of 1 to 4 mg/L was chosen arbitrarily for lamotrigine as a basis for the initial clinical trial program (23,24). However, no good correlation has been reported between lamotrigine levels and its efficacy or toxicity (25). In a recent prospective study of lamotrigine therapy (26), 32 patients became seizure-free at widely varying daily doses (median, 200 mg; range, 25 to 850 mg) and plasma concentrations (median, 3.6 mg/L; range, 1.4 to 18.7 mg) (Fig. 1). Like-

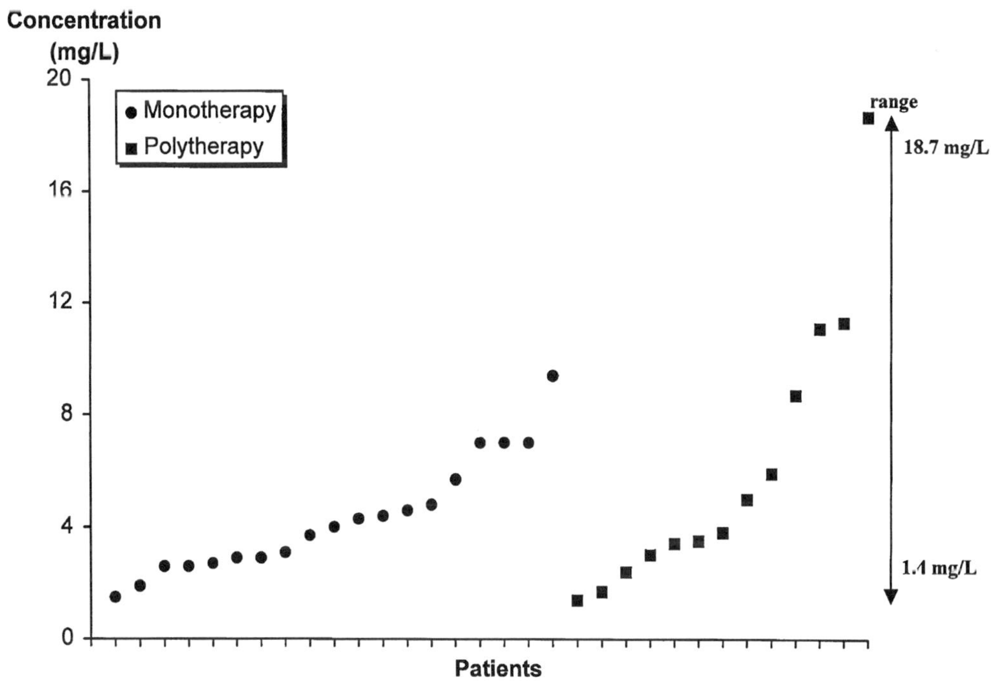

FIG. 1. Lamotrigine concentrations in 32 seizure-free patients. (From Kilpatrick et al., ref. 26, with permission.)

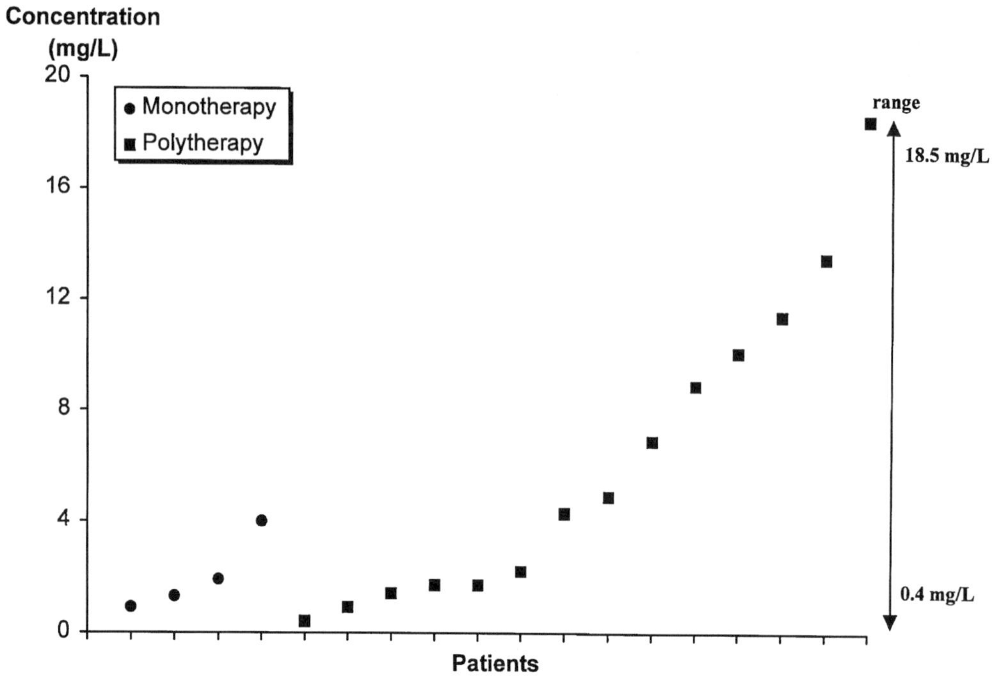

FIG. 2. Lamotrigine concentrations in 18 patients with side effects abating on dose reduction. (From Kilpatrick et al., ref. 26, with permission.)

wise, in 18 patients who experienced intolerable side effects that abated with a reduction in dosage, there were similar substantial variations in daily lamotrigine doses (median, 300 mg; range, 100 to 900 mg) and circulating concentrations (median, 4 mg/L; range, 0.4 to 18.5 mg/L) (Fig. 2). It is therefore unlikely that an isolated concentration of lamotrigine will be of any clinical value in predicting optimal seizure control or the development of side effects.

Gabapentin

Although structurally related to GABA, gabapentin does not appear to have a primary GABAergic mechanism of action (27). Recent evidence suggests that it may act by blocking calcium channels in the brain (28). Like vigabatrin, gabapentin is excreted unchanged by the kidney and has a short elimination half-life of 5 to 7 hours (29). Variable absorption at high dosage together with substantial interindividual variation during a dosage interval results in a wide range of concentrations in different patients treated according to similar dosage schedules (Fig. 3). The situation is further complicated by the suggestion that this absorptive process may be saturable (30).

Data with gabapentin on concentration-effect-toxicity relationships are sparse (31). A dose-related improvement in seizure control and a linear correlation between gabapentin dose and plasma concentration were found in one study (32). In the U.K. Gabapentin Study (33), mean concentrations were higher (not surprisingly!) in responders than in nonresponders, and increased efficacy was associated with higher concentrations of the drug. Sivenius and colleagues (34) observed a therapeutic effect only when plasma gabapentin levels exceeded 2 mg/L. In our own patients, a 50% or greater response has been noted in some patients with gabapentin concentrations exceeding 10 mg/L (35). One patient with renal impairment reported a 67% reduction in seizure numbers without side effects while tak-

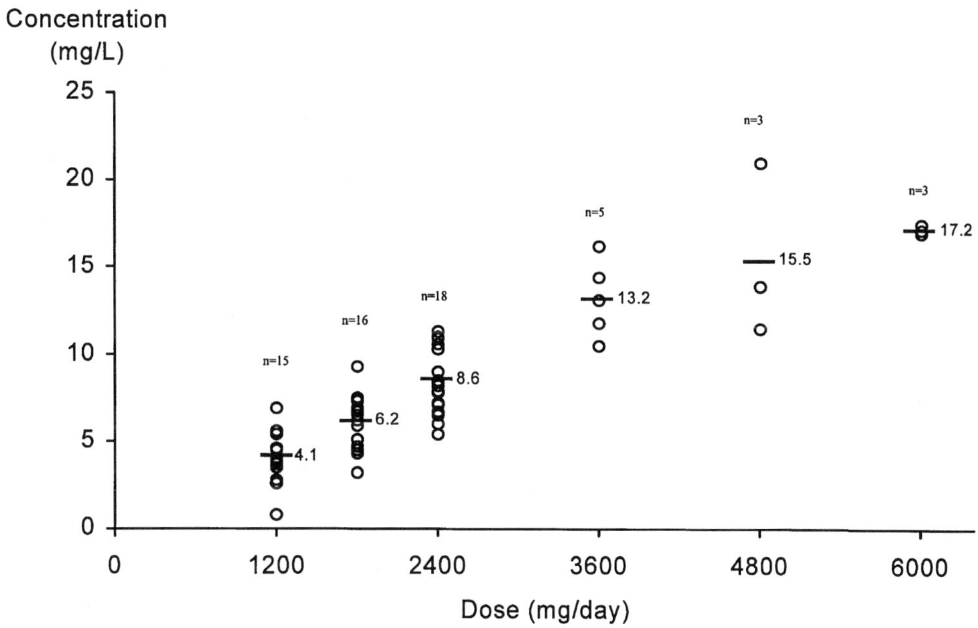

FIG. 3. Gabapentin concentrations at the same time since dosing in patients on different treatment schedules.

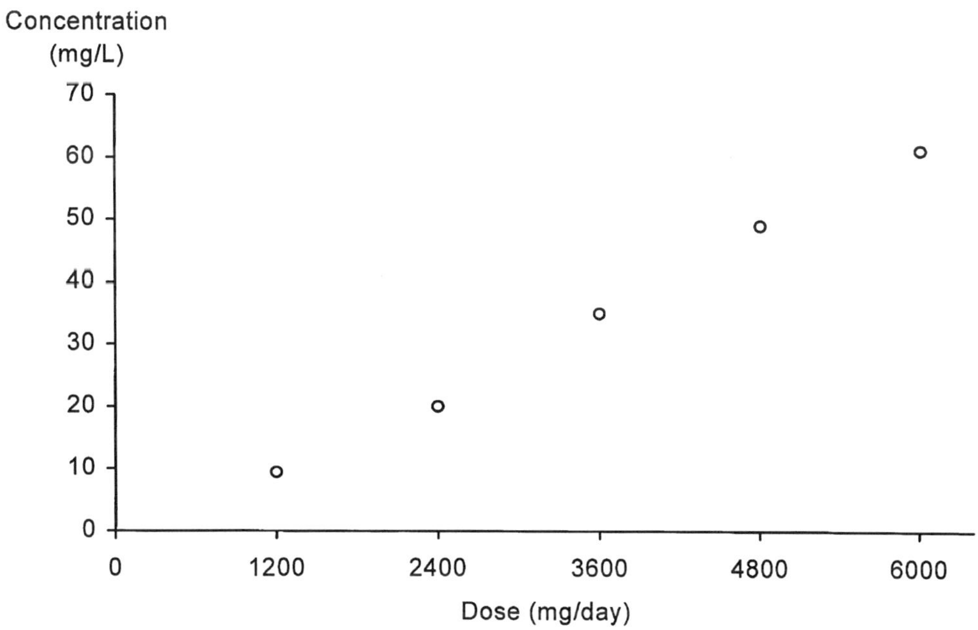

FIG. 4. Gabapentin concentrations at the same time since dosing in a patient with renal impairment.

ing 6000 mg of gabapentin daily. On this dose, the plasma gabapentin level was 61.2 mg/L (Fig. 4). Because of its short elimination half-life, circulating gabapentin concentrations during a dosage interval can be expected to exceed 100% (Fig. 5). In addition, Ben-Menachem (36) and colleagues could find no linear relationship between plasma and cerebrospinal fluid gabapentin levels in patients receiving long-term treatment. In rodents, disequilibrium between plasma and brain concentrations of gabapentin has been reported (37). Not surprisingly, therefore, gabapentin concentrations have not been shown to be clinically useful in predicting efficacy or toxicity with the drug (31). All these factors make the identification of a useful target range for plasma gabapentin highly unlikely.

DISCUSSION

Unless a drug has a long elimination half-life exceeding 24 hours, such as phenobarbital, it is usually necessary to stipulate the timing of blood sampling in relation to the previous dose if the clinical benefits of therapeutic drug monitoring are to be maximized. A trough concentration is usually employed for drugs with short elimination half-lives, although the evidence in support of this approach is weak (6). If the concern is toxicity, a peak concentration is likely to be more helpful. At the very least, any symptoms should be related to the time since the last dose was taken. No such data are currently available for any of the three drugs considered in this chapter.

In Table 2, the suitability of vigabatrin, lamotrigine, and gabapentin for therapeutic monitoring according to the criteria discussed in Table 1 is considered. All three drugs fall far short of fulfilling these requirements. Vigabatrin, a racemate, has a much longer duration of effect than would be predicted from its half-life. No good correlation between its concentration and efficacy or side effects has

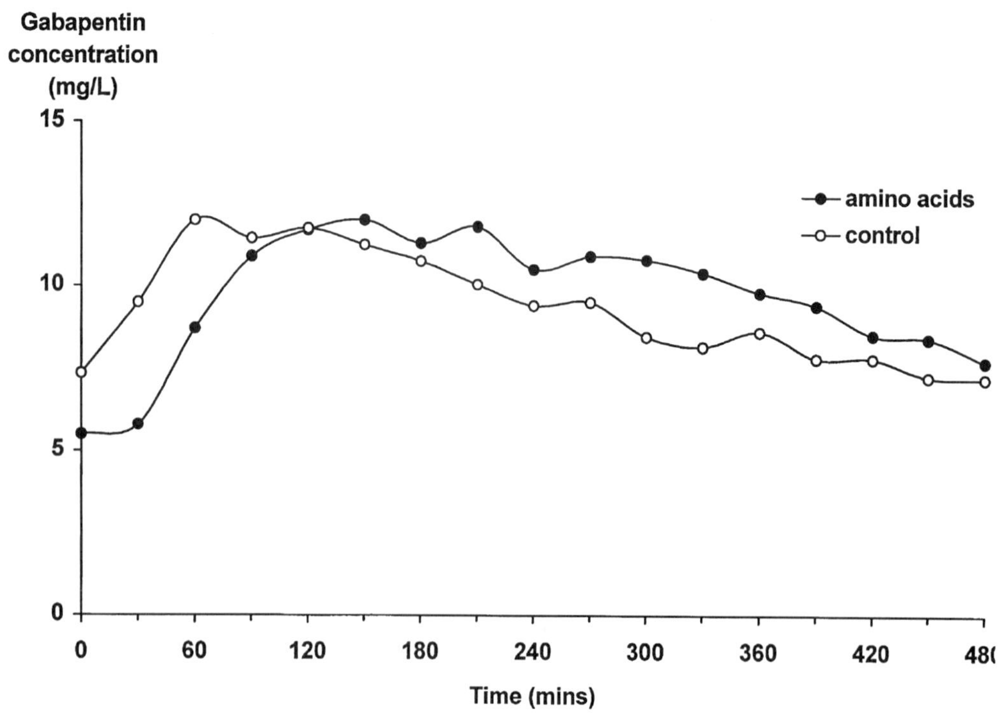

FIG. 5. Gabapentin concentrations during a dosing interval in a patient taking 2 g three times daily with or without amino acid supplementation.

TABLE 2. *Criteria for therapeutic monitoring in relation to three new antiepileptic drugs*

	Vigabatrin	Lamotrigine	Gabapentin
Kinetics well worked out	No	Yes	No
Wide pharmacokinetic variability	Yes	Yes	Yes
Little pharmacodynamic variability	No	No	No
Established target range	No	No	No
Easy, cheap, reliable assay	No	No	No
Percentage of "correct" answers	20%	40%	20%

been identified. Lamotrigine, on the face of it a better bet for therapeutic monitoring, is well tolerated by some patients at concentrations above 10 mg/L, whereas headache, nausea, and dizziness inexplicably develop in others at levels below 2 mg/L. Gabapentin has a short elimination half-life that may or may not mirror its duration of action. There is no good correlation between plasma and cerebrospinal fluid concentrations. Some patients benefit from doses as high as 6000 mg daily with high circulating concentrations. No useful relationship has been shown between gabapentin levels and the clinical response to the drug.

Even as a measure of compliance, a plasma level of any of these drugs is likely to tell the clinician only whether or not the patient has taken it recently. Some notion of whether the levels are "high" or "low" will also be obtained, perhaps hinting at the likely leeway for an increment in dose. Nevertheless, dosage can be adjusted perfectly adequately on clinical grounds alone. The patient will tell the doctor whether the dose is "therapeutic" or "toxic," not the biochemist. Finally, although chromatographic assays are available for all three compounds, these are complex and do not fulfill the criteria of simplicity, ease of use, and cheapness. An immunofluorometric assay for lamotrigine has been published (14), but is not yet in widespread use.

CONCLUSION

Although it is early days yet, it seems likely that routine monitoring of vigabatrin, lamotrigine, and gabapentin at the epilepsy clinic will not prove clinically useful except in a very few patients. Assaying these drugs should currently be undertaken only as a research tool. Alternate approaches are needed to monitor the efficacy and toxicity of new antiepileptic drugs (38).

REFERENCES

1. Brodie MJ, Dichter MA. Antiepileptic drugs. *N Engl J Med* 1996;334:168–175.
2. Chadwick DW. Overuse of monitoring of blood concentrations of antiepileptic drugs. *Br Med J* 1987;2: 723–724.
3. Brodie MJ, Feely J. Practical clinical pharmacology. Therapeutic drug monitoring and clinical trials. *Br Med J* 1988;296:1110–1114.
4. Dodson WE. Level off. *Neurology* 1989;39:1009–1010.
5. Commission on Antiepileptic Drugs, International League Against Epilepsy. Guidelines for therapeutic monitoring of antiepileptic drugs. *Epilepsia* 1993; 34: 585–587.
6. McKee PJW, Brodie MJ. Therapeutic drug monitoring. In: Engel J, Pedley TA, eds. *Epilepsy: a Comprehensive Textbook*. New York: Lippincott-Raven Publishers; 1997: 1181–1194.
7. Walker MK, Patsalos PN. Clinical pharmacokinetics of new antiepileptic drugs. *Pharmacol Ther* 1995;67: 351–384.
8. Tsanaclis LM, Wicks J, Williams J, Richens A. Determination of vigabatrin in plasma by reverse-phase high-performance liquid chromatography. *Ther Drug Monit* 1991;13:251–253.
9. Löscher W, Fassbender CP, Gram L, Kramer M, Hostermann D, Zahner B, Stefan H. Determination of GABA and vigabatrin in human plasma by a rapid and simple HPLC method: correlation between clinical response to vigabatrin and increase in plasma GABA. *Epilepsy Res* 1993;14:245–255.
10. Cohen AF, Land GS, Breimer DD, Yuen WC, Winton C, Peck AW. Lamotrigine, a new anticonvulsant: pharmacokinetics in normal humans. *Clin Pharmacol Ther* 1987;42:535–541.
11. Cociglio M, Alric R, Bouvier O. Performance analysis of a reversed-phase liquid chromatographic assay of lamotrigine in plasma using solvent-demixing extraction. *J Chromatogr* 1991;572:269 276.
12. Hengy H, Kolle EU. Determination of gabapentin in plasma and urine by high-performance liquid chromatography and pre-column labelling for ultraviolet detection. *J Chromatogr* 1985;341:473–478.
13. Forrest G, Sills GJ, Leach JP, Brodie MJ. Determination of gabapentin in plasma by high-performance liquid chromatography. *J Chromatogr* 1996;681:421–425.

14. Sailstad JM, Findlay JWA. Immunofluoromatic assay for lamotrigine (Lamictal) in human plasma. *Ther Drug Monit* 1991;13:433–442.
15. Sabers A, Gram L. Pharmacology of vigabatrin. *Pharmacol Toxicol* 1992;7:237–243.
16. Leach JP, Brodie MJ. Novel antiepileptic drugs: an explosion of activity. *Seizure* 1995;4:5–17.
17. McKee PJW, Blacklaw J, Friel E, Thompson GG, Gillham RA, Brodie MJ. Adjuvant vigabatrin in refractory epilepsy: a ceiling to effective dosage in individual patients? *Epilepsia* 1993;34:937–943.
18. Ben-Menachem E, Persson L, Mumford J. Long-term evaluation of once-daily vigabatrin in drug-resistant partial epilepsy. *Epilepsy Res* 1990;5:240–246.
19. Grant SM, Heel RC. Vigabatrin. *Drugs* 1991;41: 839–926.
20. Xie X, Lancaster B, Peakman T, Garthwaite J. Interaction of the antiepileptic drug lamotrigine with recombinant rat brain type Iia Na^+ channels and with native Na^+ channels in rat hippocampal neurones. *Pflugers Arch Eur J Physiol* 1995;430:437–440.
21. Brodie MJ. Lamotrigine. *Lancet* 1992;339:1397–1400.
22. Brodie MJ. Lamotrigine versus other antiepileptic drugs: a star rating system is born. *Epilepsia* 1994;35 (Suppl 5):S41–S46.
23. Leach JP, Brodie MJ. Lamotrigine: clinical use. In: Levy RH, Mattson RH, Meldrum BS, eds. *Antiepileptic Drugs*. 4th ed. New York: Raven Press; 1995: 889–895.
24. Brodie MJ, Richens A, Yuen AWC, the UK Lamotrigine/Carbamazepine Monotherapy Trial Group. Double-blind comparison of lamotrigine and carbamazepine in newly diagnosed epilepsy. *Lancet* 1995;345: 476–479.
25. Rambeck B, Wolf P. Lamotrigine clinical pharmacokinetics. *Clin Pharmacokinet* 1993;25:433–443.
26. Kilpatrick ES, Forrest G, Brodie MJ. Concentration-effect and concentration-toxicity relations with lamotrigine—a prospective study. *Epilepsia* 1996;37:534–538.
27. Goldlust A, Su T-Z, Welty DF, Taylor CP, Oxender DL. Effects of anticonvulsant drug gabapentin on the enzymes in metabolic pathways of glutamate and GABA. *Epilepsy Res* 1995;22:1–11.
28. Gee NS, Brown JP, Dissanayake VUK, Offord J, Woodruff GN. The novel anticonvulsant drug, gabapentin (Neurontin), binds to the $alpha_2$ delta subunit of a calcium channel. *J Biol Chem* 1996;271:5768–5776.
29. Chadwick D. Gabapentin. *Lancet* 1994;343:89–91.
30. Dichter MA, Brodie MJ. New antiepileptic drugs. *N Engl J Med* 1996;334:1583–1590.
31. McLean MJ. Clinical pharmacokinetics of gabapentin. *Neurology* 1994;44(Suppl 6):S17–S22.
32. Crawford P, Ghadiali E, Lane R, Blumhardt L, Chadwick D. Gabapentin as an antiepileptic drug in man. *J Neurol Neurosurg Psychiatry* 1987;50:682–686.
33. UK Gabapentin Study Group. Gabapentin in partial epilepsy. *Lancet* 1990;335:1114–1117.
34. Sivenius J, Kalviainen R, Ylingen A, Riekkinen P. Double-blind study of gabapentin in the treatment of partial seizures. *Epilepsia* 1991;32:539–542.
35. Wilson EA, Forrest G, Brodie MJ. High-dose gabapentin is absorbed and can be effective. *Epilepsia* 1996; 37(Suppl 4):127.
36. Ben-Menachem E, Soderfelt B, Hamberger A, Hedner T, Persson LI. Seizure frequency and CSF parameters in a double-blind, placebo-controlled trial of gabapentin in patients with intractable complex partial seizures. *Epilepsy Res* 1995;21:231–236.
37. Welty DF, Schielke GP, Vartanian MG, Taylor CP. Gabapentin anticonvulsant action in rats: disequilibrium with peak drug concentrations in plasma and brain microdialysate. *Epilepsy Res* 1993;16: 175–181.
38. Mattson RH. Antiepileptic drug monitoring: a reappraisal. *Epilepsia* 1995;30(Suppl 5):S22–S29.

Antiepileptic Drug Development.
Advances in Neurology, Vol. 76,
edited by J. French, I. Leppik, and M. A. Dichter.
Lippincott–Raven Publishers, Philadelphia © 1998.

23

Cognitive and Behavioral Assessments in AED Trials

Kimford J. Meador

Department of Neurology, Medical College of Georgia, Augusta, Georgia 30912.

INTRODUCTION

Although a variety of factors may affect cognition and behavior in patients with epilepsy (1), the effects of antiepileptic drugs (AEDs) are of particular concern to the clinician. Even though the untoward effects of AEDs generally are modest compared with the effects of other factors (e.g., pre-existing brain damage) (2,3), AEDs are the major therapeutic modality employed to treat seizures and so their side effects are iatrogenically induced. Furthermore, as many AEDs are equivalent in efficacy for the most common seizure types (4), differences in side effects become an important factor in determining which AED to use. To make such clinical decisions based on the relative risks and benefits of AEDs, physicians have to have adequate and reliable data concerning the magnitude and relative effects of the various AEDs on cognition and behavior.

It is well accepted that polytherapy and higher AED doses increase the risk for cognitive side effects (3). The risks associated with increased doses occur primarily at anticonvulsant blood levels (ABLs) above the standard therapeutic ranges. In contrast, marked effects may occur with polytherapy even when all ABLs are within the standard therapeutic ranges. However, the individual patient may not only tolerate polytherapy or an ABL above the standard therapeutic range, but even obtain the best risk-to-benefit ratio. More controversial are the issues of differential AED effects and the clinical significance of these untoward effects. These controversies can be attributed in large part to the common occurrence of methodologic flaws in studies examining the cognitive and behavioral effects of AEDs (see refs. 3 and 5 for reviews).

METHODOLOGIC ISSUES

A randomized, controlled trial is the most reliable method for assessing not only a drug's efficacy but also its side effects, the operant word being "controlled" (6). A variety of confounding factors must be adequately controlled in the design if valid conclusions are to be drawn. Furthermore, the resulting publication must include sufficiently detailed information about the design, conduct, and analysis of the study if the reader is to have confidence that the conclusions are warranted (7). Unfortunately, a great deal of the literature on the cognitive effects of AEDs does not meet these criteria.

Experimental Design

Five components of the experimental design that must be controlled include the following: (a) selection bias, (b) inadequate power, (c) nonequivalence on critical clinical variables, (d) nonequivalence on dependent measures, and (e) lack of sensitivity and validity of dependent variables (3). One purpose of randomization is to control for selection bias; however, many studies examining the effects of AEDs on cognition have violated this criterion by evaluating patients from their clinical population who have already been assigned AEDs based on other factors. To demonstrate how this might affect neuropsychologic results, Dodrill (8) compared two groups of patients from his clinical population. The patients were on various AEDs, but only one group was receiving valproate. When he compared IQ scores in the two groups, he found that the mean IQ of the valproate group, which was 87, was statistically lower ($p < .02$) than the mean IQ the group on other AEDs, which was 99. One might conclude that valproate was particularly detrimental to cognition. However, Dodrill had tested the same two groups of patients 5 years previously, when none of the patients was receiving valproate. The magnitude of IQ difference ($p < .01$) was exactly the same between the group that subsequently received valproate (IQ of 85) and the other group (IQ of 97). Thus, the differences were caused by selection bias and not by the effects of valproate. Even if subjects are randomized, the sample size must be large enough to avoid selection bias if a parallel group design is employed. This problem is avoided by crossover designs, but then one must obtain adequate control of carryover effects. With either design, sample size must be adequate to provide sensitivity and, it is hoped, a basis for generalization to other patients.

Nonequivalence on critical clinical variables may invalidate a study (3). Clinical variables of particular concern include AED dose, ABLs, treatment duration, concomitant drugs, clinical response (e.g., frequency and severity of seizures), underlying disease state (e.g., seizure type or etiology), age, and sex. The 1977 study by Dodrill and Troupin (9) can be considered as an example. Using a double-blind, randomized, crossover study, they reported that carbamazepine produced fewer cognitive side effects than phenytoin. However, the mean ABLs were 9.3 μg/mL for carbamazepine (standard range, 6 to 12 μg/mL) and 31.2 μg/mL for phenytoin (standard range, 10 to 20 μg/mL). Thus, they had actually compared one drug in midtherapeutic ABL range with another AED in the grossly toxic range. When they reanalyzed their data in 1991 controlling for ABLs, they found no differences (10).

Nonequivalence on dependent measures may occur if there is no assurance of comparable group performance levels for the variables of interest. For example, nonorthogonal contrasts have been conducted in some studies comparing the performance of controls tested only once with that of patients tested on multiple occasions, thereby confounding test-retest effects with drug effects (11). As another example, the study by Scolnik el al. (12) compared children exposed *in utero* to carbamazepine with children exposed to phenytoin. However, some children were tested at 2 years of age and some at 3 years of age with two different measures of IQ. Furthermore, the magnitude of difference in IQ between the two groups of children exposed to AEDs was the same as that in their mothers, suggesting that the observed differences in the groups of children might be based on genetics rather than exposure to drugs. Thus, without assurance that the two groups of children were similar except for differences in drug exposure, one is left with concern regarding comparability independent of AED exposure.

The characteristics of the cognitive and behavioral measures are important. As the main dependent measures, the neuropsychologic variables must be sensitive to the effects of AEDs. As AEDs cause diffuse membrane effects across multiple brain regions, one might expect that they would affect multiple types of cognitive function. However, the effects of AEDs are most readily apparent on a subset of neuropsychologic tasks. Tests involving vigilance, divided attention, psychomotor speed, complex eye-hand coordination, mood, and subjective symptoms appear to be particularly sensitive to AED effects (13). The dependent measures must be reliable. If repeated measure designs are used, test-retest effects must be known or controlled. Finally, measures should have ecologic validity relative to problems encountered by patients in the real world.

Statistical Issues

In addition to inadequate experimental designs, several errors in statistical analysis can obscure the interpretation of results. Statistical issues include the following: (a) type I error (i.e., concluding that the drugs are different when they are not); (b) type II error (i.e., concluding that the drugs are not different when they are); (c) comparing studies with nonequivalent designs and statistics, and (d) determining clinical versus statistical significance (3). As the number of statistical comparisons increases, the likelihood is greater that statistically significant differences will be caused by chance rather than by genuine performance differences between the AEDs. In the past, this has been a common error in the AED literature on cognition. Differential cognitive effects have been inferred inappropriately from a few statistical differences out of many comparisons. Type I errors can be controlled by an *a priori* plan for Bonferoni correction or by delineation of primary outcome variables. However, this approach has to be balanced against the risk for producing type II errors. Alternately, an *a priori* plan may be made not to control statistically for type I errors, but to interpret the statistical results appropriately. For example, if a statistically significant result is obtained, other variables measuring the same cognitive construct should also differ in the same direction between the two groups, even if they do not reach statistical significance. Of course, the point is mute if a large percentage of variables reach statistical significance in the same direction. No single study can answer such questions conclusively, and one would be most confident of AED differences if the same pattern recurs over a series of studies. Finally, the magnitude of differences must be assessed to determine whether the statistically significant findings are clinically significant. This requirement necessitates that the simple unadjusted summary data of the primary outcomes be presented with means and appropriate measures of variability (e.g., confidence intervals). Several AED cognition studies in the past have presented only transformed data, making it impossible for the reader to assess the clinical significance of the findings.

REVIEW OF PAST STUDIES

Several detailed reviews of prior studies are available (3,5). The present review focuses on a few select studies. A large Veterans Administration cooperative study compared the cognitive effects of carbamazepine, phenobarbital, phenytoin, and primidone in patients with new-onset epilepsy using a parallel group design (2). In a comparison of the four drug groups, no consistent pattern emerged. Furthermore, few differences were noted from the nondrug baseline to the end of 1 month of AED treatment. Similarly, a second Veterans Administration cooperative study comparing the cognitive effects of carbamazepine and valproate revealed no overall differences (14). One might conclude from these studies that the standard AEDs cause no cognitive effects, much less differential effects. However, the cognitive effects of AEDs in monotherapy are modest and were likely obscured in the Veterans Administration studies by test-retest effects, beneficial effects of seizure reduction, and the parallel group design.

In a series of studies, we have compared the effects of the standard AEDs using double-blind, randomized, crossover, monotherapy trials in patients and healthy volunteers, controlling for confounding variables (e.g., ABLs). The first study compared carbamazepine, phenobarbital, and phenytoin in a small group of patients with epilepsy (15). Only one statistically significant difference for 15 variables was found, with worse performance for phenobarbital on a graphomotor coding task (i.e., Digit Symbol Substitution Task). However, an overall pattern across most of the variables suggested worse performance on phenobarbital compared with both carbamazepine and phenytoin.

The second study compared carbamazepine and phenytoin in healthy volunteers using 12 tests yielding 21 variables (16,17). For the direct comparisons between the two AEDs, only two statistically significant differences were found, one in favor of carbamazepine (i.e., Finger Tapping) and one in favor of phenytoin (i.e., Stroop). Overall, the simple means were equal on three variables, favored carbamazepine in five, and favored phenytoin in 13. Thus, no overall consistent differences were found between the two AEDs. In contrast, comparison of the AED states with the nondrug conditions revealed statistically significant differences on half of the variables (i.e., 11 of 21), with better performance off drug than on either AED.

The third study compared the effects of phenobarbital, phenytoin, and valproate in healthy volunteers (18). Statistically significant differential AED effects were found on seven of the 22 variables, with worse performance on phenobarbital compared with either phenytoin or valproate. Similarly, simple means were worse for phenobarbital than either of the other AEDs on 17 of 22 variables. One statistically significant difference was found between phenytoin and valproate. However, the magnitude of the difference was small, with mean performances on Stroop of 46 for phenytoin and 48 for valproate. Furthermore, comparisons of simple means revealed no overall pattern of differences, with 11 favoring phenytoin and 11 favoring valproate. Again, performance on the nondrug conditions was superior compared with the AED conditions on half of the variables statistically (i.e., 11 of 22), and simple means for the nondrug conditions were better than for any of the three AEDs for 17 of the 22 variables.

In summary, these results reveal greater adverse cognitive effects for phenobarbital, but no clinically significant differences between carbamazepine, phenytoin, and valproate. All four AEDs exhibited adverse effects compared with the nondrug conditions. Although the statistical differences between nondrug and AED states were robust, the magnitudes of the differences were modest. For example, the latency of the P3 event-related potential is an index of cognitive processing speed. In our studies of healthy volunteers, the P3 latency was prolonged 25 milliseconds for phenobarbital and about 15 milliseconds for carbamazepine, phenytoin, and valproate compared with the nondrug conditions. Thus, the cognitive slowing produced by these AEDs after 1 month of therapy is approximately equal to the acute effects of over-the-counter antihistamines (19). Although one would expect that the effects of antihistamines would be less after 1 month of the therapy, the point is that the effects of these AEDs in monotherapy within the standard therapeutic ABL ranges are not dramatic. In clinical practice, the effects may also be offset in part by the beneficial effects of reduced seizure activity. However, the relatively modest cognitive effects of AEDs may be clinically significant in certain situations. For example, patients who particularly require vigilance or psychomotor speed in their daily activities may find the effects of AEDs especially problematic.

ANTIEPILEPTIC DRUG EFFECTS AT THE EXTREMES OF AGE

The effects of AEDs on cognition at the extremes of age are less clear. The elderly are more susceptible to the cognitive effects of a variety of drugs, for both pharmacokinetic and pharmacodynamic reasons. However, only one study has specifically examined the cognitive effects of AEDs in the elderly. Craig and Tallis (20) found few differences between phenytoin and valproate in elderly patients with epilepsy, and few effects of the two AEDs compared with the nondrug baseline.

Given the potentially cumulative effects of even modest AED effects over the long term during neurodevelopment, children might be at increased risk for sequelae. In the only double-blind, randomized, crossover, monotherapy study in children, performance on phenobarbital was worse than on valproate (21). Consistent with these findings, greater adverse effects of phenobarbital have been found compared with placebo in children with febrile convulsions (22) and compared with carbamazepine and valproate in children with new-onset epilepsy (23). In the later study, P3 latency was delayed in the phenobarbital group by the same order of magnitude as in the previously mentioned adult studies. Comparisons of carbamazepine, phenytoin, and valproate in children with epilepsy have yielded few differences (24).

Exposure to AEDs *in utero* would in theory create the greatest risk to neurodevelopment. Animal studies have revealed dose-dependent neurobehavioral deficits from AED exposure *in utero* at doses below those that commonly cause anatomic teratogenic abnormalities (25,26). However, the magnitude of adverse effects and the presence of differential AED effects remain unresolved. Two recent clinical studies deserve comment. In one study, the authors claimed differential effects of carbamazepine and phenytoin for exposure *in utero* (12). However, conclusions from the study were invalidated by numerous flaws, including inappropriate statistical analyses and inequalities in mean AED doses, sex of subjects, outcome measures of IQ, matching to controls, and percentages of women without epilepsy in the AED groups. Maternal IQ is the single most potent predictor of a child's IQ. In the above study, the magnitude of IQ differences between mothers and children was the same for the two AED groups, suggesting that the observed differences in the children might be based on genetic factors rather than a drug effect. The other recent study involved children of women without epilepsy who received phenobarbital during pregnancy (27). Their children exhibited decreased IQ, especially if the pregnancy was unwanted and the maternal socioeconomic status was low. Further studies are required to resolve this important controversy and fully delineate the effects of *in utero* exposure on neurodevelopment.

NEW ANTIEPILEPTIC DRUGS

To date, more studies on cognitive effects have been conducted on vigabatrin than any of the other new AEDs. When compared with placebo, vigabatrin has produced few adverse effects on cognition or quality-of-life measures (28–31). Preliminary studies have also been conducted comparing vigabatrin with two other AEDs. A small study in epileptic patients showed fewer effects for vigabatrin compared with carbamazepine, but the study had an open-label design and there were a sizable number of dropouts (32). Despite its effects on τ-aminobutyric acid (GABA), vigabatrin caused fewer effects than the benzodiazepine lorazepam in healthy volunteers, but this study employed single doses, so that the full effects of vigabatrin on GABA were not obtained (33). A small, randomized, double-blind study comparing oxcarbazepine and phenytoin revealed no differences in the cognitive measures employed (34). Positive effects on patients' perception of quality of life have been demonstrated for lamotrigine (35), but cognitive performance has not been adequately assessed. Initial reports are also available for gabapentin and tiagabine. Positive effects were suggested for gabapentin in a dose-response study, but there was no placebo or control group for test-retest effects (36). Compared with placebo, tiagabine exhibited no statistical differences (37). However, the absence of a statistical difference is not proof of the absence of effects. If the same criteria were applied to the Veterans Administration studies, then we would have to conclude that none of the older AEDs caused cognitive effects either. Therefore, the differential effects of the new AEDs compared with the older AEDs, much less with each other, remain uncertain. Future studies directly comparing the new AEDs with each other and with the older AEDs will be required to clarify this issue. Until such studies are conducted, the relative risk-to-benefit ratios of the new AEDs cannot be fully assessed.

SUMMARY OF THE PRESENT STATE OF KNOWLEDGE

1. All the well-tested AEDs have been shown to cause some cognitive side effects. It remains unclear whether an AED can be developed that reduces neuronal irritability without reducing neuronal excitability and thus affecting normal neuronal function to at least some extent.

2. The risks for cognitive side effects are increased with polypharmacy and with increasing doses/ABLs, although individual patients may well tolerate polypharmacy or ABLs above the standard therapeutic range.

3. The magnitude of the cognitive effects produced by AEDs is generally modest and may be offset in part by reduced seizure frequency and severity. However, the effects can be clinically significant in some patients.

4. Differential effects of AEDs on cognition do exist (e.g., phenobarbital), but some claims of differential effects appear unfounded.

5. The differential effects of the new AEDs in comparison with each other and with the older AEDs remain uncertain.

6. Age-specific effects at both extremes of age remain unclear, especially the long-term effects on neurodevelopment of *in utero* exposure.

DESIGN RECOMMENDATIONS FOR FUTURE STUDIES OF COGNITION AND BEHAVIOR

1. It is essential to employ double-blind, randomized paradigms.
2. Preferably, studies should be designed specifically to examine cognitive and behavioral effects. Cognitive studies appended to studies primarily designed to assess efficacy are more prone to confounding effects (e.g., dropouts, seizures).
3. Ensure equivalence for critical clinical variables.
   A. To control for seizure effects, use patients with well-controlled seizures or study AED effects in healthy adults.
   B. Use AED doses (and if possible ABLs) that are equivalent in therapeutic efficacy. This issue may be problematic for the new AEDs, for which data directly comparing efficacy with other AEDs are limited.
   C. Monotherapy studies are preferable to avoid pharmacokinetic and pharmacodynamic interactions that could complicate interpretation of results. However, well-designed polytherapy studies can be informative in certain circumstances.
   D. If a parallel group design is used, ensure equivalent baseline performances across groups.
4. Utilize repeated measures design. If a parallel group design is used, consider obtaining at least two baseline assessments to establish a stable baseline and to control in part for test-retest effects; this is particularly important if there is no placebo control group.
5. Consider the strengths and weaknesses of crossover and parallel group designs.
6. Employ a sample size large enough to ensure adequate power (e.g., .80).
7. Consider the use of nontreatment controls. In healthy volunteer studies or add-on treatment studies in patients, this should be accomplished with a placebo treatment arm. The use of nontreatment patient controls in monotherapy studies may help in the assessment of test-retest effects but will likely introduce nonrandom treatment assignment elements into the design.
8. Choose behavioral assessments that are sensitive to domains expected to be affected by AEDs and that have some ecologic validity.
9. Compose the neuropsychologic battery to define the pattern of AED effects on cognitive performance and on subjective measures, such as mood and quality of life.
10. Follow accepted guidelines in the analysis and reporting of the data.
    A. Appropriately balance the design and discussion to avoid type I and type II errors.

B. Present sufficient unadjusted summary data on the primary outcome variables, including untransformed means and appropriate measures of variability (e.g., confidence intervals).

11. Interpret and discuss the results, differentiating clinical versus statistical significance.

REFERENCES

1. Lennox WG. Brain injury, drugs and environment a cause of mental decay in epilepsy. *Psychiatry* 1942:99: 174–180.
2. Smith DB, Mattson RH, Cramer JA, et al. Results of a nationwide Veterans Administration cooperative study comparing the efficacy and toxicity of carbamazepine, phenobarbital, phenytoin, and primidone. *Epilepsia* 1987;28:S50–S58.
3. Meador KJ, Loring DW. Cognitive effects of antiepileptic drugs. In: Devinsky O, Theodore WH, eds. *Epilepsy and Behavior*. New York: Wiley-Liss; 1991; 151–170.
4. Mattson RH, Cramer JA, Collins JF, Smith DB, et al. Comparison of carbamazepine, phenobarbital, phenytoin, and primidone in partial and secondarily generalized tonic-clonic seizures. *N Engl J Med* 1985;313: 145–151.
5. Vermeulen J, Aldenkamp AP. Cognitive side effects of chronic antiepileptic drug treatment: a review of 25 years of research. *Epilepsy Res* 1995;22:65–95.
6. Sacks H, Chalmers TC, Smith H. Randomized versus historical controls for clinical trials. *Am J Med* 1982; 72:233–240.
7. The Standards of Reporting Trials Group. A proposal for structure reporting of randomized controlled trials. *JAMA* 1994;272:1926–1931.
8. Dodrill CB. Problems in the assessment of cognitive effects of antiepileptic drugs. *Epilepsia* 1992;33(Suppl 6):S29–S32.
9. Dodrill CB, Troupin AS. Psychotropic effects of carbamazepine in epilepsy: a double-blind comparison with phenytoin. *Neurology* 1977;27:1023–1028.
10. Dodrill CB, Troupin AS. Neuropsychological effects of carbamazepine and phenytoin: a reanalysis. *Neurology* 1991;41:141–143.
11. Gallassi R, Morreale A, Lorusso S, Procaccianti G, et al. Cognitive effects of valproate. *Epilepsy Res* 1990;5: 160–164.
12. Scolnik D, Nulman I, Rovet J, Gladstone D, et al. Neurodevelopment of children exposed *in utero* to phenytoin and carbamazepine monotherapy. *JAMA* 1994;271: 767–770.
13. Meador KJ. Cognitive side effects of antiepileptic drugs. *Can J Neurol Sci* 1994;21(Suppl 3):S12–S16.
14. Prevey ML, Delaney RC, Cramer JA. Valproate versus carbamazepine: comparison of cognitive functioning. *Epilepsia* 1992;33:110.
15. Meador KJ, Loring DW, Huh K, Gallagher BB, King DW. Comparative cognitive effects of anticonvulsants. *Neurology* 1990;40:391–394.
16. Meador KJ, Loring DW, Huh K, et al. Comparative cognitive effects of carbamazepine and phenytoin in healthy adults. *Neurology* 1991;1:1537–1540.
17. Meador KJ, Loring DW, Abney OL, et al. Effects of carbamazepine and phenytoin on EEG and memory in healthy adults. *Epilepsia* 1993:34:153–157.
18. Meador KJ, Loring DW, Moore EE, et al. Comparative cognitive effects of phenobarbital, phenytoin, and valproate in healthy subjects. *Neurology* 1995;45: 1494–1499.
19. Meador KJ, Loring DW, Thompson EE, Thompson WO. Differential cognitive effects of terfenadine and chlorpheniramine. *J Allergy Immunol* 1989;84:322–325.
20. Craig I, Tallis R. The impact of sodium valproate and phenytoin on cognitive function in elderly patients: results of a single-blind randomized comparative study. *Epilepsia* 1994:35:381–390.
21. Vining EPG, Mellitis ED, Dorsen MM, et al. Psychologic and behavioral effects of antiepileptic drugs in children: a double-blind comparison between phenobarbital and valproic acid. *Pediatrics* 1987;80:165–174.
22. Farwell JR, Lee YJ, Hirtz DG, Sulzbacher SI, Ellenberg JH, Nelson KB. Phenobarbital for febrile seizures—effects on intelligence and on seizure recurrence. *N Engl J Med* 1990;322:364–369.
23. Chen Y, Kang W, Chin-Min So W. Comparison of antiepileptic drugs on cognitive function in newly diagnosed epileptic children: a psychometric and neurophysiological study. *Epilepsia* 1996;37:81–86.
24. Forsythe I, Butler R, Berg I, McGuire R. Cognitive impairment in new cases of epilepsy randomly assigned to carbamazepine, phenytoin, and sodium valproate. *Dev Med Child Neurol* 1991;33:523–534.
25. Finnell RH, Dansky LV. Parental epilepsy, anticonvulsant drugs, and reproductive outcome: epidemiologic and experimental findings spanning three decades. 1: Animal studies. *Reprod Toxicol Rev* 1991;5: 281–299.
26. Fisher JE, Vorhees C. Developmental toxicity of antiepileptic drugs: relationship to postnatal dysfunction. *Pharm Res* 1992;26:207–221.
27. Reinisch JM, Sanders SA, Mortensen EL, Rubin DB. *In utero* exposure to phenobarbital and intelligence deficits in adult men. *JAMA* 1995;274:1518 1525.
28. Dodrill CB, Arnett JL, Sommerville KW, et al. Evaluation of the effects of vigabatrin on cognitive abilities and quality of life in epilepsy. *Neurology* 1993;43: 2501–2507.
29. Gillham RA, Blacklaw J, McKee PJW, et al. Effect of vigabatrin on sedation and cognitive function in patients with refractory epilepsy. *J Neurol Neurosurg Psychiatry* 1993;56:1271–1275.
30. Grunewald RA, Thompson PJ, Corcoran R, et al. Effects of vigabatrin on partial seizures and cognitive function. *J Neurol Neurosurg Psychiatry* 1994;57: 1057–1063.
31. Dodrill CB, Arnett JL, Sommerville KW, et al. Effects of differing dosages of vigabatrin (Sabril) on cognitive abilities and quality of life in epilepsy. *Epilepsy* 1995; 36.164–173.
32. Kalviainen R, Aikia M, Sankkonen AM, et al. Vigabatrin versus carbamazepine monotherapy in newly diagnosed patients with epilepsy: a randomized controlled study. *Arch Neurol* 1995;52:989–996.
33. Saletu B, Grunberge J, Linzmayer L, et al. Psychophysiological and psychometric studies after manipu-

lating the GABA system by vigabatrin, a GABA-transaminase inhibitor. *Int J Psychophysiol* 1986;4:63–80.
34. Aikia M, Kalviainen R, Sivenius J, et al. Cognitive effects of oxcarbazepine and phenytoin monotherapy in newly diagnosed epilepsy: 1-year follow-up. *Epilepsy Res* 1992;11:199–203.
35. Smith D, Baker G, Davies G, et al. Outcomes of add-on treatment with lamotrigine in partial epilepsy. *Epilepsia* 1993;34:312–322.
36. Dodrill CB, Arnett JL, Hayes AG, et al. Evaluation of quality of life during a double-blind multicenter study of gabapentin (GBP; Neurontin) monotherapy in patients with medically refractory partial seizures. *Epilepsia* 1995;36(Suppl 4):88.
37. Dodrill CB, Arnett JL, Mercante D, et al. Changes in mental abilities and adjustment with conversion to tiagabine monotherapy. *Neurology* 1996;46(Suppl): A277.

Antiepileptic Drug Development.
Advances in Neurology, Vol. 76,
edited by J. French, I. Leppik, and M. A. Dichter.
Lippincott–Raven Publishers, Philadelphia © 1998.

24

Economic Factors in the Development of New Antiepileptic Drugs

Roger J. Porter

Wyeth-Ayerst Laboratories, Radnor, Pennsylvania 19101.

INTRODUCTION

The quest for new drugs for epilepsy is not only scientific and clinical, it is also related to a number of other, nonscientific issues. This chapter outlines those issues that determine not only whether a promising lead will be pursued and developed, but whether the lead will even be uncovered. Our system of drug development largely depends on the marketplace, and only in unusual circumstances can a new drug avoid, even temporarily, the dictates of the market. This discussion will not enlighten those already exposed to an industrial setting, but it may be of value to others who have not had such experience.

ISSUES AT THE CORPORATE LEVEL

Although many of the early drugs used to treat epilepsy were discovered by serendipity and good fortune, most of the more recent drugs have been uncovered by deliberate programs. Such programs search, in one of several ways, for substances that might meet certain specifications for antiepileptic drugs. One of the oldest and most successful of these approaches has been the screening method, in which thousands of compounds are evaluated in simple tests and models to seek at least a minimal level of activity. More sophisticated screens are targeted against specific receptors, again hoping for a certain level of activity. Another approach is the rational design of a molecule that will act on a specific target (e.g., τ-aminobutyric transaminase) to alter cellular/synaptic function and, one would hope, affect the epileptic process in a positive way.

This all seems so straightforward and simple. Why, then, are more drugs not available for testing? There are several answers. First, as shown in Fig. 1, most new drugs are developed by the pharmaceutical industry and not through academic or government research (1). This is true for many reasons, but perhaps the most important is that drug discovery is a very labor-intensive and complex interdisciplinary undertaking requiring substantial long-term capital investment. Of the structures in society that are most capable of sustaining such an effort, large, corporate pharmaceutical companies are clearly the most effective. Discovery efforts outside industry have been directed at only a few disorders. The quest for medicines to treat cancer has benefited enormously from the efforts of the National Cancer Institute of the National Institutes of Health, which spends many tens of millions of dollars each year to search for new compounds. The search for drugs to treat AIDS is similarly blessed. And, on a much smaller scale, the screening program of the Epilepsy Branch serves a critical, albeit relatively financially limited, role in supporting industry's search for antiepileptic drugs.

If, then, the problem is in the industry, why are more antiepileptic drugs not in the dis-

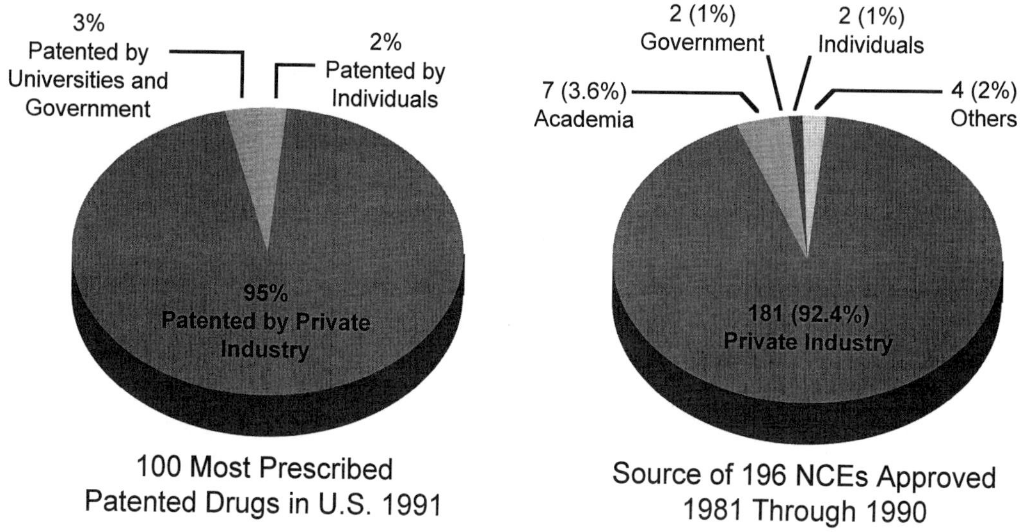

Source: PMA Survey; Center for the Study of Drug Development, Tufts University (1991)

FIG. 1. The sources of drug discovery in the United States. (Information compiled by the Pharmaceutical Manufacturers' Association and Tufts University.)

covery pipeline? The answer to this question lies in the priorities of two disparate parts of the corporation, the discovery department and the marketing department. Discovery groups are organized to support the expectations of the company for new drugs in the future. In many cases, drugs currently in the discovery pipeline will not become generally available for patient use for 6 to 10 years. So discovery requires a long-term investment. It also entails a substantial risk. One must assume that the compounds currently in the pipeline will be embraced by the market in the future, and that they will not be obsolete on arrival. It is not only the discovery department that is concerned with this issue; the marketing department speaks with a strong voice on the same subject. The problem of a new drug that sells poorly is, after all, the burden of the marketing group. Therefore, powerful forces are at play to ensure that the discovery resources available are targeted to the company's best estimate of what a successful drug will look like 8 to 10 years in the future.

Unfortunately, few companies have targeted discovery programs seeking new antiepileptic drugs. The mechanisms of epileptogenesis and seizure discharge in humans are complex and probably quite heterogeneous, and pharmaceutical industry management has not encouraged investment in this area. Such a dilemma makes all the more important, for those who advocate the discovery of new antiepileptic drugs, the continuing support of the Epilepsy Branch programs—programs that serve, in part, as a surrogate for industry discovery and early development of new antiepileptic drugs.

If the first hurdle is overcome, that is, if a company has identified a compound that looks favorable as a potential antiepileptic drug, what criteria are then applied to make a decision on further development? A brand new treatment for an important disorder with no existing therapy is clearly optimal, but such an event is unusual. The next most attractive compound is one that represents a new therapeutic class and will be the first of this class to reach the market. After that would be a drug in the same class as the competition but with a significant advantage. Examples of such advantages include an improved side ef-

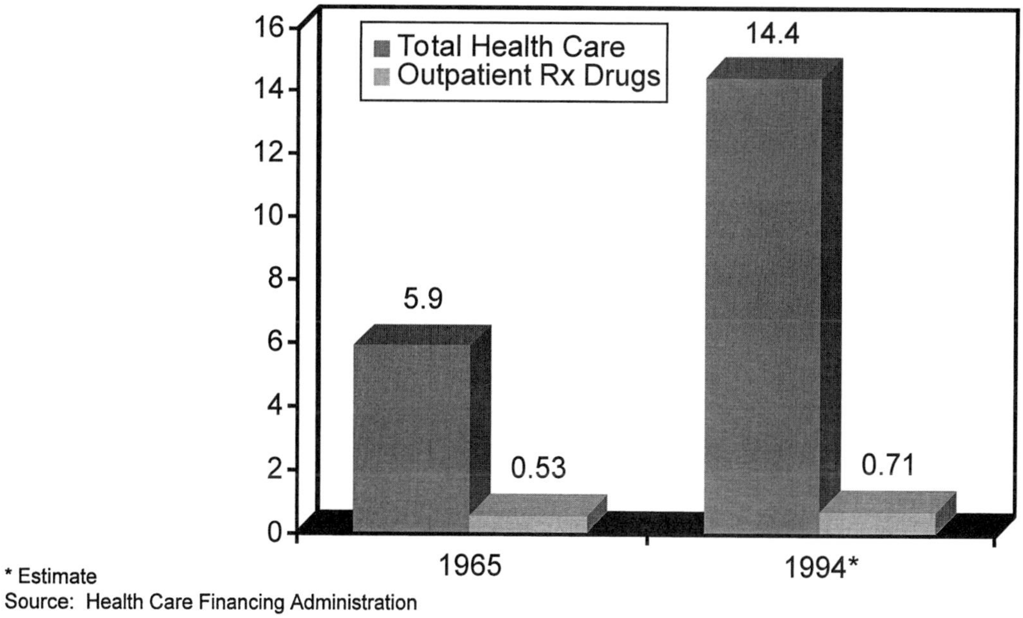

FIG. 2. The escalation of health care expenses as percent of GDP and the minimal contribution of outpatient drugs to this dramatic increase. (From Norris and Fox, ref. 2.)

fects profile or a more convenient dosing regimen. The issue of whether a new drug makes a unique contribution or is really a "me too" compound is complex, especially when subtle adverse effects are considered. Ultimately, however, the marketplace makes a judgment on the value of a new drug and determines the success or failure of the product.

THE HEALTH CARE ENVIRONMENT

The costs of health care are escalating rapidly and consuming an ever larger percentage of the gross domestic product (GDP), as shown in Fig. 2. Even though the costs of drugs have contributed very little to this rise, as is documented in the figure, the counterforces attempting to control the overall cost increases find pharmaceutical companies an inviting target. Price increases for drugs have greatly diminished as a result of such pressure, placing corporations in the dilemma of needing to please their stockholders while maintaining a research presence. The results are corporations that run lean, often contracting out sizable portions of their work (partly in anticipation of potential shrinkage in the *future* workload).

The problems of health care costs will not soon diminish. With the aging of the generation of baby boomers, health costs will inevitably rise. Even though the pharmaceutical industry considers itself part of the *solution* rather than part of the problem, price consciousness will remain. According to Norris and Fox (2), managed care companies (the leaders in cost control) now account for approximately 50% of the U.S. prescription drug market, a figure expected to rise to 90% by the year 2000. Also, the use of cheaper generic drugs has increased, so that whereas these accounted for 15% of the prescription drug market in 1983 and 30% in 1989, they represent 50% at present (2).

THE RISING COST OF DRUG DEVELOPMENT

All the while that downward pressure is being exerted on drug prices, the cost of developing a new compound continues to escalate. The estimate of cost per approved new chem-

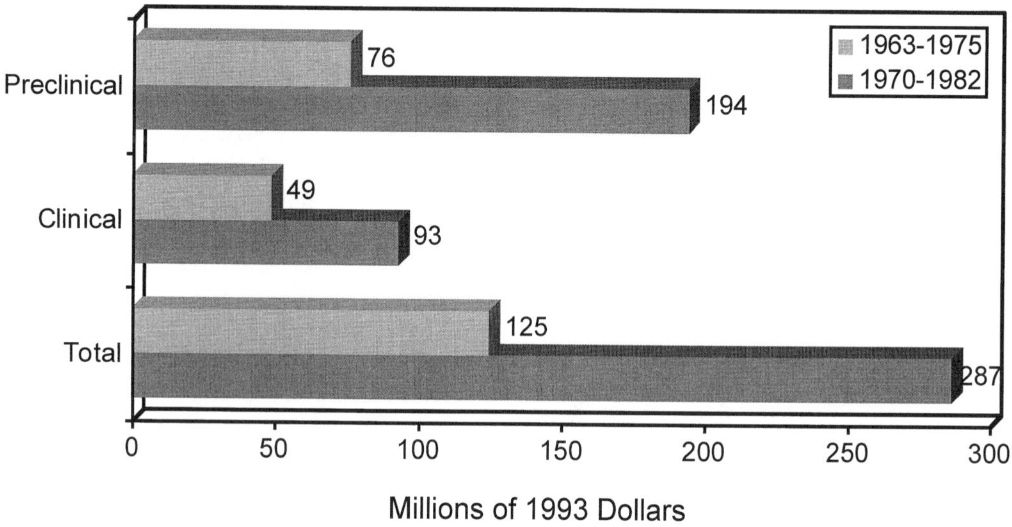

Preclinical, Clinical, and Total Capitalized Cost Per Approved New Chemical Entity for NCEs First Tested in Humans During 1963-1975 and 1970-1982. Source of Data: Hansen (1); DiMasi et al. (2).

FIG. 3. The escalation of drug development costs. (From DiMasi, ref. 3.)

ical entity has risen from $125 million for drugs first tested in humans during 1963–1975 to $287 million for the period 1970–1982 (Fig. 3). From these figures, DiMasi (3) concludes that clinical costs nearly doubled in inflation-adjusted dollars between the two study periods.

As shown in Fig. 4, the costs of research can be documented by the research and development expenditures for the industry, in which costs are clearly escalating more rapidly than are the number of approved new chemical entities (NCEs) (3). Not only has cost increased; the time required for develop-

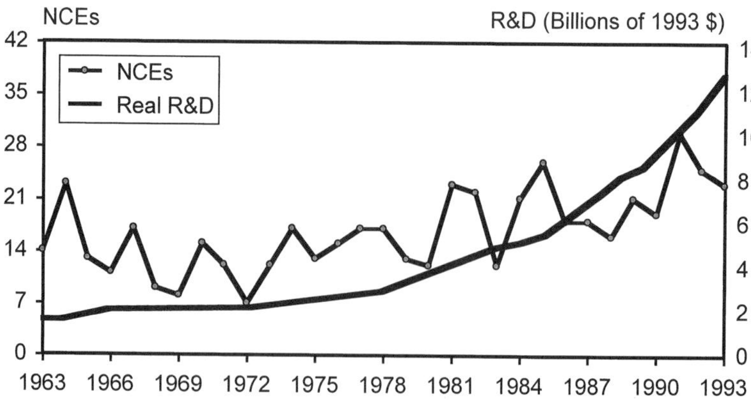

FIG. 4. U.S. pharmaceutical industry R&D expenditures in constant dollars and the number of new chemical entities approved in the United States from 1963–1993. R&D expenditures are for pharmaceutical research and Manufacturers of America member firms and were deflated using the GDP implicit price deflator.

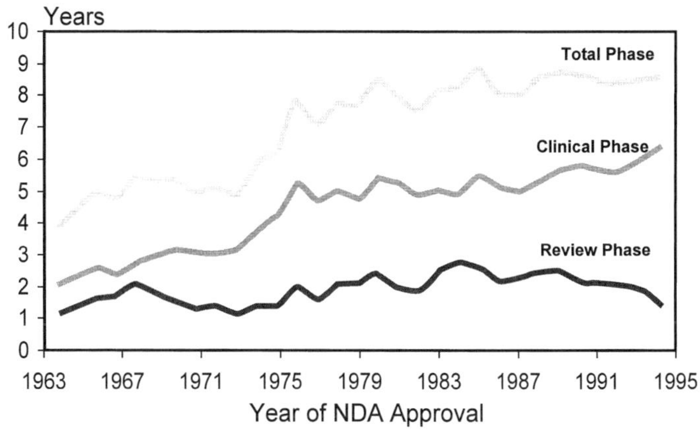

FIG. 5. The escalating time needed for drug regulatory approval. (From Kaitin, ref. 4.)

ment and review has also lengthened considerably. From a total of approximately 4 years in 1963, the development time lengthened to more than 8 years by 1995 (4). As can be seen in Fig. 5, although the review phase has been shortened somewhat in the past few years, a lengthening of the clinical phase has offset this gain (4).

COSTS OF DEVELOPING ANTIEPILEPTIC DRUGS

One of the negative factors in the development of new antiepileptic drugs is the perception that such drugs are costly and difficult to develop. The charge of the original Surgeon General's Advisory Committee in the 1960s to the National Institutes of Health was to evaluate this perception and lower the barrier. The studies by the Epilepsy Branch showed that few pharmaceutical companies had programs to discover drugs and that virtually no compounds were in clinical development. Even though new drugs are now actually appearing in the marketplace and more are in the late phases of development, the notion persists that these compounds are more difficult and time-consuming to develop than most other drugs. The scene is clearly better than in the 1960s, when few qualified investigators could be found, but the lack of industrial discovery programs in antiepileptic drugs does not bode well for the future.

THE WORLD MARKET FOR ANTIEPILEPTIC DRUGS

If the lack of current industrial discovery programs is discouraging for those who wish to advance new antiepileptic drugs into development, the data available on the burgeoning market allow for offsetting optimism. The worldwide market has grown from just under $1 billion in 1991 to an estimated $1.8 billion in 1996 (5) (Fig. 6). These figures are of considerable interest to the pharmaceutical industry, and the double-digit growth rate is a potential stimulus to those who would consider bringing new entities into the market. The reasons for such growth include better diagnosis and more effective therapies—especially the recently approved new drugs.

However, from the standpoint of industrial enthusiasm, there is at least a short-term downside to the recent arrival of a series of new and novel antiepileptic drugs to the market. Companies are concerned that all the new drugs will dilute the market and make later entries—especially if they are not novel—less likely to succeed. In fact, only if the market is satisfied are these fears justified. If not, a new

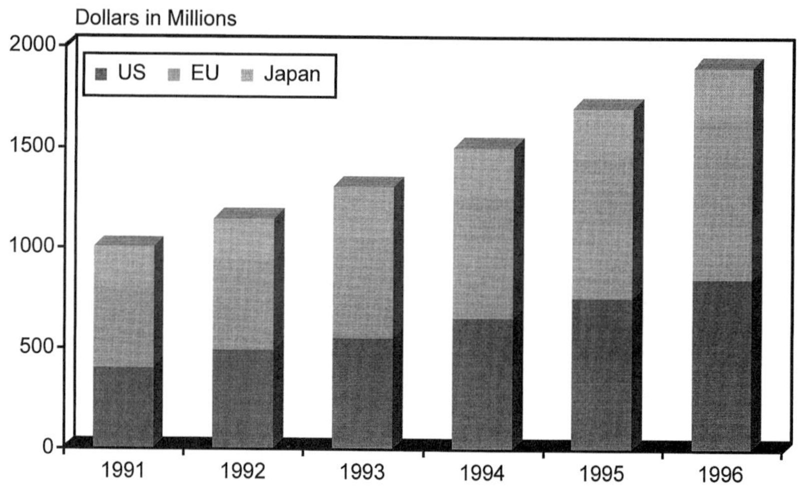

FIG. 6. The world market for antiepileptic drugs. The figures are the moving annual totals, calculated in the first quarter of 1996. (From IMS, ref. 5.)

entry will surely succeed—especially if it is novel, effective, and less toxic.

SUMMARY

The development of new antiepileptic drugs is closely linked to a series of economic factors and perceptions. Industrial interest in such drugs continues to be relatively low, and few companies presently have active discovery programs. The market, however, is large and growing and should encourage more industrial interest in the future.

REFERENCES

1. Pharmaceutical Research and Manufacturers' Association, Washington DC.
2. Norris T, Fox MJ. All ethical pharmaceuticals—pharmaceutical product development in the health care reform movement. In: Smith R, ed. *Medical and Health Care Marketplace Guide.* 11th ed. Philadelphia: IDD Enterprises LP; 1995.
3. DiMasi JA. Trends and drug development: costs, times, and risks. *Drug Info J* 1995;29:375–384.
4. Kaitin KI. Trends in drug development: the center's review of recent new drug approvals. In: *Syllabus of the Annual Corporate Sponsors and Advisory Board Meeting*, May 1, 1996, Somerville, MA.
5. IMS. First Quarter Statistics.

Antiepileptic Drug Development.
Advances in Neurology, Vol. 76,
edited by J. French, I. Leppik, and M. A. Dichter.
Lippincott–Raven Publishers, Philadelphia © 1998.

25

Recent Issues and Considerations in the Regulation of Antiepileptic Drugs

Russell G. Katz*

Division of Neuropharmacological Drug Products, Food and Drug Administration, Rockville, Maryland 20857.

INTRODUCTION

A number of recent changes in some of the regulations governing drug development as well as in the approach to several other important issues have had, or are expected to have, a significant impact on the development of new drugs intended to treat patients with various forms of epilepsy. The first part of this chapter focuses on some of the recent actions taken by the Food and Drug Administration relevant to antiepileptic drug (AED) development. In the second portion of the chapter, some of the issues raised by the development of dosage forms other than immediate-release oral preparations, the most commonly available dosage form for AEDs, are discussed.

ESTABLISHING PEDIATRIC CLAIMS

On December 13, 1994, the Food and Drug Administration published final regulations detailing the kinds of data that it will consider when deciding whether a drug approved for a particular indication in adults should be approved for children. To approve a treatment for use in children when adequate and well-controlled trials are available only in adults, the Agency must conclude that the disease and the effects of the drug, both beneficial and adverse, are sufficiently similar in adults and children to permit extrapolation of the adult effectiveness data to children. In addition, other data may be required, including pharmacokinetic data that will permit adequate dosing recommendations to be written for pediatric patients.

On September 27, 1994 (before the regulations cited above were officially in effect, but a considerable time after they had been published for comment), the Peripheral and Central Nervous Systems Drugs Advisory Committee, a panel of expert consultants to the Agency, took up the question of the use of Tegretol in children below the age of 6 years (previously approved labeling had limited dosing recommendations to patients >6 years old). Because the application did not contain the results of adequate and well-controlled studies in this population, the argument for effectiveness had to address the three critical issues described above.

First, to establish that the disease to be treated (specifically, partial seizures) was similar in adults and children, the sponsor demonstrated that the effect of the drug is on seizures, not on epilepsy as a global condition, and that the mechanism of seizure development is similar in adults and children, as shown in studies on cortical tissue taken at surgery in pediatric and adult patients with epilepsy.

*The views expressed are those of the author and are not official views of the Food and Drug Administration.

Next, to establish the similarity of the effect of the drug in adults and children, the sponsor was able to demonstrate that voltage-dependent, use-dependent sodium channel binding of carbamazepine occurs in adult and fetal neurons, and that this binding is capable of aborting abnormal, repetitive neuronal firing.

Finally, the establishment of an appropriate dosing regimen in children was accomplished in the following way. In the clinical trials that had been performed in children (which were not adequate by design to demonstrate effectiveness), the vast majority of patients were successfully titrated to achieve plasma levels of the parent compound of between 4 and 12 μg/mL, the accepted therapeutic range for carbamazepine. These levels were achieved at doses between 10 and 20 mg/kg in most patients. The sponsor was able to show that the antiseizure effects of the drug occurred at a concentration of about 8.5 μmol in in vitro studies, which corresponds to the levels of unbound carbamazepine achieved at the dosing regimen cited above in the clinical trials. In this way, the sponsor demonstrated that the range of doses given in the clinical trials resulted in plasma levels of unbound parent compound associated with effectiveness in in vitro systems designed to evaluate antiseizure effect, and the sponsor therefore argued that this dosing regimen would result in therapeutic levels of carbamazepine in children.

The Advisory Committee found this line of reasoning persuasive (along with the finding that adverse events in children were considered acceptable), and recommended that the use of Tegretol in children under the age of 6 years be included in labeling (this has subsequently occurred). However, a few important results of this decision are worth noting.

The Committee explicitly stated that the conclusion applied to Tegretol specifically, and that in general a finding of effectiveness in children based on adequate and well-controlled trials in adults must be made with appropriate data on the specific drug under question in each case.

Having said this, however, it is obvious that acceptance of the argument presented in this case *does* establish the important general finding that partial seizures are, for purposes of establishing drug effectiveness, sufficiently similar in adults and children, a finding that clearly cannot be considered to be drug-specific.

RESEARCH IN EMERGENCY SITUATIONS

A final regulatory issue of note that is likely to be of interest to the epilepsy community is the recently approved regulation pertaining to the study of investigational treatments in emergency situations in which valid informed consent (either from the patient or the patient's legally authorized representative) cannot be obtained before the use of the test article. These regulations will permit research into treatments for several types of seizures (e.g., treatment of status epilepticus, treatment and/or prevention of posttraumatic seizures) that otherwise would be extremely burdensome or, perhaps, impractical.

Regulations published in final form on October 2, 1996, address the circumstances under which such research can proceed. In brief, research may proceed in the absence of informed consent if the Institutional Review Board determines that the patient is faced with a life-threatening situation for which available treatments are inadequate and for which the collection of adequate scientific information is necessary to determine the safety and effectiveness of particular interventions. In such a case, the Institutional Review Board must find that obtaining informed consent is not feasible because the patient's medical condition precludes it, the treatment must be given before consent can be obtained, and there is no reasonable way to identify patients eligible for the trial prospectively. A finding must be made that participation in the research may benefit the patient directly (because the patient is faced with a life-threatening situation, available evidence suggests that the treatment may be useful, and the risks of the treatment are acceptable) and that the trial could not be carried out without the waiver of the requirement for informed consent. Additional safeguards include requirements for the investigators to make efforts, within prescribed time frames, to obtain consent from a legally authorized representative before the treatment is initiated, or, failing this, an attempt to contact a family member who is not an authorized representative and ask whether this family member objects; consultation with representatives of the community in which the research is to be performed before it is carried out, and the inclusion of requirements for the Institutional Review Board to inform patients and/or their legally authorized representatives as soon as possible after the treatment is given. Further, any protocol in which this mechanism is proposed must be submitted under a separate Investigational New Drug application (IND) and may not be submitted as an amendment to an existing IND. Relevant aspects of these new regulations as they pertain to interventions with investigational drugs are in Title 21, Code of Federal Regulations, Parts 50, 56, 312, and 314, and the interested reader is referred to the *Federal Register* of October 2, 1996, pages 51498–41533, for a description of the new regulations and additional relevant background material.

ESTABLISHING EFFECTIVENESS FOR SECONDARILY GENERALIZED SEIZURES

Most commercial sponsors develop AEDs to treat partial seizures, with a focus on complex partial seizures, presumably because these seizures are those most commonly refractory to available treatments. Ordinarily, however, sponsors wish to make a claim that their treatment is effective against the secondarily generalized tonic-clonic seizures that not infrequently follow partial seizures. There has recently been a change in the requirements for demonstrating such an effect.

By definition, a *secondarily* generalized seizure must follow a *primary* event—in this case, a partial seizure. It would be expected, therefore, that any treatment that decreases the frequency of the primary event must also, perforce, decrease the frequency of the secondary events. With this understanding, it could be considered that any effective treatment for partial seizures is also effective against secondarily generalized seizures.

However, it has recently become clear that a claim for an effect in preventing secondarily generalized seizures carries with it a different implication. The implication of such a claim is that the drug has a specific effect on the process of generalization, independent of its effect on prevention of the primary event. Given this understanding of the proposed claim, then, it is clear that any claim for an effect on secondary generalization must be supported by an analysis that is *conditional on the occurrence of the primary event.*

ALTERNATE DOSAGE FORMS

In recent years, there has been considerable interest and activity in the development of dosage forms other than the traditional oral, immediate-release forms. These dosage forms (e.g., delayed-release and extended-release oral forms and intravenous, rectal, transdermal, and buccal forms) each provide, in specific clinical settings, advantages (and potential disadvantages) over the same drug given via an immediate-release tablet or capsule. In the past year, the Agency has evaluated at least three novel dosage forms intended for the treatment of various forms of epilepsy and/or seizures, and a discussion of these applications provides insight into the issues that arise when decisions about the effectiveness of such treatments are necessary. In each case, the treatment is either a new dosage form of an already approved drug or is closely related to an already available treatment.

When a dosage form other than an approved oral, immediate-release form is proposed, the fundamental question that must be answered is whether additional adequate and well-controlled trials must be performed with the new dosage form, or whether the effectiveness of the original dosage form can be extrapolated to the new product. In general, new products can be assumed to be effective (and safe) only if they are strictly bioequivalent, defined as having the same rate [as assessed by maximal concentration (C_{max}) and time to maximal concentration (t_{max})] and extent [as assessed by area under the curve (AUC)] of absorption as the original product, within certain prespecified limits of variability. This test of bioequivalence is ordinarily what is applied to a generic copy of an innovator drug when the proposed generic is similar to the innovator (for example, both are immediate-release capsules). When the two products are not strictly bioequivalent (e.g., if the two products have a similar extent but different rates of absorption), whether or not there is a change in dosage form, the question of the effect of these differences in kinetics on the effectiveness of the new product must be addressed.

The sponsor of an application for a new dosage form may attempt to submit an application based solely on a comparison of the kinetic performance of the new dosage form to the available dosage form, without safety data or effectiveness data from adequate and well-controlled clinical trials. Such an application, called an Abbreviated New Drug Application (ANDA), the sort ordinarily required for generic drugs, must first be reviewed by a Petitions Committee, which decides if an ANDA is the appropriate mechanism for filing. Changes in dosage forms, routes of administration, dosage strengths, and active ingredients in a fixed-combination product are all eligible for approval through the ANDA route if judged appropriate. In reality, however, the first product for a particular drug that represents a change of the type listed above is usually submitted in what is known as a 505(b)(2) application. A 505(b)(2) application is an NDA that contains less than the full panoply of studies (either clinical or preclinical) ordinarily required, but it does contain more data than are ordinarily contained in an ANDA. What specific additional data are required is decided by the appropriate new drug review division and will vary from case to case. The data required may be derived from controlled trials, but when such data are not required, evidence that the differences in kinetics between the old and new dosage forms will not affect the clinical effectiveness of the new dosage form is ordinarily required.

Oral Dosage Forms

There are two common types of oral dosage form that differ from the immediate-release form: the delayed-release and the extended-release oral dosage forms. Delayed-release oral products delay the release of drug compared with immediate-release products, but once release begins, the same pattern is followed as with the immediate-release product. In other words, the time-concentration curve for such products is shifted to the right of that for immediate-release products. The most common example of this type of product is the enteric coated tablet, designed to withstand degradation in the stomach and release its contents more distally in the gastrointestinal tract.

Extended-release products permit at least a twofold reduction in dosing frequency compared with immediate-release products. These products release drug more slowly than immediate-release products and are designed to offer several advantages over immediate-release products. Most commonly, they are designed to deliver an amount of drug to the system comparable with that delivered when the same daily dose is given more frequently via immediate release, but with less fluctuation in drug levels throughout the dosing interval (e.g., lower C_{max} and higher C_{min}). These altered kinetics are intended to decrease the occurrence of adverse events, maintain or increase effectiveness, and increase compliance, as a consequence of the decreased frequency of dosing.

The equivalent effectiveness of extended-release products compared with immediate-release products is often assumed but rarely proved. The decreased fluctuations in plasma levels seen with these products is ordinarily considered preferable to the peaks and valleys associated with the immediate-release products, and evidence establishing that these fluctuations are not necessary for effectiveness is often deemed unnecessary. This is particularly true in the case of drugs administered on a long-term basis, such as AEDs. However, unless there is a well-defined relationship between plasma concentration and desired pharmacologic effect and toxicity, especially when there is essentially no time lag between drug administration and effect (as is the case, perhaps, with airway resistance and inspired aerosolized bronchodilators), there is little reason *a priori* to conclude in any given case that kinetics have no effect on outcome. In certain circumstances, controlled trials may be necessary to establish the effectiveness of an extended-release dosage form, as when the clinical effect is indirect (e.g., mediated through complex mechanisms), when there is evidence of tolerance with repeated exposure, when fluctuations in plasma levels are large, and/or when there is a lack of knowledge of the relationship between plasma concentration and clinical effect. This last point is of particular importance in regard to AEDs, because a link between plasma levels and effectiveness has not been established for any of the newer AEDs. Further, whereas so-called therapeutic ranges exist for a number of the older AEDs commonly used, these ranges have not been adequately or rigorously established.

Recently, the Agency undertook the review of an extended-release form of Tegretol, designed to be administered twice a day. This product was not strictly bioequivalent to the immediate-release product. As with all extended-release products, it was *designed* not to be bioequivalent, because absorption was delayed compared with that of the then available Tegretol dosage form. The sponsor argued that because absorption of drug was equivalent for the two products, additional evidence of effectiveness was unnecessary. However, examination of the data revealed that the C_{min} of the active 10,11-epoxide was (minimally) lower than the C_{min} of the metabolite derived from the immediate-release product. Because a trough level of one of the active moieties was *lower* with the extended-release dosage, it was not certain that seizure control would be maintained throughout the dosing interval. For this reason, the Agency relied on an analysis that examined the combined plasma levels of the parent and active metabolite (the two chemical species being considered equipotent, based on ancillary data) to compare the relevant kinetic parameters of the two products. With this approach, the values for AUC, C_{max}, and C_{min} of the two products were seen to be equivalent. Because of the essential identity of the plasma levels derived from the two products, the Agency was willing to accept that differences in t_{max} for the products was likely clinically meaningless. Had there been significant differences between the actual levels of the combined active species (even in the face of equivalent AUCs), the question of what additional data, if any, would be required to establish the effectiveness of the extended-release product would not have been a trivial matter.

Intravenous Dosage Forms

A recent example of the issues raised when an intravenous dosage form is developed to substitute for one that is already available is the case of fosphenytoin. This prodrug, when given intravenously, is rapidly (within minutes) converted to phenytoin. One important issue, from a regulatory viewpoint, was that the determination of whether this new drug was effective depended on the specific indication for which it was being given.

Intravenous phenytoin is approved for a number of indications that can be considered "chronic" or nonemergent (e.g., in perioperative or other settings in which oral phenytoin cannot be taken) and for other indications that require acute dosing (e.g., status epilepticus).

For indications that can be considered chronic, or substitutes for prophylactic oral phenytoin, approval of this product relied on the sponsor's ability to identify a dosing regimen that resulted in plasma levels considered to be within the commonly accepted therapeutic range for phenytoin. (This represents one of the very few times a determination of effectiveness has been based on such a consideration for AEDs and is derived from the extremely extensive experience available for phenytoin).

The approval of fosphenytoin as an acute treatment for status epilepticus posed additional problems. Here, the judgment was made that appropriate plasma levels had to be achieved rapidly and sustained for a reasonable time. In this setting, appropriate plasma levels meant those that were at least as great as those resulting from the maximally permitted infusion rate of phenytoin (i.e., 50 mg/min). Plasma levels lower than these could not be considered to confer benefit reliably in an acute setting. With this standard, the sponsor was able to identify an infusion rate of fosphenytoin that resulted in plasma levels of unbound phenytoin at least as high as those achieved after intravenous administration of phenytoin; these levels were achieved rapidly (compared with intravenous phenytoin) and persisted for appropriate periods of time. The sponsor initially had difficulty identifying an infusion rate of fosphenytoin that resulted in levels of total phenytoin comparable with those achieved with intravenous phenytoin, but then noted that fosphenytoin itself displaces phenytoin from plasma protein binding sites, thereby giving rise to unbound levels of phenytoin that are appropriate. The decision to rely on the levels of unbound phenytoin was based on the belief that unbound drug is the entity giving rise to the pharmacologic effect desired.

Rectal Dosage Forms

Sometimes, the existence of an alternate dosage form gives rise to difficult questions entirely unrelated to its kinetic performance, as happened in the case of a proposed rectally administered diazepam product, recently approved at the time of this writing.

Although both oral and parenteral dosage forms of diazepam have been approved for various epileptic indications, no rectally administered AED had previously been approved for marketing in the United States. Although the kinetics of the rectal dosage form would be expected to differ from those of either the oral or parenteral forms (the kinetic values of rectal dosage forms would, in general, be expected to be between those of oral and parenteral dosage forms), these kinetic considerations do not figure primarily in the issues posed by this application.

The availability of a rectally administered AED makes possible the treatment of conditions previously untreatable. In particular, the availability of such a product permits an acute episode to be treated outside a formal health care environment (e.g., an emergency room). That is, a rectal dosage form creates the potential for treatment of an acute seizure at home by a caregiver. Although diazepam is, of course, already frequently administered rectally (using specially prepared parenteral diazepam), the submission of an NDA raises for the first time the regulatory question of the appropriate indication for this product. This is of fundamental importance from a regulatory point of view, because a product may be approved for a condition only if labeling can clearly and unambiguously describe the condition to be treated.

With this in mind, the sponsor of the application has attempted to define an entity previously undefined, or idiosyncratically defined—acute repetitive seizures. According to the sponsor, an episode of acute repetitive seizures is distinct from the patient's other seizures. Acute repetitive seizures are stereotypic and easily identified, and they have a natural history that is relatively predictable. The episodes, according to the sponsor, are variously referred to in the literature as flurries or clusters.

The existence of the new dosage form, therefore, has prompted the establishment of an entirely new diagnostic entity, or at least one that has never been adequately defined before, and thereby poses unique problems for both the regulatory body and the treating community. The existence of a diagnosis or condition cannot simply be posited. For an indication to be acceptable, the condition must be verified and found to be legitimate by the relevant expert community. Detailed diagnostic criteria must be developed, validated (and in this case be able to be applied by the lay public), and the course of the illness should be documented. At the time of this writing, these issues have not been settled, although they are to be discussed at a meeting of the Advisory Committee late in 1996.

Buccal Dosage Forms

Buccal dosage forms, which are designed to be placed in the oral cavity and be absorbed through the buccal mucosa, are not at this time actively being developed for the treatment of epilepsy. However, they are being actively developed for other conditions, and a brief comment about some issues surrounding their approval may be worthwhile.

Although these dosage forms are designed to be absorbed through the oral mucosa, some drug may be swallowed. In these cases, the metabolism will be a combination of what ordinarily occurs with oral products (the portion that is swallowed) and what takes place after the administration of parenteral products (the portion that is absorbed directly across the mucosa). Ordinarily, then, if either an oral or a parenteral dosage form is already available (but not both), controlled trials might be required to establish the effectiveness of the buccal form, as in most cases there might be significant differences in kinetics between the buccal form and whichever dosage form is already marketed.

However, in the special case of a product that is already available as an oral *and* a parenteral product, a kinetic approach may be acceptable. Specifically, if it can be demonstrated that the plasma levels of all the active chemical species generated from the buccal dosage form *fall between the levels of these species generated by the oral and parenteral products at all times during the dosing interval*, it would be reasonable to infer the efficacy of the buccal drug, because the plasma levels would always be bracketed between levels of species known to be effective. Of course, such an approach is acceptable only if all the active moieties are known and measurable, a situation that does not always exist.

Antiepileptic Drug Development.
Advances in Neurology, Vol. 76,
edited by J. French, I. Leppik, and M. A. Dichter.
Lippincott–Raven Publishers, Philadelphia © 1998.

26

Ethical and Institutional Review Board Issues

Brett E. Skolnick

Department of Neurology, Pennsylvania Hospital, Philadelphia, Pennsylvania 19107.

HISTORICAL, ETHICAL, AND LEGAL FOUNDATIONS

Concerns about ethics in the practice of medicine have a long history, but until the middle of this century they were mostly centered around the practice of medicine, not clinical research. In 1946, 23 Nazi physicians went on trial at Nuremberg for crimes committed against prisoners of war. These crimes included exposure of humans to extremes of temperature, performance of mutilating surgery, and deliberate infection with lethal pathogens. During the trial, fundamental ethical standards for the conduct of research involving humans were codified into the Nuremberg Code (1), which set forth 10 conditions that must be met to justify research involving human subjects. The two most important conditions were the need for voluntary informed consent of subjects and a scientifically valid research design that could produce results for the good of society. The Nuremberg Code was reflected in the Declaration of Human Rights and accepted in principle by each of the 51 original signatory nations of the Charter of the United Nations. At that time, however, most countries, including the United States, had no mechanism for implementing the provisions of the Nuremberg Code.

Federal policy for the protection of human subjects was first developed at the National Institutes of Health (NIH) in 1953. This policy was consistent with the Nuremberg Code in that it gave special emphasis to the protection of healthy, adult research volunteers for whom participation in research offered little direct gain. The policy of the NIH was innovative in providing a mechanism for the *prospective* review of research conducted by individuals who had no direct involvement or intellectual investment in the research. This was the beginning of the research review mechanism, the Institutional Review Board (IRB), that is now fundamental to the current system of protections of human subjects throughout the United States. In the 1960s, clinical research expanded, with a concomitant increase in the number of individuals participating as subjects. Interest in the rights of research subjects grew not only because of a general increase in attention to human rights, but also because of a number of highly publicized abuses in clinical research. In 1966, Henry Beecher (2), a highly respected physician-investigator from Harvard University, shocked the medical community with his report of unethical or questionably ethical practices that were common in the conduct of human subjects research in many research institutions. Investigators were reported to have injected elderly indigent people with live cancer cells, without their consent, to learn more about the human immune system. The investigators were cited for fraud, deceit, and unprofessional conduct, although no apparent harm to subjects occurred. The World Health Organization recognized a need for guidelines that were broader in scope than the Nuremberg Code and the Declaration of Helsinki, and "Recommendations Guiding Medical Doctors in Biomedical Research Involving Human Subjects" was adopted by the World Medical Society in 1964. These guidelines have been revised a number of times, most recently in 1989, and currently are in use throughout the world (3,4,5). The first Public Health Service Policy on the Protection of Human Subjects was issued in 1966. At first, the policy applied to federally funded extramural research activities, but it was later expanded to cover all human subjects research conducted or supported by the Department of Health, Education, and Welfare. It required prospective review of human subjects research, taking into account the rights and welfare of the subjects involved, the appropriateness of the methods used to secure informed consent, and the risks and potential benefits of the research. The elements of informed consent included the requirement that consent be documented and signed by subjects or their representatives.

Several events in the early 1970s led to renewed and intense efforts in the United States to protect human subjects. Most notable was the revelation that since the 1930s, approximately 400 black men in Tuskegee, Alabama, had been involved, without their knowledge, in a lengthy study (the Tuskegee Syphilis Study) on the natural history of syphilis. These men were systematically denied penicillin, even after its introduction as the standard treatment for the disease (6,7). The Senate Committee on Labor and Human Resources held hearings on this study and on other alleged health care abuses of prisoners and children. The outcomes of these hearings were (a) enactment of the National Research Act of 1974 (8), requiring a codification of current policy for the protection of human subjects into Federal regulations, which was done in 1974, and (b) formation of the National Commission for the Protection of Human Subjects of Biomedical and Behavioral Research. The National Commission for the Protection of Human Subjects of Biomedical and Behavioral Research, which functioned from 1974–1978, evaluated the existing system, recommended improvements to the Secretary of Health, Education, and Welfare and issued reports on research involving pregnant women, live human fetuses, prisoners, children, the mentally disabled, and on the use of psychosurgery. It also issued "The Belmont Report: Ethical Principles and Guidelines for the Protection of Human Subjects of Research" (9). A major advancement in the development of public policy, the Belmont Report provided guidance for distinguishing therapeutic medicine from research, identified three fundamental ethical principles for the protection of human subjects, and illustrated how the ethical principles should be applied to the conduct of human subjects research.

In 1979, the process of revising the 1974 regulations was started, but it was not until 1981 that final approval (by the Department of Health and Human Services) was given to Title 45, Code of Federal Regulations, Part 46, Protection of Human Subjects (45.CFR.46) (10). Initially, these regulations were applicable only when research was conducted or supported by the Department of Health and Human Services, but in June 1991, 45.CFR.46 was revised and became the basic policy that now governs all federally supported research.

ETHICAL PRINCIPLES OF THE BELMONT REPORT

The Belmont Report, which was published in 1979, provides the philosophical underpinnings for the current laws governing human subjects research. Unlike the Nuremberg Code and the Helsinki Declaration, which consist of "guidances" or "rules," the Belmont Report establishes three fundamental ethical principles that are relevant to all research involving human subjects: Respect for Persons, Beneficence, and Justice. Although other important principles sometimes apply to research, these three provide a comprehensive framework for ethical decision making in research involving human subjects. The principle of Respect for Persons acknowledges the dignity and autonomy of individuals, and requires that people with diminished autonomy be provided special protection. This principle requires that subjects give informed consent to participation in research. Because of their potential vulnerability, certain subject populations are provided with additional protections. These include live human fetuses, children, prisoners, the mentally disabled, and people with severe illnesses. The principle of Beneficence requires the protection of individuals by maximizing anticipated benefits and minimizing possible harms. Therefore, it is necessary to examine carefully the design of any study and its risks and benefits; this includes, in some cases, identifying alternate ways to obtain the benefits sought from the research. Research risks must always be justified by the expected benefits of research. Finally, the principle of Justice requires that all subjects be fairly treated. For example, subjects should be carefully and equitably chosen to ensure that certain individuals or classes of individuals—such as prisoners, elderly people, or financially impoverished people—are not systematically selected or excluded without scientifically or ethically valid reasons. Also, unless there is careful justification for an exception, research should not involve persons from groups that are unlikely to benefit from subsequent applications of the research.

Each of these principles carries strong moral force, and difficult ethical dilemmas arise when they conflict. A careful and thoughtful application of the principles of the Belmont Report will not always achieve a clear resolution of ethical problems. However, it is important to understand and apply the principles, because doing so helps to ensure that people who agree to be experimental subjects will be treated in a respectful and ethical manner. These regulations apply to all research involving human subjects. Such activities include "hands-on" involvement with patients or subjects and also indirect involvement, such as analysis of data or human samples (e.g., blood or tissue). The Belmont Commission early in its deliberations understood the importance of distinguishing between research and practice. Although it may not appear to be difficult to distinguish between the two entities, this has been an area of some legitimate concern. The term "research" is defined in the Code of Regulations as "a systematic investigation designed to develop and contribute to generalized knowledge." Any study in which the data obtained are intended for publication or public presentation or that involves the use of an investigational drug, device, or procedure constitutes research and must undergo the IRB review process. "Practice" refers to the class of activities engaged in to enhance the well-being of an individual patient.

45.CFR.46 is not a set of rules that can be applied rigidly to make determinations of whether a proposed research activity is ethically "right" or "wrong." Rather, these regulations provide a framework in which investigators and others can ensure that serious efforts have been made to protect the rights and welfare of research subjects. Each institution holding a Multiple Project Assurance (MPA) has a qualified IRB that oversees the implementation of 45.CFR.46 for all research. The Office for the Protection of Research Rights (OPRR) requires each institution that conducts or supports research involving human subjects to set forth the procedures it will use to protect human subjects in a policy statement called an assurance of compliance, commonly referred to as an assurance. The MPA covers all research involving human subjects conducted by investigators, or in which investigators collaborate, regardless of the site.

Multiple Project Assurance

Overall responsibility for the protection of human subjects rests with the institution and its legal designee, who establishes and implements policies and procedures in accord with 45.CFR.46. Everyone who shares this responsibility is expected to be familiar with the MPA. The MPA includes policies and procedures regarding (a) the responsibilities of investigators who conduct, support, or collaborate in basic or clinical research activities involving human subjects; (b) the responsibilities of the IRB for the review and approval of research activities involving human subjects; and (c) responsibilities for protecting human subjects.

Responsibilities of Investigators

Investigators are responsible for protecting the rights and welfare of the human subjects who participate in their research. They must also understand the ethical standards and regulatory requirements governing their research activities. All investigators who conduct or collaborate in a research activity are responsible for knowing whether or not their research involves human subjects. A "human subject" is a living individual about whom an investigator obtains either (a) data through interaction or intervention with the individual, or (b) identifiable private information. In many cases, the determination of whether a particular research activity involves human subjects is not difficult, but in some cases the line is blurred. When it is not clear to an investigator whether research activities involve human subjects, they are encouraged to seek the advice of the IRB and its representatives. In questionable cases, final responsibility for determining whether human subjects are involved rests with the IRB.

Specific Research Activities Not Subject to Multiple Project Assurance

Certain research activities are not subject to the requirements of an MPA. These include the collection and study of (a) samples from deceased individuals, (b) samples collected for diagnostic purposes only, (c) samples or data that are available from commercial or public repositories or registries. However, investigators should be aware that even though research with these types of materials is not covered by the MPA, it may be subject to other requirements, such as rules governing technology transfer.

Exempt Activities

Six categories of research, although they involve human subjects, are exempt from the requirements of the MPA. These are listed in 45.CFR.46. One example is the study or collection of existing records (e.g., pathologic specimens), if these sources are publicly available or if the information is recorded by the investigator so that subjects cannot be directly identified or through identifiers linked to the subjects. Other exemptions include research involving taste testing of food, surveys, interviews, use of educational tests, and observation of public behavior. The general rationale behind exempting the six categories is that although the research involves human subjects, it does not expose them to physical, social, or psychologic risks.

The IRB is authorized to determine whether a research activity is exempt from the requirements of 45.CFR.46. Investigators who think their research activity fits into one of the exempt categories should complete the necessary forms for their IRB and request in writing that the protocol be reviewed as possibly exempt. Investigators should not make determinations about exemptions without consulting the IRB.

ELEMENTS OF A RESEARCH PROTOCOL

Investigators conducting or collaborating in research involving human subjects must receive approval by an IRB before they begin their study. Generally, an investigator provides the IRB with a research protocol, which is a written description of, and scientific rationale for, the proposed research activity. It includes a discussion of the human subject protection issues relevant to the study and addresses, at a minimum, the following issues: risks to subjects; all procedures that are experimental; anticipated benefits to subjects, if any; anticipated number of subjects; the proposed consent document and consent process to be used, and appropriate additional safeguards if potentially vulnerable subjects are to be enrolled. Potentially vulnerable subjects may include the elderly, prisoners, children, cognitively impaired persons, or people who are economically or educationally disadvantaged. More information on how to prepare a research protocol may be obtained directly from the responsible IRB.

RESPONSIBILITIES OF INSTITUTIONAL REVIEW BOARDS

Research investigators have a fundamental responsibility to safeguard the rights and welfare of the subjects participating in their research activities. In addition, our society has decided by law that an objective review of research activities involving human subjects by a group of diverse individuals is most likely to protect human subjects and promote ethically sound research. IRBs are generally composed of members with expertise in science, ethics, and other nonscientific areas. This diversity fosters a comprehensive approach to safeguarding the rights and welfare of subjects. In their deliberations about proposed research activities, IRB members should take into account the ethical principles of the Belmont Report, the requirements of 45.CFR.46, and the MPA of their institution, as well as the nature and content of the proposed research. IRBs evaluate proposed research activities using the following criteria: (a) The design of the study is consistent with sound scientific principles and ethical norms; (b) the protocol meets the MPA criteria necessary for approval; (c) the necessary elements of informed consent have been fulfilled; (d) additional appropriate safeguards have been provided if potentially vulnerable subjects are to be studied. In exercising their authority, IRBs may approve, disapprove, or table research protocols. Most often, the IRB approves a research study with required changes, often referred to as stipulations. However, IRBs are obliged to disapprove any protocol that does not meet the above criteria. In addition, IRBs conduct continuing review of each approved research protocol or activity at least yearly, although an IRB may request earlier evaluations or updates if it determines that the research presents significant physical, social, or psychologic risks to subjects. The IRB may modify, suspend, or terminate approval of research that has been associated with serious harm to subjects or is not being conducted in accord with the MPA or the decisions, stipulations, and requirements of the IRB.

Local IRBs have the additional function of ensuring that local factors (community and institutional perspectives) are given appropriate consideration. Particular concern is directed to the process of informed consent of the participant or research subject, to ensure that full disclosure of the research procedures and relative risks and benefits are adequately presented. The safety and welfare of the research participants is of utmost concern. The IRB serves as an independent assessor of the overall risks and benefits of the investigational study and ensures that patient are informed of all necessary aspects of the study so as to be able to make an informed decision to participate or not to participate.

Problems in Consent Documents

The most frequent deficiency in clinical trial consent forms is the failure to identify persons to contact in the event of injury or to ask questions on research or patients' rights. Consent forms may name the same person as the contact for more than one of these areas, but it is of key importance that all be addressed in the documents. It is suggested that the contact for patients' rights be unaffiliated with the study. The deficiency cited second most frequently is an inadequate confidentiality statement. Consent forms should describe who has access to the study records and, if appropriate, patients' medical records. The Food and Drug Administration in clinical trials involving new drugs or even approved drugs will require access to patients' records. The Food and Drug Administration may not be able to ensure that these medical records will not be released, as required by law. In the case of a court order, or if Congress wants records, an individual's medical records could be released. The third most frequent omission is an incomplete description of the research procedures. A full description of the study plan should be included in a consent document. In the case of investigational agents (drug, device, biologic), unless there is a reason to the contrary, the investigator should indicate that one of the reasons for the study is to determine the safety and efficacy of the agent. Reviews of the alternate procedures that patients may be afforded, if they choose not to participate in the trial, are frequently omitted or incompletely described. These may often be "standard" approved therapies, with their respective risks and known benefits; alternatively, patients/subjects can decide to seek no further treatment for their medical condition. Patients/subjects must know that these options are available and understand that they will not be deprived of proper medical treatment if they refuse to consent. This raises the issue of the "investigator/physician" dichotomy. In much of clinical research, the most knowledgeable and experienced physician may also be the investigator who has either designed the research protocol or recognizes a clinical need for alternate interventions. As such, these investigators/ physicians present a dilemma to prospective subjects who also are patients currently under their care. Such situations require careful discussion with the subject/patient so that all elements of possible coercion are minimized. In the ideal research environment, the physician would be the patient's advocate and not also be a potential beneficiary of the research effort.

The last and most essential, from an economic perspective, element of the consent document is a complete description of treatment for research-related injuries and compensation for such injury. The Food and Drug Administration does not clearly describe boundaries for this statement, stipulating only that the consent document should include information regarding issues related to the treatment of injury and compensation for such injury. Many IRBs have taken the position that treatment of injury is typically the responsibility of sponsors (pharmaceutical companies) and that their responsibilities should be adequately described in the consent form. In certain circumstances, it may be impossible to separate injury related to the agent (drug, device, biologic) from progression of the underlying disease process. In these circumstances, it is important to state clearly how proper assignment of such responsibility will be determined. This is particularly important in the current health care climate, in which health maintenance organizations and other indemnity programs may deny payment for injury resulting from participation in research. This becomes a particular problem during treatment with new drug regimes comprising approved agents (e.g., oncology patients); the drugs under study are approved but are being studied in an off-label dose regime or in a different disease entity. It is also a problem when dose-escalation studies are performed with currently prescribed drugs. It is important to provide a clear description of the costs of injuries that may be incurred and of what additional risks are being assumed as a result of any additions to clinically indicated therapy.

Institutional Review Board Perspective

Consent forms often fail to clarify the difference between "standard" therapy and research, so that patients may not truly understand the experimental nature of their participation. Subjects should be informed in advance that treatment decisions may be made by adhering to the specifications of a protocol, and that these decisions may not necessarily be based on an individual patient's needs. It is also important to note that often such adherence to a protocol may result in improved long-term medical care with better risk management for society. This, however, is not always achieved. Patients and investigators believe that experimental therapy will be better than what is already available, when in fact the therapy may be worse. It is important to discuss the general aspects of clinical research as well as the specifics of each trial. It is the investigator's responsibility to ensure that the consent form is written at an appropriate reading level and does not contain technical and scientific or medical jargon that is impossible for the average study subject to comprehend.

To improve the adequacy and speed of review of research protocols, investigators should have and exhibit a full understanding of the protocol they submit. Sponsor protocols are generally adequate, but investigators are often not as familiar with the protocol as they should be, and that lack of familiarity raises alarms with the IRB. Investigators should spend the necessary time to prepare their application to the IRB so as to eliminate correspondence addressing IRB concerns. If IRB perceived risks are not addressed, the investigator will be questioned regarding the application. Thus, investigators must show that they understand all the safety implications of the work they are undertaking.

Coercion

Rules of the Food and Drug Administration rules prohibit the coercion of subjects into either participating or staying in a clinical trial, but the Agency sets no precise monetary figure on what would or would not be considered coercive payment. It is often difficult to know whether subjects are being paid too little, too much, or just enough. One way to keep payment from being coercive is to keep it low. For a typical outpatient study that may require repeated visits to the physician's office, it would be reasonable to reimburse for the costs of transportation and possibly for the time. Such arrangements may include reasonable travel and parking expenses. It is understood that careful review by the IRB of these amounts is necessary, as for the financially desperate, any amount could be coercive. There are unethical means other than cash payment of attracting people into a study or maintaining their cooperation after they have agreed to participate. For example, if the consent forms offer free drug treatment with the implication that it is equal to or better than available therapy, this could be construed as inappropriate. It is important to explain carefully to the subject that the drug is experimental.

Two matters of continued debate are the withholding of part of a fee until study completion and the promise of a bonus for those who finish a trial. The first case often arises when researchers need patients for a given period each week. The dropout rate for such work can be high, because subjects have other obligations or grow tired of having the weekly study commitment. Partially withholding payment is one way to lower dropout rates. Added payment for study completion is prohibited by some IRBs. In cases in which IRBs have allowed such a bonus, it is viewed as reasonable only if the bonus is a small percentage of the overall study payment. Some IRBs see both methods, withholding payment or providing a bonus, as coercive, because they indicate that subjects who discontinue participation will incur a penalty.

Responsibilities

It is the responsibility of the IRB to (a) approve, disapprove, or approve with modifications a protocol; (b) monitor the progress and conduct of a study; (c) suspend, terminate, restrict, or request modifications to a study as necessary.

It is the responsibility of the investigators to (a) ensure that studies are not begun before final approval by the IRB; (b) not implement amendments, addenda, or revisions before approval by the IRB; (c) comply with the annual review of protocol; (d) notify the IRB promptly of any adverse events and completion of the study; (e) ensure the accuracy and completeness of all information submitted to the IRB.

Consent

The consent document itself is a written summary of the information that should be provided to each subject. Many clinical investigators use the consent document as a guide for the verbal explanation of the study. The subject's signature provides documentation of consent to participate in a study but is only one part of the consent process. The entire informed consent process involves providing a subject adequate information concerning the study, allowing an adequate opportunity for the subject to consider all options, responding to the subject's questions, and ensuring that the subject has understood the information. The final step is obtaining the subject's voluntary agreement to participate and continuing to provide information as the subject or situation requires. To be effective, the process should provide ample opportunity for the investigator and the subject to exchange information and ask questions.

Elements of Consent

Federal law requires that consent statements contain the following:

1. An explanation of the purpose of the research, the expected duration of the subject's participation, and a description of the procedure. There is no need to describe the details of the design, especially if this will affect the subject's responses in ways that jeopardize the validity of the research. It is necessary only to describe what the subject will experience in terms the subject understands. Jargon, legalistic terminology, and explanations that are irrelevant to a decision whether to participate should be avoided.
2. A description of any foreseeable risks or discomforts.
3. A description of any benefits reasonably to be expected.
4. A description of the alternatives to participation, when appropriate.
5. A description of how confidentiality or anonymity will be maintained.
6. A statement regarding the availability of compensation and medical care for injuries arising from participation in the protocol.
7. Indication of whom to contact for answers to questions about the research subject's rights, or in case a research-related injury occurs. Contact persons should include both the investigator and an appropriate administrator of the institution.
8. Indication that participation is voluntary, that refusal to participate will involve no penalty or loss of benefits to which the subject would otherwise be entitled, and that the subject may discontinue participation at any time.

Often, common sense will dictate that other elements also be included:

9. If the research is sponsored, the investigator should disclose the identity of the sponsor.
10. When appropriate, the researcher should be identified personally.

Finally, good communication and good sense require that openness and honesty characterize the ongoing relationship with subjects and others in the research setting. In field settings (e.g., workplaces, schools, hospitals), such communication may involve not only subjects but also other individuals (e.g., family members) who are part of the setting but not subjects. The researcher should be open to discussion of problems that the research raises for the various interests represented within a particular setting. Any communication with the press about the research should be cleared through the IRB and the sponsor. Food and Drug Administration regulations require minimally IRB review.

Language

The general informed consent requirements outlined in federal regulations require that consent documents be in a language understandable to study subjects. Many IRBs spends a great deal of time "translating" consent documents into lay language. A question has been raised about whether an informed consent document needs to be translated into the native language of a study subject who does not understand English. Federal regulations (21.CFR.50.20) require that "the information that is given to the subject or the representative shall be in a language understandable to [them] . . . When the study subject population will include people who do not understand English and the clinical investigator or the IRB anticipates that the consent process is likely to be conducted in a language other than English, . . . a translated consent document is prepared . . . [that] accurately conveys the information as approved by the IRB." As required by federal regulations, each subject is to receive a copy of the consent document. Although a translator may be helpful in facilitating conversation with a non–English-speaking subject, routine *ad hoc* translations of the consent document should not be substituted for a written translation. Any translated version of an informed consent document must be forwarded to the IRB and receive IRB approval. All amendments to the informed consent document also must be translated into the appropriate language.

If a non–English-speaking subject is unexpectedly encountered, enrollment is imminent, and time does not permit review of a translated document, oral translation of the English language version may be permissible. If subjects are enrolled without an IRB-approved translated consent document, a statement in the study records (and on the English language consent form) should indicate that the translation took place, identify the translator, and document that the witness affirms that the subject understands the study and consent process. Every effort should be made to secure written translation of the vital emergency contact information for the study subject.

An occasional subject who understands English, but does not read or write English, may participate in a research study, but again an impartial witness should document that "informed consent" did take place and that the subject understands the essential elements of consent.

Most IRBs prefer that documents not in English be submitted with English language versions. An explanation regarding the source of translations and the technical expertise of the translator is helpful for IRB review. In some cases, the IRB may consult with language experts or require a "back-translation" to ensure an accurate representation of study risks and benefits. These steps are always taken to ensure that the rights and welfare of study subjects are held to the highest standard. Studies conducted in this country with non–English-speaking subjects as well as studies conducted in foreign countries must meet these requirements. Exclusion of study subjects solely on the basis of language or cultural barriers is prohibited.

SPECIAL CIRCUMSTANCES

Approved Drugs Versus Investigational Drugs

There are situations in which currently approved drugs, although well accepted as a "standard" of care, may also be associated with known and sometimes unacceptably high risks for significant adverse effects. Physicians/investigators are then faced with the dilemma of determining the point in time when the various approved agents have been adequately evaluated and when investigational agents may be introduced. An example from the field of epilepsy may be given. In this field, frequent use of polytherapy is the norm. Epilepsy researchers, faced with the difficulties of withdrawing possibly effective agents, have made use of innovative study designs that avoid dealing with drug washouts. Patients, with a baseline seizure frequency, are provided with access to adjuvant therapy with a new agent, which enables the relative clinical benefits to be assessed. This design, however, is confounded by possible drug interactions that may not enable an optimal dose to be achieved or may result in unacceptable side effects caused by potentiation of the original antiepileptic drug. Careful consideration needs to be given to the study of new drugs in clinical areas in which numerous older alternatives exist. Exhaustive evaluation of all approved drugs before initiating a therapeutic trial of a new investigational drug is not necessarily best management. These studies may pose an inherently greater risk but may provide greater long-term benefit to both the patient and society. Careful deliberation of these critical issues is necessary before determining the appropriateness of such designs.

Emergency Procedures

IRBs in executing their responsibilities have allowed that the benefit to society should always be contrasted with the benefit to the patient. Although always a consideration, it now would appear that societal benefits may, in certain carefully defined conditions, outweigh the benefit to the individual. For example, a new regulation is intended to facilitate the conduct of research trials in patients who are gravely ill or injured with heart attacks, strokes, or head injuries, for whom time is of the essence, when available treatments are unproven or unsatisfactory and relatives cannot be found in time to give permission for experimental treatments. It is important in these circumstances that the risks and benefits of the investigational treatment be reasonable in the light of what is known about the medical condition and the risks and benefits of other therapies.

SUMMARY

IRBs provide an important role in the protection of research subjects/patients. Research investigators have an inherent potential conflict of interest as health care professionals; as physicians, they are dedicated to promoting the welfare of individual patients, whereas as researchers, they seek knowledge that can be generalized and is applicable to persons other than the individual patient under study. The second goal may be in conflict with the first. IRBs have the paramount responsibility of protecting the rights and welfare of human research subjects. Although the IRB system is not perfect, conscientious IRBs reassure the public that the rights and welfare of human subjects are seriously considered by people who do not have a vested interest in the outcome of the research.

By exercising their responsibilities, IRBs promote the protection of human subjects. IRB approval provides a significant affirmation of the scientific and ethical qualities of research, and therefore offers important validation to research and research investigators. IRBs, acting in accordance with the guiding principles of the Belmont Report and within the regulatory guidelines of 45.CFR.46, are intended to provide balance between society's interest in advancing scientific knowledge and the mandate to protect the rights and welfare of human subjects.

REFERENCES

1. Trials of War Criminals Before the Nuremberg Military Tribunals Under Control Council Law No. 10. Washington, DC: US Government Printing Office; 1949: 181–182 (vol 2).
2. Beecher HK. Ethics and clinical research. *N Engl J Med* 1966;274:1354–1360.
3. World Medical Association Declaration of Helsinki. Adopted by the 18th World Medical Assembly, Helsinki, Finland, June 1964.
4. World Medical Association Declaration of Helsinki. Amended by the 29th World Medical Assembly, Tokyo, Japan, October 1975.
5. World Medical Association Declaration of Helsinki. Amended by the 41st World Medical Assembly, Hong Kong, September 1989.
6. Curran WJ. The Tuskegee Syphilis Study. *N Engl J Med* 1973;289(14):730–731.
7. Brandt AM. Racism and research: the case of the Tuskegee Syphilis Study. *Hastings Center Report* 1978; 8:21–29.
8. National Research Act, Publication L, No. 93-348, 1974.
9. The National Commission for the Protection of Human Subjects of Biomedical and Behavioral Research. The Belmont Report: Ethical Principles and Guidelines for the Protection of Human Subjects in Research. Federal Register Doc 79-12065, 1979.
10. Department of Health and Human Services. Protection of Human Subjects. Federal Register 56, 28003, Doc O-307-551, 1991.

Antiepileptic Drug Development.
Advances in Neurology, Vol. 76,
edited by J. French, I. Leppik, and M. A. Dichter.
Lippincott–Raven Publishers, Philadelphia © 1998.

27

Postmarketing Studies

Neil M. Sussman

Department of Neurology, Yale University School of Medicine, New Haven, Connecticut 06520.

Postmarketing studies are clinical trials conducted after an investigational drug has been approved and launched in a market. That means a company is selling the drug in a particular country. Drugs are approved by the regulatory bodies in a particular country, and launch of the new drug is a company activity. With launch, the company expects to sell the drug in that market. Occasionally, a drug is approved but never launched in a particular market because the foreseeable sales are so low. Once launched and selling, the sales force has the opportunity to listen to physicians' comments about the new drug, to find out whether new side effects are emerging or there are any anecdotes about the new drug being used to treat another indication.

New studies are usually designed by the postmarketing or phase IV research group at the request and cooperation of a company's marketing group. The marketing group may be a part of the sales division or may be a separate, free-standing budgetary branch. It is unlikely that marketing will be part of the development group. However, the budget of the phase IV research group may be attached to sales, marketing, or development. The outlook of the phase IV group is to perform studies to enhance the position of the drug within its competitive milieu so as to increase sales.

The purposes of postmarketing studies are as follows:

1. Determine new indications
2. Expand the indication to include more aspects of a particular disease
3. Provide information on treatment comparisons
4. Detect rare side effects
5. Determine more efficient dosing schedules
6. Satisfy regulatory requirements—that is, Food and Drug Administration requirements set forth at the time of drug approval

As required by the Food and Drug Administration, the sales force may discuss the drug (this includes advertising and direct physician contact) only within the context of approved labeling. As the sales force becomes familiar with the drug and the needs of physicians (physicians as the spokespersons and representatives of patient needs), nuances of the use and prescription requirements of the drug will be voiced by the sales representatives. The marketing group digests the requests of the sales representatives and proposes a postmarketing strategy to the postmarketing research group. Within the labeling indications, the postmarketing research group will design the studies to answer the questions that marketing has posed. For instance, at Johnson & Johnson the phase IV group is studying how quickly the dose of topiramate should be raised—in essence, the titration schedule (information from Ortho McNeil).

The defining characteristics of postmarketing studies are indicated above, but drug development is a more seamless process in which the boundaries between phase III and IV are not crisp. As investigators gain experience with an investigational drug, new areas of clinical research emerge and programs are planned to facilitate new studies to enhance the profile of the new drug. In phase III, the clinical research associates and the medical monitor serve as an advanced corps of personnel who interact with the physician/investigator to discuss new ideas, as the sales force, marketing group, and phase IV medical group do with marketed products.

If the marketing plan indicates that disorders other than that approved in labeling need to be studied to enhance sales, the development group or phase II-III group may become involved and direct such studies. These studies might be for a new indication, and to change the labeled indication would require that an abridged New Drug Application (ANDA) be submitted to the Food and Drug Administration. The studies would then be for registrational purposes and could fit within the framework of the development group. The new indication might be for an entirely different disease state, such as use of the anesthetic propofol to treat status epilepticus (1,2). Approval would require at least two positive, adequate, and well-controlled studies and enough patient exposure to ensure a general safety profile of the drug within the new disease state (1,2). Also, studies might be needed to define drug-drug interactions with the most commonly used antistatus drugs, such as diazepam, lorazepam, phenytoin, and phenobarbital, and perhaps several of the antiepilepsy drugs used chronically.

On the other hand, a company may not wish to register the new indications but may want the information to appear in peer-reviewed literature only. This would not help the sales force in its discussions about the drug, but it would help inform physicians using the drug for individual circumstances. Again, studies for journals may be performed by the development research group under the auspices and budget of the company. However, another scenario may occur in which individual investigators or a group of investigators want to study the effects of the new drug on a different disease state. The academic research group prescribes the drug for the new indication and observes its effects in an open-label manner as pilot-type studies. The group may then petition the company for support for a larger, controlled trial. The support might be as little as donated drug and/or placebo or as much as a fully supported trial. The trial would be designed and monitored by the academic investigative group or might be managed by the company, either the phase II-III group or the phase IV group.

The new indication may be within the broader indication, as occurred in postmarketing studies for butorphanol nasal spray (Stadol®). Butorphanol is indicated for the relief of moderate to severe pain when an opioid analgesic is warranted (package insert). The recent postmarketing trials by Bristol-Myers Squibb have centered around use of butorphanol in migraine headache (3,4). Indeed, because of these specific studies within the broad indication, the principal use of butorphanol nasal spray is for migraine headache. This is an example of enhancement of the use of a drug within indication by targeting one specific disease within that indication.

The time period in which to study other indications within the life cycle of a drug has varied greatly from drug to drug and company to company, depending on company culture, budgeting, personnel commitment, and speed of the development program. First, the life cycle of a drug must be defined. Briefly, the compound either is created to some specification, such as receptor modulator, neurotransmitter, or neuroprotective agent, or has been found serendipitously. The compound is studied physiologically and then pathophysiologically. It undergoes animal toxicology studies. A disease-specific formulation is created (intravenous, oral, patches, nasal spray, or some other form). It then is administered to humans, first normal subjects, then diseased persons. At this point, the drug can be given to people with a wide variety of disease states in pilot trials, and the positive trials are then analyzed by marketing and development to determine which diseases to study in the phase III, large-scale, registrational trials.

The vigabatrin development program followed this pattern; extensive pilot work was performed before registrational trials were begun in subjects with such diverse diseases as Huntington's chorea (5), Friedreich's ataxia (6), cerebellar ataxia (7), spasticity (8), tardive dyskinesia (9,10), Parkinson's disease (11,12), schizophrenia (13), and various types of epilepsy, including absence (14), complex partial seizures (15), and infantile spasms (16).

Once the NDA has been filed, new trials can be started pending approval. With vigabatrin, trials for complex partial seizures in children were initiated in the United States. The phase III B program and postmarketing program blend together, and goals for the drug become similar. The phase III B and early postmarketing period are the time in the life cycle of the drug when budget and personnel needs may be greatest.

The other method of drug development is exemplified in the gabapentin program, in which gabapentin was rapidly developed to registrational approval for epilepsy. Pilot trials are now being conducted in diverse indications, including amyotrophic lateral sclerosis and neuropathic pain. These trials were started based on the results of preclinical studies (17,18,19). Other areas of interest for the marketing group are ways to demonstrate effectiveness, which essentially broadens the population that would respond to the new drug. Efficacy is the measure of improvement in a disease or symptoms observed in comparison with another agent, usually placebo but sometimes an active comparator. Efficacy is confined to the population studied in the clinical trials. Effectiveness often incorporates a wider population—patients excluded from clinical trials because they are of unsuitable weight or age, have concomitant disease, or are taking concomitant medications.

Inclusion criteria are less stringent in effectiveness trials. Postmarketing studies are a way to relax the inclusion criteria to broaden the population base and gain more information about the drug in large numbers of patients. Weight is not restricted. Concomitant drug use, simultaneous presence of other diseases, and wider age ranges are allowed. In postmarketing epilepsy trials, patients with such comorbid conditions as depression, psychosis, heart disease, renal and liver disease, and migraine will be entered into trials.

Active drug comparator trials are usually reserved for phase III B and postmarketing periods. Active drug comparator trials are required for pricing reimbursement in Canada and Australia. Comparator trials are useful but are not yet required in Europe for registration. These trials are not part of the U.S. registrational process, but they are used to generate peer-reviewed articles.

Quality-of-life and pharmacoeconomic data are usually generated by late phase III and III B studies. Considerable information about the drug is necessary to design quality-of-life and pharmacoeconomic trials that will demonstrate an advantage for the drug. Side effect profiles, optimal dosing, and any positive idiosyncracies of the drug need to be known. For example, nefazodone entered the market recently, competing with the serotonin reuptake inhibitors to treat depression. Nefazodone was similar to these drugs in efficacy and side effect profile, except that it showed improvement in sleep (20) and sexual function (17). Quality-of-life questions concerning sexual dysfunction were added to the next series of trials, and nefazodone was vastly superior to the serotonin reuptake inhibitors in the area of retaining or restoring sexual function in depressed patients. Here then is an advantage for nefazodone for marketing.

The need for pharmacoeconomic data is increasing, and the requirements in many countries are changing rapidly. In many countries in Europe, pharmacoeconomic data are needed not for registration but for promotion, formulary approval, and reimbursement. Belgium and Spain require pharmacoeconomic data for promotion; Italy and the United Kingdom for formulary approval; Austria, Portugal, and Scandinavia for promotion and formulary approval. Australia and Canada require such data for reimbursement. In the United States, hospital formularies and managed care (managed cost) organizations are asking pharmaceutical companies to provide pharmacoeconomic data.

In epilepsy, most of the recent drugs are used as add-on therapy. With postmarketing, monotherapy trials are being pursued with lamotrigine, gabapentin, topiramate, and vigabatrin. The registrational trials are usually restrictive in regard to dosage recommendations. In post-NDA studies, new dosage schedules, optimal frequency, and dose ranges can be explored more fully. The topiramate phase IV program entails the evaluation of frequency of dosing.

Unusual side effects can be explored in large, open trials, as efficacy is no longer an issue. As an example, the cough that is a side effect of angiotensin-converting enzyme (ACE) inhibitors was seen in efficacy trials with an incidence ranging from 0.2% up to 30%. In a large postmarketing trial, however, the cough side effect was specifically studied and was found to occur in 7.3% (18). It may be possible to determine whether adverse events are side effects or idiosyncratic and which populations are at risk (19).

Post marketing and phase III B studies provide a good opportunity for companies to expand knowledge of the new drug. Expanding the information base provides marketing and the sales force with information to guide physicians, provide better service, and ultimately increase market share and sales.

REFERENCES

1. McBurney JW, Teiken PJ, Moon MR. Propofol for treating status epilepticus. *J Epilepsy* 1994;7:21–22.
2. Mackenzie SJ, Kapadia F, Grant IS. Propofol infusion for control of status epilepticus. *Anesthesia* 1990;45: 1043–1045.
3. Diamond S, Freitag RG, Diamond ML, Urban G. Transnasal butorphanol in the treatment of migraine headache pain. *Headache Quarterly, Current Treatment and Research* 1992;3:160–167.
4. Hoffert MJ, Couch JR, Diamond S, et al. Transnasal butorphanol in the treatment of acute migraine. *Headache* 1995;35:65–69.
5. Scigliano G, Giovannini P, Girotti F, et al. Gamma-vinyl GABA treatment of Huntington's Disease. *Neurology* 1995;34;94–96.
6. DeSmet Y, Mera JY, Tell G, et al. Effect of gamma-vinyl GABA in Friedreich's ataxia. *Can J Neurol Sci* 1982;9: 171–173.
7. Bonnet AM, Esteguy M, Tell G, et al. A controlled study of oral vigabatrin (gamma-vinyl GABA) in patients with cerebellar ataxia. *Can J Neurol Sci* 1986;13: 331–333.
8. Data on file, Hoechst Marion Roussel.
9. Gerlach J. Tardive diskinesia. Pathophysiological mechanisms and clinical trials. *Encephale* 1988;14:227–232.
10. Tamminga CA, Thaker GK, Ferraro TN, Hare TA. GABA agonist treatment improved tardive dyskinesia. *Psychiatry Res* 1983;8:261–269.
11. Korsgaard S, Casey DE, Gerlach J. Effect of gamma-vinyl-GABA in tardive dyskinesia. *Psychiatry Res* 1983;8:261–269.
12. Lambert PA, Cantiniaux P, Chabannes JP, et al. Essai thérapeutique du gamma-vinyl GABA, un inhibiteur de la GABA- transaminase, dans les dyskinésies tardives induites par les neuroleptiques. *Encephale* 1982;8: 371–376.
13. Lambert PA, Chabannes JP, Cantiniaux P, et al. Effects du gamma-vinyl GABA per os dans cinq cas de schizophrénie hébéphreno-catatonique. *Encephale* 1983;9: 145–149.
14. Dulac O, Chiron L, Luna D, et al. Vigabatrin in childhood epilepsy. *J Child Neurol* 1991;6(Suppl 2): 530–537.
15. Data on file, Hoechst Marion Roussel.
16. Chiron C, Dulac O, Beaumont D, et al. Therapeutic trial of vigabatrin in refractory infantile spasms. *J Child Neurol* 1991;6(Suppl 2):552–559.
17. Feiger A, Kiev A, Shrivastava R, Wisselink PG, Wilcox CS. Nefazodone versus sertraline in outpatients with major depression: focus on efficacy, tolerability, and effects on sexual function and satisfaction. *J Clin Psychiatry* 1996;57(Suppl): (*in press*).
18. Strocchi E, Valtancoli G, Ricci C, et al. Post-marketing studies of subjective side effects. A case for strict methodological criteria and careful analysis of data. *Pharmacol Res* 1992;25(Suppl 1):79–80.
19. Smart AJ, Walters L. The importance of post-marketing drug surveillance. *S Afr Med J* 1992;82:383–384.
20. Armitage R, Rush AJ, Trivedi M, Cain J, Roffwarg HP. The effects of nefazodone on sleep architecture in depression. *Neuropsychopharmacology* 1994;10:123–127.

Subject Index

Subject Index

Page numbers followed by *f* refer to figures and page numbers followed by *t* refer to tables